Stedman's

POCKET MEDICAL
ABBREVIATIONS

Stedman's

POCKET MEDICAL

ABBREVIATIONS

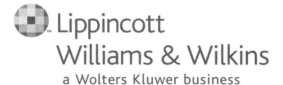

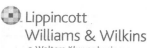

Lippincott
Williams & Wilkins
a Wolters Kluwer business

Publisher: Julie K. Stegman
Senior Product Manager: Eric Branger
Associate Managing Editor: Cecilia González
Typesetter: Brighid Willson
Printer & Binder: RR Donnelley

Copyright © 2006 Lippincott Williams & Wilkins
351 West Camden Street
Baltimore, Maryland 21201-2436

Printed in the United States of America

ISBN 0–7817-6694–X

01
1 2 3 4 5 6 7 8 9 10

Contents

Acknowledgments

An important part of our editorial process is the involvement of medical transcriptionists—as advisors, reviewers, and/or editors.

We extend special thanks to Ellen Atwood for editing the manuscript and for helping to resolve many difficult questions. We also thank Ellen for performing the final prepublication review. As always, Barb Ferretti played an integral role in the process by reviewing the content files for format, updating the database, and providing a final quality check.

As with all our Stedman's word references, this resource incorporates the suggestions and expertise of our many contacts in the medical transcriptionist community. Thanks to all of our advisory board participants, reviewers, and editors; AAMT meeting attendees; and others who have written us with requests and comments—keep talking, and we'll keep listening.

Editor's Preface

Abbreviations, acronyms, and symbols are such an integral part of science, and particularly medical science, that it is difficult to imagine these short forms disappearing completely. In the name of patient safety, the Joint Commission on Accreditation of Healthcare Organizations (JCAHO) and the Institute for Safe Medical Practices (ISMP) have published lists of abbreviations, acronyms, and symbols that are not to be used in handwritten or printed patient documentation. These lists are remarkably short and do not support the erroneous contention that all abbreviations are bad and should never be used under any circumstances. Some healthcare institutions have published in-house lists of acceptable abbreviations, but this is neither universal nor required. Journals, textbooks, and spoken medical language will likely not only continue to rely on abbreviations, but will also continue to add to the stockpile of existing short forms as a result of growth and change. Scientific and mathematical notation will continue to use short forms and symbols.

The need for comprehensive and understandable lists of the acceptable short forms has actually increased dramatically over the past five or so years. It is now even more critical that transcriptionists, students, allied health personnel, and records and billing technicians have clear, understandable reference to appropriate usage and expansion of abbreviations.

Research and discoveries in genetics, disease processes, therapies, organisms, medical equipment, testing, and analysis, as well as the vernacular of terrorism and the "new" warfare, have provided an abundance of new words with corresponding abbreviations. Many of these new abbreviations already exist, but with different expansions. Applying the correct expansion to an abbreviation is a matter of context. Other than the JCAHO Do Not Use list, usage and style are not universal. This may be governed by a publisher, institution, hospital, or practitioner, and may differ widely. Some allow abbreviations, some only the expanded form, while others require both abbreviation and expansion in varying combinations or styles.

The publisher has a duty to provide a well-researched, accurate, and useful product. This handbook, *Stedman's Pocket Medical Abbreviations*, is the result of carefully reviewing existing databases, evaluating usage, winnowing out terms that are confusing, obscure, or frank error, and keeping the most commonly used and agreed-upon expansions for medical specialties. Of necessity, general science and mathematical abbreviations are included, limited to those most likely to occur in clinical medical settings. Dangerous, error prone, and JCAHO's prohibited abbreviations are clearly identified with the use of red color.

We trust that this publication will be a valuable tool to assist in the practical application of medical information.

Ellen Atwood

Publisher's Preface

Stedman's Pocket Medical Abbreviations offers a concise, authoritative reference to medical abbreviations and their meanings, providing the assurance of quality and accuracy to the healthcare community, including practitioners, educators, students, and to the wordsmiths of the healthcare professions—medical transcriptionists, medical editors and copyeditors, health information management personnel, and court reporters. In addition, this reference offers valuable abbreviations, acronyms, symbols, and their meanings to those who work with or are exposed to medical terminology and medical documentation in many other areas, such as insurance and law.

We received many requests to create a pocket version of *Stedman's Abbreviations, Acronyms & Symbols*. To that end, we have published this book to meet our customers' needs for a comprehensive, yet concise, portable format, enabling our readers to quickly find the many common abbreviations, acronyms, and symbols used in the healthcare setting along with their meanings. Special consideration has been given to the Joint Commission on Accreditation of Healthcare Organizations (JCAHO) and to the Institute for Safe Medical Practices (ISMP) published lists of abbreviations, acronyms, and symbols that are not to be used in handwritten or printed patient documentation. These "dangerous" abbreviations, as well as those identified by both organizations and others as "do not use" or "error prone," are highlighted in the text in red type.

A major focus of the development of this pocket reference, from the design to the format and style of the individual entries, was to present sought-after information in a format that would facilitate easy lookup and quick comprehension. Novices as well as seasoned professionals are encouraged to read the descriptions of this reference's organization, format, and style in the Explanatory Notes to make the most of its features.

We at Lippincott Williams & Wilkins strive to provide you with the most up-to-date and accurate word references available. We welcome your suggestions for improvements, changes, corrections, and additions—whatever will make this *Stedman's* product more useful to you. Please complete the postage-paid card in this book, or contact us by email at stedmans@lww.com.

Explanatory Notes

Terms identified by the Joint Commission on Accreditation of Healthcare Organizations (JCAHO) and the Institute for Safe Medical Practices (ISMP) and others as Do Not Use, Error Prone, or Dangerous are distinguished by red type.

Abbreviations as well as their expansions are listed in alphabetical order, letter by letter. See Format and Style for details. Refer to Greeks, Scientific Notation, and Amino Acid Abbreviations for relevant information.

FORMAT AND STYLE

Preferences and Style: Stedman's collects current examples from the literature, and this book, as do others in the series, reflects preferences and usage across a wide spectrum of users and organizations in English-speaking countries. Institutions, regulatory agencies, personal preferences, and non-United States English language usage may differ in style or rules. Please follow the guidelines of your governing agency should conflicts arise.

Organization and Order: All types of terms follow the same alphabetical sequence, with no distinction or identification of the various types of abbreviations, initialisms, acronyms, or symbols. For simplicity, all the examples and explanations herein are referred to as "abbreviation."

Each entry consists of a boldface short form (abbreviation), its "expansions" or meaning(s) following, listed alphabetically, indented, and in lightface. When there is more than one expansion, each resides on its own line, letter-by-letter in alphabetical order, with the above-noted consideration to special characters. Standard type face is followed by italics. Upper case precedes lower case. See below for Numerals.

ABG
    air-bone gap
    aortoiliac bypass graft
    arterial blood gas
    axiobuccogingival

If the expansion requires more space, it wraps to the next line with extra indentation.

POEMS

polyneuropathy, organomegaly, endocrinopathy, M protein,
  and skin changes (syndrome)
polyneuropathy, organomegaly, endocrinopathy,
  monoclonal gammopathy, and skin changes

Numerals: Arabic numerals, preceding, within, or following an abbreviation, are ignored in the alphabetical letter-by-letter order. Series of sequential numerals will secondarily be in numerical order. Roman numerals are treated the same as Arabic numerals.

Symbols: The following typographical symbols in common usage are ignored in determining alphabetical order. See below for further information on special characters usage.

ampersand	&
colon	:
comma	,
diacritic	(accent marks)
hyphen	-
period	.
semicolon	;
slash (virgule)	/
spaces	

Capital Letters and Mixed Case: For reasons of clarity and space, we have not included every possible combination of the abbreviations with variations such as all capitals, all lower case, and initial capital letter. However, if your workplace or supervisor prefers initial capitals on particular terms, it is not "wrong" to follow that style. Simply find the lower case abbreviation and make the first letter capital.

abd hyst   **Abd hyst**

Some terms are normally mixed case:

pH
mmHg
EtOH

Plurals: We have retained plural expansions only when more than one, or plurality, is described by the expansion. Plural forms of singular abbreviations have been discarded. To make a plural, simply add a lower case "s" to the abbreviation.

ABG (singular)   **ABGs** (plural)

SPECIAL CHARACTERS

Greeks: Greek characters used alone as symbols are found in Appendix 3 along with their expansions, meanings, and English translations. Appendix 3 also contains a list of abbreviations beginning with the Greek character mu (μ) that are identified as **Dangerous** by JCAHO and ISMP and should never be used.

If a Greek letter begins an abbreviation, it is ignored and the term is alphabetized by the first letter of the English alphabet in the abbreviation.

AQMS
  acute quadriplegic myopathy syndrome
βAR
  beta-adrenergic receptor
AR
  Achilles reflex

If a Greek letter ends an abbreviation, that term will be alphabetized following the upper case abbreviation and expansions and before the upper case abbreviations with numerals.

M
  blood group system
  chin
MΩ
  megohm
M1
  left mastoid

Periods: Periods are used in lower case English or Latin abbreviations if the shortened version is also a regular word.

add.   **addict.**   **anal.**

Periods are no longer used in upper case English degrees or titles.

MD   **RN**   **BS**

Mixed case terms usually have periods in the United States, but not in other English-speaking countries. This style can be highly variable, so please follow your institution's guidelines.

Mr.   **Dr.**   **Jr.**

Periods are used in most lower case Latin abbreviations, but never upper case.

b.i.d.	**BID**
q.d.	**QD**
p.o.	**PO**

Brackets: Brackets contain information about a term's origin (etymology), and immediately follow the expanded form. Enclosed within the brackets are the language of origin and the foreign word of origin in italics. The languages are signified.

L., Latin; G., Greek; Ger., German; Fr., French; Sp., Spanish; It., Italian

HD
   hard corn [L. *heloma durum*]

Colons: The preferred scientific notation to express ratio is the colon.

S:N
   signal to noise ratio

Parentheses: Parentheses used within the abbreviation are ignored in ordering.

PAA
P(A-aDO2)
p(A-a)O2
pAAT

Used with the expansion, parentheses have several functions.

1. Enclose explanatory material to provide further information:

A
    absolute (temperature)
    (start of) anesthesia

2. Clarify usage that otherwise might be ambiguous:

BEPTI
    bionomics, environment, *Plasmodium*, treatment, and immunity
    (malaria epidemiology)

3. Provide a mini-definition:

Gy
    gray (unit of absorbed dose of ionizing radiation)

4. Identify the generic name of a drug:

CAM
    cyclophosphamide, Adriamycin (doxorubicin), and methotrexate

Brackets, parentheses, and the material they contain are ignored in alphabetization.

Slang: Slang terms are inappropriate in formal documents. Some hospitals and institutions do allow a limited number of abbreviations to be used in place of the expansion, such as **LAD** rather than **left anterior descending**. Unless otherwise specified in your particular circumstance, slang terms should always be expanded.

appy
    appendectomy
crit
    hematocrit
DTs
    delirium tremens

We have taken great care to remove derogatory, racist, sexist, and other insulting terms from this edition.

Scientific Notation: Certain units of measure, scientific notation, amino acids, and elements have universally recognized or preferred abbreviations, although multiple forms may be encountered in print. We have reserved (or limited) the expansions of these abbreviations to the universally accepted meanings.

UNITS OF MEASURE

Initial Capital and Upper Case Abbreviations

ampere	A	gray	Gy
becquerel	Bq	henry	H
celsius	C	hertz	Hz
coulomb	C	newton	N
curie	Ci	pascal	Pa
Fahrenheit	F	siemens	S
farad	F	tesla	T
joule	J	volt	V
liter	L	watt	W

Amino Acid Abbreviations: Each amino acid has two recognized abbreviations, a trivial name, and a letter symbol. Again, there are variations to be found in print, not universally recognized.

Amino Acid	Name	Symbol	Amino Acid	Name	Symbol
alanine	Ala	A	arginine	Arg	R
asparagine	Asn	N	aspartic acid	Asp	D
cysteine	Cys	C	glutamine	Gln	Q
glutamic acid	Glu	E	glycine	Gly	G
histidine	His	H	isoleucine	Ile	I
leucine	Leu	L	lysine	Lys	K
methionine	Met	M	phenylalanine	Phe	F
proline	Pro	P	serine	Ser	S
threonine	Thr	T	tryptophan	Trp	W
tyrosine	Tyr	Y	valine	Val	V

References

In addition to the lists of our MT Editorial Advisory Board members (from their daily transcription work), we used the following sources for new terms in *Stedman's Pocket Medical Abbreviations*.

Books

The AAMT Book of Style, 2nd Edition. Modesto, CA: AAMT, 2002.

Davis, N., MEDical ABBREViations, 12th ed. Warminster, PA: Neil M. Davis Associates, 2005.

Delong, M., Medical Acronyms, Eponyms, & Abbreviations. Los Angeles: Practice Management Information Corporation, 2002.

Haber, K., Common Abbreviations in Clinical Medicine. New York: Raven Press, 1988.

Jablonski S., Dictionary of Medical Acronyms & Abbreviations. Philadelphia, PA: Elsevier Saunders, 2005.

Lance, L.L., Quick Look Drug Book 2006. Baltimore: Lippincott Williams & Wilkins, 2006.

Stedman's Abbreviations, Acronyms & Symbols, 3rd Edition. Baltimore: Lippincott Williams & Wilkins, 2003.

Stedman's Alternative and Complementary Medicine Words, 2nd Edition. Baltimore: Lippincott Williams & Wilkins, 2005.

Stedman's Anatomy & Physiology Words, 2nd Edition. Baltimore: Lippincott Williams & Wilkins, 2002.

Stedman's Cardiovascular & Pulmonary Words, 4th Edition. Baltimore: Lippincott Williams & Wilkins, 2004.

Stedman's Dermatology & Immunology Words, 3rd Edition. Baltimore: Lippincott Williams & Wilkins, 2005.

Stedman's Endocrinology Words, 2nd Edition. Baltimore: Lippincott Williams & Wilkins, 2005.

Stedman's GI & GU Words, 4th Edition. Baltimore: Lippincott Williams & Wilkins, 2005.

Stedman's Internal Medicine & Geriatric Words. Baltimore: Lippincott Williams & Wilkins, 2002.

Stedman's Medical Dictionary, 28th Edition. Baltimore: Lippincott Williams & Wilkins, 2006.

Stedman's Medical Dictionary for the Health Professions and Nursing, Illustrated, 5th Edition. Baltimore: Lippincott Williams & Wilkins, 2005.

Stedman's Medical and Surgical Equipment Words, 4th Edition. Baltimore: Lippincott Williams & Wilkins, 2004.

Stedman's OB-GYN & Genetics Words, 3rd Edition. Baltimore: Lippincott Williams & Wilkins, 2001.

Stedman's OB-GYN & Pediatric Words, 4th Edition. Baltimore: Lippincott Williams & Wilkins, 2005.

Stedman's Oncology Words, 5th Edition. Baltimore: Lippincott Williams & Wilkins, 2006.

Stedman's Ophthalmology Words, 3rd Edition. Baltimore: Lippincott Williams & Wilkins, 2004.

Stedman's Organisms & Infectious Disease Words. Baltimore: Lippincott Williams & Wilkins, 2002.

Stedman's Orthopaedic & Rehab Words, 4th Edition. Baltimore: Lippincott Williams & Wilkins, 2003.

Stedman's Pathology & Lab Medicine Words, 4th Edition. Baltimore: Lippincott Williams & Wilkins, 2005.

Stedman's Plastic Surgery, ENT, & Dentistry Words, 4th Edition. Baltimore: Lippincott Williams & Wilkins, 2005.

Stedman's Pocket Abbreviations, Acronyms & Symbols, for PDA. Baltimore: Lippincott Williams & Wilkins, 2004.

Stedman's Psychiatry Words, 3rd Edition. Baltimore: Lippincott Williams & Wilkins, 2003.

Stedman's Radiology Words, 5th Edition. Baltimore: Lippincott Williams & Wilkins, 2006.

Stedman's Surgery Words, 2nd Edition. Baltimore: Lippincott Williams & Wilkins, 2002.

Vera Pyle's Current Medical Terminology, 10th Edition. Modesto, CA: Health Professions Institute, 2005.

Journals

Latest Word. Philadelphia: Saunders, 1999–2005.

Perspectives on the Medical Transcription Profession. Modesto, CA: Health Professions Institute, 1999–2005.

A
 absolute
 acetum (vinegar)
 acromion
 activity (radiation)
 alanine (*See also* Ala)
 alveolar gas (subscript)
 anisotropic (band in striated muscle)
 blood group in the ABO system
 ear [L. *auris*]
 mass number
 (start of) anesthesia
 subspinale (point A in cephalometrics)
 year [L. *annum*]
A angstrom
A+ blood type A positive
A- blood type A negative
a
 arterial blood (subscript)
 atto-
a. artery [L. *arteria*]
a specific absorptivity
A₁
 aortic first sound
 first auditory area
A₂
 aortic second sound
 second auditory area
A>B air greater than bone (conduction)
AA
 acetic acid
 achievement age
 active avoidance
 acupuncture analgesia
 alcohol abuse
 amino acid
 amplitude of accommodation
 anterior apical
 aortic arch
 atlantoaxial
 audiologic assessment
 autoanalyzer

A&A
 aid and attendance
 arthroscopy and arthrotomy
 awake and aware
A:A arm to ankle (pulse ratio)
Aa
 alveolar to arterial (gradient)
 aortic artery
aA
 abampere
 arterial to alveolar (gradient)
aa. arteries [L. *arteriae*]
AAA
 abdominal aortic aneurysm
 acquired aplastic anemia
AABCC alertness (consciousness), airway, breathing, circulation, and cervical spine
AABR automated auditory brainstem response
AAC augmentative and alternative communication
AACD
 abdominal aortic counterpulsation device
 age-associated cognitive decline
AAD
 acid-ash diet
 acroangiodermatitis
 antiarrhythmic drug
 antibiotic-associated diarrhea
 atlantoaxial dislocation
AAE annuloaortic ectasia
AAF
 acetic acid-alcohol-formalin (fixative)
 altered auditory feedback
 ascorbic acid factor
aAG autoantigen
AAI
 acute adrenal insufficiency
 atrial demand-inhibited (pacemaker)
 axial acetabular index

AAL anterior axillary line
AAMI age-associated memory impairment
AAN
   AIDS-associated nephropathy
   analgesic-associated nephropathy
AAO awake, alert, oriented
AAOx3 alert, awake, and oriented to time, place, and person
AAR Australia antigen radioimmunoassay
AAROM active-assisted range of motion
AAS
   acid aspiration syndrome
   alcoholic abstinence syndrome
   androgenic-anabolic steroid
   aortic arch syndrome
   atlantoaxial subluxation
   atomic absorption spectrophotometer
   atypical absence seizure
AASH adrenal androgen-stimulating hormone
AAT
   Aachen aphasie test
   activity as tolerated
   alanine aminotransferase
   alkylating agent therapy
   androgen ablation therapy
   animal-assisted therapy
   auditory apperception test
AB
   abdominal
   abnormal
   abortion
   active bilaterally
   Alcian blue
   antibiotic (*See also* ABx)
   apex beat
   asthmatic bronchitis
   axiobuccal
   blood group in ABO system
A&B apnea and bradycardia
A:B acid to base ratio
Ab antibody
a-b air-bone (conduction)

ABAER automated brainstem auditory evoked response
A band the dark-staining zone of a striated muscle
ABBI Advanced Breast Biopsy Instrumentation
abbr, abbrev abbreviation
ABC
   absolute bone conduction
   acalculous biliary colic
   acid balance control
   airway, breathing, circulation
   all but code (resuscitation order)
   antigen-binding capacity
   apnea, bradycardia, and cyanosis
   applesauce, bananas, and cereal (diet)
   argon beam coagulator
   aspiration biopsy cytology
   atomic, biological, chemical
   axiobuccocervical
ABC and C&C airway, breathing, circulation, cervical spine, and consciousness level
ABCD
   airway, breathing, circulation, disability
   asymmetry, border, color, and diameter (of melanoma)
ABCDE
   airway, breathing, circulation, disability, exposure
   pentavalent botulism toxoid
ABCDES alignment, bone mineralization, calcifications, distribution (of joints), erosion, soft tissue/nails (x-ray features in arthritis)
ABCIC airway, breathing, circulation, intravenous crystalloid
ABD
   abdomen
   aged, blind, and disabled
   aggressive behavioral disturbance
   autologous blood donation
   average body dose

abd hyst abdominal
hysterectomy
ABE acute bacterial endocarditis
ABEP auditory brainstem-evoked
potential
ABER abducted and externally
rotated
ABF aortobifemoral (bypass)
ABG
air-bone gap
aortoiliac bypass graft
arterial blood gas
axiobuccogingival
ABI
ankle-brachial index
atherothrombotic brain
infarction
auditory brainstem implant
ABK aphakic bullous
keratopathy
ABL
abetalipoproteinemia
African Burkitt lymphoma
antigen-binding lymphocyte
axiobuccolingual
ABLB alternate binaural
loudness balance
ABM
adjusted body mass
alveolar basement membrane
autologous bone marrow
ABMA antibasement membrane
antibody
ABMTx autologous bone
marrow transplant
ABN
abnormality
advance beneficiary notice
ABO blood group system
(groups A, AB, B, and O)
ABP
ambulatory blood pressure
arterial blood pressure
AB/PAS Alcian blue and
periodic acid-Schiff (stain)
ABR
abortus Bang ring (test)
auditory brainstem response
abr abrasion

ABS
abdominal surgery
abnormal brainstem
absent
absorbed
absorption
acute brain syndrome
aging brain syndrome
amniotic band sequence
antibody screen
anti-B serum
arterial blood sample
at bedside
AB-SAAP autologous blood
selective aortic arch perfusion
ABSR auditory brainstem
response
ABT
alcohol breath tester
autologous bone marrow
transplantation
ABV arthropod-borne virus
ABx antibiotic (*See also* AB)
ABY acid bismuth yeast
(medium)
AC
accommodative convergence
acetate
acetylcysteine
acidity
acromioclavicular
activated charcoal
adherent cell
adrenal cortex
adrenocorticoid
air conduction
alcoholic cirrhosis
alternating current
anesthesia circuit
antecubital
anterior chamber (of eye)
anterior commissure
anticoagulant
anticomplement
aortic closure
aortocoronary
assist control (ventilation)
axiocervical
before meals [L. *ante cibum*]

Ac
acetyl
actinium
aC abcoulomb
ACA
acrodermatitis chronica
atrophicans
aminocaproic acid
anterior cerebral artery
anterior choroidal artery
anterior communicating artery
(*See also* ACoA)
anticytoplasmic antibody
automatic clinical analyzer
AC:A accommodative
convergence to
accommodation ratio
ACAD atherosclerotic coronary
artery disease
ACAN acanthocyte
ACAT
acyl coenzyme A to
cholesterol acyltransferase
ratio
automated computerized axial
tomography
ACB arterialized capillary blood
AC&BC air conduction and
bone conduction
ACBG aortocoronary bypass
graft
ACC
acalculous cholecystitis
accident
amylase/creatinine clearance
anterior central curve
aplasia cutis congenita
articular chondrocalcinosis
automated cell count
AcCoA acetylcoenzyme A
accum accumulated
accur. accurately [L.
accuratissime]
ACD
absolute cardiac dullness
active compression-
decompression
advanced care directive
allergic contact dermatitis
alpha-chain disease

anemia of chronic disease
angiokeratoma corporis
diffusum
anterior cervical discectomy
anterior chamber diameter
anticonvulsant drug
arrhythmia control device
AC-DC alternating current or
direct current
ACE
aerosol cloud enhancer
alcohol, chloroform, and ether
(mixture)
angiotensin-converting enzyme
acetyl-CoA acetylcoenzyme A
ACF
acute care facility
anterior cervical fusion
area correction factor
asymmetric crying facies
ACFS anterior cervical plate
fixation system
ACG
angiocardiogram
angle-closure glaucoma
aortocoronary graft
apexcardiogram
AcG accelerator globulin (factor
V)
ACH
achalasia
adrenocortical hormone
amyotrophic cerebellar
hypoplasia
arm girth, chest depth, and
hip width (nutritional index)
ACh acetylcholine
AChA anterior choroidal artery
AChE acetylcholinesterase
ACHOO autosomal dominant
compelling helioophthalmic
outburst (syndrome)
AC&HS before meals and at
bedtime [L. *antecibum* +
horasomni]
ACI
acoustic comfort index
adrenocortical insufficiency
anticlonus index

AC IOL, ACIOL anterior
  chamber intraocular lens
ACIS automated cellular
  imaging system
ACJ acromioclavicular joint
ACL
  accessory collateral ligament
  anterior cruciate ligament
aCL anticardiolipin
ACLA anticardiolipin antibody
ACLS advanced cardiac life
  support
ACM
  anticardiac myosin
  Arnold-Chiari malformation
ACMV assist-control mechanical
  ventilation
ACOA adult child of alcoholic
ACoA anterior communicating
  artery (*See also* ACA)
acor apex cornea
acous acoustic
ACP
  accessory conduction pathway
  anterior cervical plate
AC-PC anterior commissure-
  posterior commissure
AC-PH, ac phos acid phosphatase
ACPS acrocephalopolysyndactyly
acq acquired
ACR
  absolute catabolic rate
  adenomatosis of colon and
  rectum
ACS
  abdominal compartment
  syndrome
  acrocallosal syndrome
  acrocephalosyndactyly (type
  I–V)
  anterior compartment
  syndrome
ACT
  acid clearance test
  activated clotting time
  allergen challenge test
  anticoagulant therapy
  asthma care training
  atropine coma therapy

act.
  active
  activity
Act Ex active exercise
ACTH adrenocorticotropic
  hormone (corticotropin)
ACTH-RF adrenocorticotropic
  hormone releasing factor
ACTN adrenocorticotropin
ACV assist/control ventilation
ACVB aortocoronary venous
  bypass
ACVD atherosclerotic
  cardiovascular disease
acyl-CoA acylcoenzyme A
AD
  abdominal diameter
  absorbed dose
  acetate dialysis
  active disease
  addict(ion)
  admitting diagnosis
  advanced directive
  affective disorder
  after discharge
  alcohol dehydrogenase
  alveolar duct
  Alzheimer dementia (disease)
  analgesic dose
  antidepressant
  aortic diameter
  aortic dissection
  atopic dermatitis
  autonomic dysreflexia
  autosomal dominant
  average deviation
  axiodistal
  axis deviation
A&D
  alcohol and drugs
  ascending and descending
  vitamins A and D
A.D. right ear [L. *auris dexter*]
  (*See also* RE)
a.d.
  alternating days (every other
  day) [L. *alternis dies*]
  as desired

ad
   adrenal
   anisotropic disc
ad. let there be added [L. *addetur*]
ADA
   Americans with Disabilities Act
   anterior descending artery
   approved dietary allowance
ADA # American Diabetes Association diet number
ADAS Alzheimer Disease Assessment Scale
ADAS-Cog Alzheimer Disease Assessment Scale, cognitive subscale
ADC
   Aid to Dependent Children
   AIDS dementia complex
   albumin, dextrose, and catalase (medium)
   average daily census
   axiodistocervical
ADD
   adduction
   attention deficit disorder
   average daily dose
ADDU alcohol and drug dependence unit
adeq adequate
AD/FHD acetabular depth to femoral head diameter
ADFN albinism-deafness (syndrome)
ADG axiodistogingival
ADH
   adhesion
   antidiuretic hormone
ADHD attention deficit hyperactivity disorder
ad hoc for this (purpose) [L. *ad hoc*]
ADI
   acceptable (allowable) daily intake
   atlantodens interval
   axiodistoincisal
ADI-R Autism Diagnostic Interview-Revised

adj
   adjacent
   adjoining
   adjunct
   adjuvant
ADK
   adenosine kinase (gene)
   automated disposable keratome
ADL
   adrenoleukodystrophy
   Amsterdam Depression List
ad lib. as desired [L. *ad libitum*]
ADLs activities of daily living
ADM
   abductor digiti minimi (muscle)
   admission
   admit
AdM adrenal medulla
ADME absorption, distribution, metabolism, and excretion
admin
   administer
   administration
ADMR average daily metabolic rate
ADMX adrenal medullectomy
adn
   adenoid
   adenoidectomy
ADNase antideoxyribonuclease
ad naus. to the point of producing nausea [L. *ad nauseam*]
ADO
   adolescent medicine
   axiodistoocclusal
Ado adenosine
ADOD arthrodentoosteodysplasia
adol adolescent
ADP
   adenosine diphosphate
   approved drug product
ADPase adenosine diphosphatase
ADPL average daily patient load
ADQ
   abductor digiti quinti (muscle)
   adequate

ADR
   acceptable dental remedies
   actual death rate
   adverse drug reaction
   airway dilation reflex
Adr adrenaline
ADRS Alzheimer Disease
   Rating Scale
ADS
   Alcohol Dependence Scale
   anatomical dead space
   anonymous donor sperm
   anterior drawer sign
ADT
   accepted dental therapeutics
   adenosine triphosphate
   agar diffusion test
   alternate day therapy
   androgen deprivation therapy
   Auditory Discrimination Test
ADV
   adenovirus
   advanced
   adventitia
   advice
   advise
ADW assault with deadly
   weapon
AE
   above elbow
   acrodermatitis enteropathica
   aftereffect
   agarose electrophoresis
   air embolism
   airplane ear
   alcoholic embryopathy
   anoxic encephalopathy
   antiembolitic
   antitoxin unit [Ger.
     Antitoxineinhei]
   atherosclerotic encephalopathy
A&E accident and emergency
   (department)
AEA
   above-elbow amputation
   alcohol, ether, and acetone
   (solution)
   allergic extrinsic alveolitis

AEB
   as evidenced by
   atrial ectopic beat
AEC
   absolute eosinophil count
   aortic ejection click
   at earliest convenience
AECD
   allergic eczematous contact
     dermatitis
   automatic external
     cardioverter-defibrillator
AECG ambulatory
   electrocardiogram
AED
   antiepileptic (anticonvulsant)
     drug
   antihidrotic ectodermal
     dysplasia
   automatic external defibrillator
AEDF absent end-diastolic
   blood flow (umbilical artery
   Doppler)
AEF auditory-evoked magnetic
   field
AEG
   air encephalogram
   atrial electrogram
AEI atrial emptying index
AEIOU TIPS alcohol, epilepsy,
   insulin, overdose, uremia,
   trauma, infection, psychiatric,
   stroke (causes of decreased
   level of consciousness)
AEM
   ambulatory electrocardiographic
     monitoring
   analytical electron microscope
AENNS Albert Einstein
   Neonatal Developmental Scale
AEP auditory evoked potential
AEq age equivalent
AER
   abduction-external rotation
   acoustic evoked response
   aided equalization response
   auditory evoked response
AERA average evoked response
   audiometry

AERP atrial effective refractory period

AES
anal endosonography
antiembolic stockings
antieosinophilic serum
antral ethmoidal sphenoidectomy
aortic ejection sound

AEST aeromedical evacuation support team

AEX aerobic exercise

AF
acid fast
adult female
amaurosis fugax
amniotic fluid
anteflex
anterior fontanelle
anterofrontal
antifibrinogen
antifungal
aortofemoral
apical foramen
arcuate fasciculus
atrial flutter
audiofrequency

A-F
air-fluid (level)
ankle-foot (orthosis)

AFA
advanced first aid
alcohol-formaldehyde-acetic acid (fixative or solution)

AFB
acid-fast bacillus
aortofemoral bypass

AFB1 aflatoxin B1

AFC acid-fast culture

AFE amniotic fluid embolism

AFF
atrial fibrillation-flutter
atrial filling fraction

aff afferent

AFFN acrofrontofacionasal

AFG
alpha-fetoglobulin
auditory figure-ground

AFI
amaurotic familial idiocy
amniotic fluid index

AFib atrial fibrillation

AFO ankle-foot orthosis

AFP
adiabatic fast passage
anterior faucial pillar
atrial filling pressure

aFP alpha-fetoprotein

AFRAX autism-fragile X (syndrome)

AFS
acid-fast smear
acromegaloid facial syndrome
aldehyde-fuchsin stain

AFT agglutination-flocculation test

AFX air-fluid exchange

AG
abdominal girth
angular gyrus
anion gap
antigen
antiglobulin
antigravity
atrial gallop
attached gingiva
axiogingival
azurophilic granule

A:G albumin-globulin ratio

Ag silver [L. *argentum*]

AGA
antiglomerular antibody
appropriate for gestational age

AG-AB antigen-antibody (complex)

AgCl silver chloride

AGCUS atypical glandular cells of undetermined significance

AGD agar gel diffusion

AGECAT automatic geriatric examination for computer assisted taxonomy

AGEPC acetyl glyceryl ether phosphorylcholine

AGG
agammaglobulinemia
aggregation

AGH amenorrhea, galactorrhea, hypothyroidism
agit. shake [L. *agita*]
AGL agglutination
agn agnosia
AgNO₃ silver nitrate
AGPT agar-gel precipitation test
AGR
　aniridia, ambiguous genitalia, mental retardation
　anticipatory goal response
AGS
　adrenogenital syndrome
　audiogenic seizures
AGT antiglobulin test
AGV aniline gentian violet
AH
　alcoholic hepatitis
　amenorrhea and hirsutism
　amenorrhea and hyperprolactinemia
　arterial hypertension
　artificial heart
　assisted hatching
　astigmatic hypermetropia
　atrium-His bundle
　autonomic hyperreflexia
　axillary hair
Ah ampere-hour
aH abhenry
ah hyperopic astigmatism
AHA
　alpha hydroxy acid
　arthritis-hives-angioedema (syndrome)
　autoimmune hemolytic anemia
AHA.SOC American Heart Association Stroke Outcome Classification
AHC
　adrenal hypoplasia congenita
　alternating hemiplegia of childhood
　antihemophilic factor C
AHD
　antihypertensive drug
　arteriosclerotic heart disease
　atherosclerotic heart disease
　autoimmune hemolytic disease

AHF
　accelerated hyperfractionation
　antihemophilic factor (factor VIII)
AHFS American Hospital Formulary Service
AHG
　aggregated human globulin
　antihemophilic globulin
　antihuman globulin
AHH anosmia and hypogonadotropic hypogonadism (syndrome)
AHHD arteriosclerotic hypertensive heart disease
AHI
　acetabular head index
　acromiohumeral interval
　active hostility index
　anterior horn index
　apnea-hypopnea index
　Arthritis Helplessness Index
AHL apparent half-life
AHLG antihuman lymphocyte globulin
AHLS antihuman lymphocyte serum
AHM
　ambulatory Holter monitor
　anterior hyaloid membrane
AHP
　afterspike hyperpolarization
　air at high pressure
　American Hand Prosthetics
AHPO anterior hypothalamic preoptic (area)
AHR
　airways hyperreactivity
　airways hyperresponsiveness
　autonomic hyperreflexia
AHS
　adaptive hand skills
　African horse sickness
　alveolar hypoventilation syndrome
AHT alternating hypertropia
AHuG aggregated human immunoglobulin G

AI

accidental injury
acetabular index
acute inflammation
adiposity index
aggregation index
allergy index
anal index
anaphylatoxin inhibitor
angiogenesis inhibitor
angiotensin inhibitor
anxiety index
aortic insufficiency
aortoiliac
apical impulse
apnea index
articulation index
artificial insemination
artificial intelligence
atherogenic index
atrial insufficiency
autoimmune
axioincisal
first auditory area

A&I allergy and immunology
AIA aspirin-induced asthma
AIB avian infectious bronchitis
AIBF anterior interbody fusion
AICA anterior internal cerebellar artery
AICD automatic implantable cardioverter-defibrillator
AICF autoimmune complement fixation
AICS artery of inferior cavernous sinus

AID

antiinflammatory drug
artificial insemination by donor
autoimmune deficiency
autoimmune disease
automatic implantable defibrillator
average interocular difference

AIDA automatic interpretation for diagnostic assistance
AIDS acquired immune deficiency syndrome

AIDS-HAQ acquired immunodeficiency syndrome health assessment questionnaire
AIDS-KS acquired immunodeficiency syndrome with Kaposi sarcoma
AIF apoptosis-inducing factor
AIG antiimmunoglobulin
AIH

anterior interhemispheric approach
aortic intramural hematoma
artificial insemination, homologous (husband)
autoimmune hepatitis

AIHA autoimmune hemolytic anemia
AII second auditory area
AIIS anterior inferior iliac spine
AIL

angioimmunoblastic lymphadenopathy
angioimmunoblastic lymphoma

AILD alveolar-interstitial lung disease
AIM

Ace intramedullary (nail)
aerosol inhalation monitor

AIMO anterior inferior mandibular osteotomy
AIMS

Abnormal Involuntary Movements Scale
Alberta Infant Motor Scale
arthritis impact measurement scale

AIN anterior interosseous nerve
AIOD aortoiliac occlusive disease
AIP

acute interstitial pneumonia
automated immunoprecipitation
average intravascular pressure

AIR average impairment rating
AIRE autoimmune regulator
AIRF alteration in respiratory function
AIROM active integral range of motion

AIS
  Abbreviated Injury Scale
  adenocarcinoma in situ
  adolescent idiopathic scoliosis
  amniotic infection syndrome
  amputation index score
  androgen insensitivity
    syndrome
  anterior interosseous nerve
    syndrome
AIS/ISS Abbreviated Injury
    Score/Injury Severity Score
AIT auditory integration training
AITP autoimmune
    thrombocytopenia
AIVR accelerated idioventricular
    rhythm
AIVV anterior internal vertebral
    vein
AJ ankle jerk
AK
  acne keloidalis
  actinic keratosis
  applied kinesiology
  artificial kidney
  astigmatic keratotomy
AKA
  above-knee amputation
  alcoholic ketoacidosis
  also known as
AKBR arterial ketone body
    ratio
AKE
  acrokeratoelastoidosis
  active knee extension
A/kg ampere per kilogram
AKR aldo-keto reductase
AKS
  alcoholic Korsakoff syndrome
  arthroscopic knee surgery
  auditory and kinesthetic
    sensation
AKU alkaptonuria
AKV acrokeratosis verruciformis
AL
  absolute latency
  adaptation level
  allergy
  anterolateral
  argon laser
  avian leukosis
  axial length
  axiolingual
  lethal antigen
Al aluminum
Al$_2$O$_3$ aluminum oxide
ALa axiolabial
Ala alanine (*See also* A)
ALAD abnormal left axis
    deviation
ALAG, ALaG axiolabiogingival
ALAL, ALaL axiolabiolingual
ALARA as low as reasonably
    achievable (radiation exposure)
ALAT alanine aminotransferase
ALAX apical long axis
ALB albumin
alb. white [L. *albus*]
ALBPSQ Acute Low Back
    Pain Screening Questionnaire
ALBUMS aldehyde-linker based
    ultrasensitive mismatch
    scanning (molecular analysis)
ALC
  alcoholic liver cirrhosis
  approximate lethal
    concentration
  axiolinguocervical
ALCA anomalous left coronary
    artery
ALCAPA anomalous origin of
    left coronary artery from
    pulmonary artery
ALCR alcohol rub
AL:CR axial length to corneal
    radius ratio
AlCr aluminum crown
ALD
  adrenoleukodystrophy
  alcoholic liver disease
  appraisal of language
    disturbances
  assistive listening device
ALE
  active life expectancy
  allowable limits of error
ALEC artificial lung expanding
    compound

11

ALG   axiolinguogingival
ALI   argon laser iridotomy
A-line   arterial line (*See also* art. line)
ALK
   alkaline
   alkylating (agent)
   automated laser keratomileusis
alk phos   alkaline phosphatase
ALL   acute lymphocytic leukemia
ALLD   arthroscopic lumbar laser discectomy
ALMCA   anomalous left main coronary artery
ALMN   adrenoleukomyeloneuropathy
ALN   alendronate
ALND   axillary lymph node dissection
ALO   axiolinguoocclusal
ALOS   average length of stay
ALP
   acute leukemia protocol
   anterior lobe of pituitary
   argon laser photocoagulation
ALPI   argon laser peripheral iridoplasty
ALPS
   alcoholism, leukopenia, pneumococcal sepsis
   anterior locking plate system
   Aphasia Language Performance Scale
ALS
   advanced life support
   amyotrophic lateral sclerosis
   androgen insensitivity syndrome
   anterolateral sclerosis
   anticipated lifespan
ALT
   alanine aminotransferase
   alanine transaminase
   anterolateral tract
   argon laser trabeculoplasty
   avian laryngotracheitis
alt
   alternate
   altitude

ALT:AST   alanine aminotransferase to aspartate aminotransferase ratio
ALV   ascending lumbar vein
alv
   alveolar
   alveolus
alv vent   alveolar ventilation (*See also* VA)
alvx   alveolectomy
ALW   arch-loop-whorl (fingerprint system)
AM
   adult male
   alveolar mucosa
   ametropia
   ammeter
   amplitude modulation
   anovular menstruation
   anterior midpapillary
   anteromeatal
   arterial malformation
   articulation manipulation
   Austin Moore (prosthesis)
   axiomesial
   before noon [L. *ante meridiem*]
   meter angle
   mixed astigmatism
   myopic astigmatism
A/m   ampere per meter
A/m^2   ampere per square meter
Am   americium
am   ammeter
AMA
   against medical advice
   antimitochondrial antibody
AMAC   adults molested as children
AMAL   amalgam
AMAP   as much as possible
AMB
   ambulate
   ambulatory
   avian myeloblastosis
amb
   ambient
   ambulance
AMBER   advance multiple beam equalization radiography

ambig ambiguous
ambul ambulate
AMC
  antibody-mediated cytotoxicity
  antimalaria campaign
  arm muscle circumference
  arthrogryposis multiplex
    congenita
  ataxia-microcephaly-cataract
    (syndrome)
  automatic mode conversion
  axiomesiocervical
AM:CR amylase to creatinine
  ratio
AMD
  acid maltase deficiency
  acromandibular dysplasia
  adrenomyelodystrophy
  age-related macular
    degeneration
  arthroscopic microdiscectomy
  articular motion device
  axiomesiodistal
AME
  aseptic meningoencephalitis
  Austin Medical Equipment
AMERIND American Indian
  Sign Language
AMES age, (distant) metastases,
  extent and size
Ameslan American Sign
  Language (*See also* ASL)
AMG
  acoustic myography
  aminoglycoside
  axiomesiogingival
AMH
  antimüllerian hormone
  automated medical history
  mixed astigmatism with
    myopia predominating
Amh mixed astigmatism with
  myopia predominating
AMHT automated multiphasic
  health testing
AMI
  acute myocardial infarction
  antibody-mediated immunity
  axiomesioincisal

AML
  acute myelogenous leukemia
  angiomyolipoma
  anterior mitral leaflet
AMLB alternate monaural
  loudness balance (test)
AMLR auditory middle-latency
  response
AMM agnogenic myeloid
  metaplasia
AMML acute myelomonocytic
  leukemia
ammon. ammonia
AMN
  adrenomyeloneuropathy
  anterior median nucleus
amnio amniocentesis
AMO axiomesioocclusal
A-mode amplitude mode
AMP
  acid mucopolysaccharide
  adenosine monophosphate
    (adenylic acid)
  amphetamine
  ampule
  amputation
  assisted medical procreation
  average mean pressure
amp
  amplification
  amputee
AMPEE acute multifocal
  placoid pigment epitheliopathy
AMPK adenosine
  monophosphate-activated
  protein kinase
AMPLE allergies, medications,
  past medical history, last
  meal, events preceding
  present condition (mnemonic
  for history taking)
AMRO Amsterdam Rotterdam
  (trial)
AMS
  accelerator mass spectrometry
  acute mountain sickness
  aggravated in military service
  altered mental status
  aseptic meningitis syndrome

13

AMS *(continued)*
    auditory memory span
    automated multiphasic screening
    automatic mode switching
AMSA anterior middle superior alveolar
AMSIT appearance, mood, sensorium, intelligence, and thought process (portion of mental status examination)
AMT air medical transportation
amt amount
amu atomic mass unit
AMV
    alveolar minute ventilation
    assisted mechanical ventilation
AMVL anterior mitral valve leaflet
AN
    acne neonatorum
    acoustic neuroma
    adult, normal
    aminonucleoside
    amyl nitrate
    aneurysm
    anorexia nervosa
    antenatal
    aseptic necrosis
    atrionodal
    autonomic neuropathy
    avascular necrosis
A_n normal atmosphere
An
    aniridia
    anisometropia
    anodal
    anode
    antigen
ANA
    antinuclear antibody
    articular/nonarticular
ANAG acute narrow angle glaucoma
anal.
    analgesia
    analysis
ANAS, anast anastomosis
anat anatomy, anatomic

ANCA antineutrophil cytoplasmic antibody
ANCOVA analysis of covariance
AND algoneurodystrophy
ANDA Abbreviated New Drug Application
anes
    anesthesia
    anesthesiology
    anesthetic
ANF antinuclear factor
ANG
    angiogram
    angiopoietin
    angiotensin
ang pect angina pectoris
anh anhydrous
ANISO anisocytosis
ann fib annulus fibrosus
annot. annotation
ANOVA analysis of variance
ANP atrial natriuretic peptide
ANS
    acanthion
    anterior nasal spine
    autonomic nervous system
AN-SIR advice nurse structured implicit review (telemedicine)
ANT acoustic noise test
antag antagonist
ant. ax anterior axillary
anticoag anticoagulant
anti-DNA anti-deoxyribonucleic acid
anti-dsDNA anti-double-stranded deoxyribonucleic acid
anti-HB$_c$ antibody to hepatitis B core antigen
anti-log antilogarithm
anti-PCNA antiproliferating cell nuclear antigen
anti-RNP antiribonucleoprotein
anti-Sm anti-Smith (antibody)
ant. sag D anterior sagittal diameter
ant. sup. spine anterior-superior spine

ANX
  anxiety
  anxious
anx neur anxiety neurosis
anx react anxiety reaction
AO
  acridine orange (dye or test)
  airway obstruction
  ankle orthosis
  anterior oblique
  aortic opening
  arthroophthalmopathy
  ascending aorta
  atlantooccipital
  atomic orbital
  average optical density
  axioocclusal
A-O
  acoustic-optic
  atlantooccipital (joint)
Ao aorta
AOA
  abnormal oxygen affinity
  average orifice area
AO:AC aortic valve opening to
  aortic valve closing ratio
AOAP as often as possible
AOB
  accessory olfactory bulb
  alcohol on breath
AoBP aortic blood pressure
AOC
  abridged ocular chart
  aortic opening click
  area of concern
AOCD anemia of chronic
  disease
AOCLD acute on chronic liver
  disease
AOD
  adult-onset diabetes (mellitus)
  alcohol and other drugs
  arterial occlusive disease
  arterial oxygen desaturation
  auriculoosteodysplasia
AOE arising out of employment
Ao-il aorta-iliac

AOL
  acroosteolysis
  anterior oblique ligament
AOM
  acute otitis media
  ambulatory oximetry
    monitoring
AOP
  aortic pressure
  apnea of prematurity
AOR auditory oculogyric reflex
Ao regurg aortic regurgitation
Ao sten aortic stenosis
A&Ox3 alert and oriented to
  person, place, and time
A&Ox4 alert and oriented to
  person, place, time, and date
AOZ anterior optical zone
AP
  abdominoperineal (resection)
  accessory pathway
  action potential
  adductor pollicis
  adenomatous polyposis
  alum-precipitated (vaccine)
  angina pectoris
  antepartum [L. *ante partum*]
  anteroposterior
  aortic pressure
  aortic pulmonary
  apical pulse
  apothecary
  appendectomy (*See also* appy)
  appendix (*See also* appx)
  area postrema
  arterial pressure
  association period
  atherosclerotic plaque
  atrial pacing
  axiopulpal
A&P
  abdominal and perineal
  active and present
  anatomy and physiology
  assessment and plan
  auscultation and percussion
A:P ascites to plasma ratio
Ap apex

APACG acute primary angle-closure glaucoma
APACHE Acute Physiology and Chronic Health Evaluation (score, system)
APB
abductor pollicis brevis (muscle)
atrial premature beat
APC
absolute plasma concentration
adenoidal-pharyngeal-conjunctival (agent or virus)
adenomatous polyposis coli
anterior-posterior compression
aperture current
apneustic center (of brain)
argon plasma coagulator
APD
action potential duration
afferent pupillary defect
airway pressure disconnect
antipsychotic drug
auditory processing disorder
APE
acute psychotic episode
acute pulmonary edema
airway pressure excursion
anterior pituitary extract
avian pneumoencephalitis
APF acidulated phosphofluoride
Apgar appearance (color), pulse (heart rate), grimace (reflex irritability), activity (muscle tone) (mnemonic built on eponym Apgar for newborn screen)
APH
adult psychiatric hospital
alcohol-positive history
antepartum hemorrhage
anterior pituitary hormone
aph aphasia
API arterial pressure index
APIB Assessment of Preterm Infants' Behavior
APL
abductor pollicis longus (muscle)
acute promyelocytic leukemia

anterior pituitary-like (hormone)
antiphospholipid
AP&L, AP&Lat anteroposterior and lateral (radiologic view)
aPL, APLA antiphospholipid antibody
APLS advanced pediatric life support
APM
acid-precipitable material
anteroposterior movement
APN average peak noise
APO
adductor pollicis obliquus (muscle)
airway peroxidase
apoprotein (apolipoprotein)
apo apoenzyme
apoth apothecary
APP
addiction-prone personality
antiplatelet plasma
automated physiologic profile
AP/PA anteroposterior/posteroanterior
appl
appliance
applicable
application
applied
applan. flattened [L. *applanatus*]
appr, approx approximate
APPT Adolescent and Pediatric Pain Tool
appt appointment
appx appendix (*See also* AP)
appy appendectomy (*See also* AP)
APQ average perturbation quotient
APR
abdominoperineal resection
acute phase reactant
anterior pituitary resection
auropalpebral reflex
aprax apraxia
APRV airway pressure release ventilation

APS
  acute physiology score
  adenosine phosphosulfate
  anterior pararenal space
  anterior plate system
  antiphospholipid antibody
    syndrome
  arterioportal vein shunting
  attending physician's statement
  autoimmune polyglandular
    syndrome
APSD aortopulmonary septal
  defect
APSQ Abbreviated Parent
  Symptom Questionnaire
APT
  alum-precipitated toxoid
  antiplatelet trial
  atopy patch test
AP-T apical transverse
APTT, aPTT activated partial
  thromboplastin time
APV
  antineutrophil cytoplasmic
    antibody-positive vasculitis
  average peak velocity
AQ
  achievement quotient
  acoustic quantification
  anxiety quotient
  any quantity
  aphasia quotient
aq.
  aqueous
  water [L. *aqua*]
AQLQ Asthma Quality of Life
  Questionnaire
AQMS acute quadriplegic
  myopathy syndrome
βAR beta-adrenergic receptor
AR
  Achilles reflex
  acoustic reflex
  acoustic rhinometry
  active resistance
  acute rejection
  adrenergic receptor
  alarm reaction
  alcohol related

aldose reductase
allergic rhinitis
alloy restoration
analytical reagent
androgen receptor
ankle reflex
anterior root
apical-radial (pulse)
Argyll Robertson (pupil)
articulare (craniometric point)
artificially ruptured
artificial respiration
atrial rate
atrial regurgitation
aural rehabilitation
autoradiography
autorefraction
autosomal recessive
A&R advised and released
Ar
  argon
  articulare (craniometric point)
ARA
  aortic root angiogram
  Axenfeld-Reiger anomaly
ARAD abnormal right axis
  deviation
ARAS ascending reticular
  activating system
ARB
  adrenergic receptor binder
  angiotensin receptor blocker
arb arbitrary (unit)
ARBD alcohol-related birth
  defect
ARC
  abnormal retinal
    correspondence
  AIDS-related complex
  anomalous retinal
    correspondence
  arcuate nucleus (of brain)
ARD
  allergic respiratory disease
  aphakic retinal detachment
  arthritis and rheumatic
    diseases
  atopic respiratory disease

17

ARDS
　　acute respiratory distress
　　　syndrome
　　adult respiratory distress
　　　syndrome
ARE
　　active-resistive exercise
　　AIDS-related encephalitis
ARF
　　acute renal failure
　　acute respiratory failure
ArF argon fluoride
ARF/CRF acute renal failure
　　and chronic renal failure
Arg arginine (*See also* R)
arg-gly-asp arginine-glycine-
　　aspartic acid
ARGO Adjustable Advanced
　　Reciprocating Gait Orthosis
ARHL age-related hearing loss
ARI
　　acute renal insufficiency
　　airway reactivity index
ARK adrenergic receptor kinase
ArKr argon-krypton [laser]
ARL
　　AIDS-related lymphoma
　　average remaining lifetime
ARM
　　aerosol rebreathing method
　　age-related maculopathy
　　alternating range of motion
ARMD age-related macular
　　degeneration
ARMS Adverse Reaction
　　Monitoring System
AROM
　　active range of motion
　　artificial rupture of
　　　membranes
ARP
　　absolute refractory period
　　assay reference plasma
　　at-risk period
ARROM active resistive range
　　of motion
ARS
　　AIDS-related syndrome
　　alizarin red S (dye)
　　antirabies serum

ART
　　accelerated recovery technique
　　Achilles (tendon) reflex test
　　acoustic reflex threshold
　　active-release technique
　　androgen replacement therapy
　　antiretroviral treatment
　　arrest-and-reversal treatment
　　assisted reproductive
　　　technology
　　asymmetry, range (of motion
　　　abnormality), tissue (texture
　　　abnormality)
arth.
　　arthritis
　　arthrotomy
arthro arthroscopy
art. line arterial line (*See also*
　　A-line)
ARV
　　AIDS-related virus
　　antiretroviral
AS
　　above scale
　　acoustic stimulation
　　Adams-Stokes (attack,
　　　breathing, disease)
　　adolescent suicide
　　aerosol steroid
　　anabolic steroid
　　anal sphincter
　　androgen suppression
　　angiosarcoma
　　ankylosing spondylitis
　　anovulatory syndrome
　　anterosuperior
　　antiserum
　　antisocial
　　antistreptolysin
　　anxiety state
　　aortic sound
　　aqueous solution (suspension)
　　arteriosclerosis
　　aseptic meningitis
　　astigmatism
　　asymmetric
　　atherosclerosis
　　atrial stenosis
　　atropine sulfate
　　audiogenic seizure

sickle cell trait (heterozygous genotype)

A.S. left ear [L. *auris sinistra*] (*See also* LE)

As arsenic

A·s ampere-second

aS absiemens

As₂O₃ arsenic trioxide

ASA
acetylsalicylic acid (aspirin)
Adams-Stokes attack
American Society of Anesthesiologists (classification)
anterior spinal artery
aspirin-sensitive asthma
atrial septal aneurysm

ASA I–V American Society of Anesthesiologists' patient classifications I to V, followed by "E" for emergency operations

ASA I healthy patient with localized pathologic process

ASA II patient with mild to moderate systemic disease

ASA III patient with severe systemic disease limiting activity but not incapacitating

ASA IV patient with incapacitating systemic disease

ASA V moribund patient not expected to live

ASAP as soon as possible

ASB
anencephaly-spina bifida (syndrome)
anesthesia standby

ASC
altered state of consciousness
ambulatory surgery center
anterior subcapsular cataract
asthma symptom checklist

asc
anterior subcapsular
arteriosclerotic
ascending

ASCAD
arteriosclerotic coronary artery disease
atherosclerotic coronary artery disease

ASCI acute spinal cord injury

ASCS autologous stem cell support

ASCT autologous stem cell transplantation

ASCUS atypical squamous cells of undetermined significance

ASCVD arteriosclerotic (atherosclerotic) cardiovascular disease

ASD
adaptive seating device
Alzheimer senile dementia
antisiphon device
arthritis syphilitica deformans
atrial septal defect

ASD2 secundum atrial septal defect

ASE axilla, shoulder, elbow (bandage)

ASES American shoulder and elbow system

ASF
aniline-sulfur-formaldehyde (resin)
anterior spinal fusion

ASH aldosterone-stimulating hormone

A & Sh arm and shoulder

AsH hypermetropic astigmatism

ASHCVD arteriosclerotic (atherosclerotic) hypertensive cardiovascular disease

ASHD atrial septal heart disease

AS/Ho antiserum, horse

ASI
addiction severity index
arthroscopic screw installation

ASIA American Spinal Injury Association (score)

ASIA-A complete spinal injury

ASIA-B incomplete spinal injury, preserved sensation

ASIA-C incomplete spinal injury, preserved motor (nonfunctional)

ASIA-D incomplete spinal injury, preserved motor (functional)

ASIA-E complete recovery from spinal injury

ASIQ Adult Suicidal Ideation Questionnaire

ASIS anterior superior iliac spine

ASL American Sign Language (*See also* Ameslan)

ASLV avian sarcoma and leukosis virus (Rous virus)

AsM myopic astigmatism

ASMI anteroseptal myocardial infarction

asmt assessment

ASN
  alkali-soluble nitrogen
  arteriosclerotic nephritis
  automatic single-needle monitor

Asn asparagine (*See also* N)

ASO
  aldicarb sulfoxide
  allele-specific oligonucleotide
  ankle stabilizing orthosis
  antistreptolysin-O
  arteriosclerosis obliterans
  atherosclerosis obliterans

ASOR asialoorosomucoid

ASO-RAD arteriosclerotic renal artery disease

ASP
  abnormal spinal posture
  amnesic shellfish poisoning
  antisocial personality
  aortic systolic pressure
  aspiration
  automatic signal processing

asp
  asparate
  aspartic acid

ASPAT antistreptococcal polysaccharide A test

AS-PCR allele-specific polymerase chain reaction

ASPD
  anterior superior pancreaticoduodenal
  antisocial personality disorder

ASPED angel-shaped phalangoepiphyseal dysplasia

asper aspergillosis

ASPG antispleen globulin

Asp-Glu-Tyr aspartic acid-glutamic acid-tyrosine

ASPI Adolescent Problem Severity Index

ASPS alveolar soft part sarcoma

ASPVD
  arteriosclerotic peripheral vascular disease
  atherosclerotic pulmonary vascular disease

ASQ
  abbreviated symptom questionnaire
  Ages and Stages Questionnaire
  anxiety scale questionnaire

ASR
  adrenal to spleen ratio
  aldosterone secretion rate
  aldosterone secretory rate
  analyte-specific reagent
  atrial septal resection

AS/Rab antiserum, rabbit

ASRD aspirin-sensitive respiratory disease

ASS
  acute serum sickness
  anterior-superior spine
  Asthma Severity Score

ASSI Accurate Surgical and Scientific Instruments (Corporation)

assn association

assoc
  associate
  association

ASSQ autism spectrum screening questionnaire

ASSR adult situational stress reaction

asst assistant

AST
    above selected threshold
    acoustic stimulation test
    alcohol sniff test
    angiotensin sensitivity test
    anterior spinothalamic tract
    antistreptolysin titer
    Aphasia Screening Test
    aspartate aminotransferase
    aspartate transaminase
    astemizole
    atrial overdrive stimulation
      rate
    audiometry sweep test
ASTA anti-alpha-staphylolysin
AS TOL as tolerated
ASV
    adaptive support ventilation
    antisiphon valve
    antisnake venom
ASVD
    arteriosclerotic vascular
      disease
    atherosclerotic vascular disease
Asx asymptomatic
AT
    abdominal tympany
    Achard-Thiers (syndrome)
    achievement test
    Achilles tendon
    activity therapy
    adjuvant therapy
    air temperature
    air trapping
    anaerobic threshold
    antithrombin
    antitrypsin
    applanation tonometry
    assistive technology
    ataxia-telangiectasia
    atraumatic
    atrial tachycardia
    attenuate
    autoimmune thrombocytopenia
    autologous transplant
    axonal terminal
at.
    atom
    atomic

AT-I, -II, -III angiotensin I–III
ATA
    antithyroglobulin antibody
    antithyroid antibody
    anti-*Toxoplasma* antibody
ata atmosphere absolute
ATC
    aerosol treatment chamber
    around the clock
ATCC American Type Culture
    Collection
ATD
    Alzheimer-type dementia
    antithyroid drug
    asphyxiating thoracic
      dystrophy
    assistive technology device
    autoimmune thyroid disease
ATG
    antithrombocyte globulin
    antithyroglobulin
ATGAM antithymocyte globulin
ATHR angina threshold heart
    rate
ATI abdominal trauma index
ATIS HIV/AIDS Treatment
    Information Service
ATLL adult T-cell leukemia-
    lymphoma
ATLS advanced trauma life
    support
ATM
    asynchronous transfer mode
    ataxia telangiectasia mutated
atm (standard) atmosphere
ATNC atraumatic, normocephalic
aTNM (at) autopsy tumor,
    nodes, and metastases (staging
    of cancer)
at. no. atomic number
ATP
    adenosine triphosphate
    ambient temperature and
      pressure
    antitachycardia pacemaker
    autoimmune thrombocytopenic
      purpura
AT-PAS aldehyde-thionine-
    periodic acid-Schiff (test)

ATPase adenosine triphosphatase

ATPD ambient temperature and pressure, dry

ATPS ambient temperature and pressure, saturated (with water vapor)

ATR
    Achilles tendon reflex
    Achilles tendon rupture
    atrial tachycardia response

atr atrophy

ATS
    antitetanus serum
    anxiety tension state

ATT
    anterior talar translation
    arginine tolerance test

ATV
    all-terrain vehicle
    anterior terminal vein
    atrioventricular

at. vol atomic volume

at. wt atomic weight

atyp atypical

ATZ anal transitional zone

AU
    antitoxin unit
    arbitrary unit
    atomic unit
    Australia antigen
    both ears [L. *aures unitas*]
    each ear [L. *auris uterque*]

Au gold [L. *aurum*]

AUA (blood concentration) area under curve

Au Ag Australia antigen

AUB abnormal uterine bleeding

AuBMT autologous bone marrow transplantation

AUD auditory

AUDEX automated urologic diagnostic expert (ultrasonographic imaging)

AUI alcohol use inventory

AUMC area under the first moment curve

AUQ Alcohol Usage Questionnaire

aur
    auricle
    auris

AUS
    artificial urinary sphincter
    auscultation

aux auxiliary

AV
    anteroventral
    anteversion
    aortic valve
    arteriovenous
    assisted ventilation
    atrioventricular
    auditory-visual
    avoirdupois

A/V
    ampere/volt
    arterial/venous
    atrial/ventricular

AVA
    antiviral antibody
    aortic valve area
    arteriovenous anastomosis
    availability

AV/AF anteverted and anteflexed

AVB atrioventricular block

AVC
    aberrant ventricular conduction
    acrylic veneer crown
    associative visual cortex
    atrioventricular conduction
    automatic volume control

AVCD atrioventricular canal defect

AVCS atrioventricular conduction system

AVD
    aortic valvular disease
    arteriosclerotic vascular disease
    arteriovenous difference
    atherosclerotic vascular disease
    atrioventricular delay

AVDP, avdp
    average diastolic pressure
    avoirdupois

AVE
  aortic valve echocardiogram
  atrioventricular extrasystole
AVF arteriovenous fistula
aVF augmented voltage unipolar
  left foot lead
  (electrocardiography)
AVG
  ambulatory visit groups
    (patient classification)
  aortic valve gradient
avg average
AVHB atrioventricular heart
  block
AVI air velocity index
AV-ICD atrial and ventricular
  implantable cardioverter-
  defibrillator
AVJ atrioventricular junction
AVJR atrioventricular junctional
  rhythm
AVJT atrioventricular junctional
  tachycardia
aVL augmented voltage unipolar
  left arm lead
  (electrocardiography)
AVM arteriovenous malformation
AVN
  arteriovenous nicking
  atrioventricular nodal
    (conduction)
  atrioventricular node
  avascular necrosis
AVNRT
  atrioventricular nodal reentrant
    tachycardia
  atrioventricular nodal reentry
    tachycardia
AVO atrioventricular opening
A-VO₂ arteriovenous oxygen
  (difference)
AVOA amorphous vascular
  occluding agent
AVP
  ambulatory venous pressure
  arginine vasopressin
AVPU alert, verbal stimulus
  response, painful stimulus
  response, unresponsive

AVR
  accelerated ventricular rhythm
  aortic valve replacement
aVR augmented voltage unipolar
  right arm lead
  (electrocardiography)
AVRP atrioventricular refractory
  period
AVS
  aortic valve stenosis
  arteriovenous shunt
  auditory vocal sequencing
AVSD atrioventricular septal
  defect
AVT
  Allen vision test
  area ventralis of Tsai
  atrioventricular tachycardia
AW
  abdominal wall
  abnormal wave
  actual weight
  alcohol withdrawal
  Anderson-Wilkins
  anterior wall
  atomic warfare
A/W able to work
A&W alive and well
aw airway
AWA
  as well as
  away without authorization
AWD alive with disease
AWG American wire gauge
AWI
  anterior wall infarction
  authorized walk-in (patient)
AWMI anterior wall myocardial
  infarction
AWO airway obstruction
AWOD alive without disease
AWOL absent without leave
AWP airway pressure
AWS
  AIDS wasting syndrome
  alcohol withdrawal syndrome
awu atomic weight unit
ax.
  axial

ax. *(continued)*
   axilla
   axis
   axon
AXB axillary block
AXBF axillobifemoral
AXC aortic crossclamp
AXT alternating exotropia
AZ acquisition zoom
AZA azelaic acid

AZF azoospermia factor
AZH assisted zonal hatching
AZO, azo indicates presence of the group -N:N-
AZT
   Aschheim-Zondek test
   azidothymidine (zidovudine)
AZTEC amplitude zone time epoch coding (in ECG)

B

bacillus
barometric (*See also* BAR)
base (chemistry, of a prism)
bel
Benoist scale
bicuspid
boils at
bone marrow-derived (cell or lymphocyte)
born
boron
bovine
bregma
buccal
Bucky (film in cassette in Potter-Bucky diaphragm)
bursa (cell)
supramentale (craniometric point)

b barn (unit of area for atomic nuclei)

b. twice [L. *bis*] (*See also* bis.)

B₀ constant magnetic field in nuclear magnetic resonance

B₁
radiofrequency magnetic field in nuclear magnetic resonance
thiamin (vitamin B₁)

B₂ riboflavin (vitamin B₂)

B₃ niacin, niacinamide, nicotinic acid (vitamin B₃)

B₅ pantothenic acid (vitamin B₅)

B₆ pyridoxine (vitamin B₆)

B₇ biotin (vitamin B₇)

B₁₂ cyanocobalamin (vitamin B₁₂)

B>A bone conduction greater than air conduction

BA
bacterial agglutination
basilar artery
best amplitude
bile acid
biliary atresia

bioactive
blocking antibody
blood agar
blood alcohol
bone age
brachial artery (pressure)
breathing apparatus
bronchial asthma
bronchoalveolar
buccoaxial

B&A
before and after
brisk and active

B<A bone conduction less than air conduction

Ba
barium
basion

BAB blood agar base

Bab Babinski (reflex, sign)

BAC
bacterial adherent colony
bacterial antigen complex
blood alcohol content
bronchoalveolar cells
buccoaxiocervical

Bac, bac.
bacillary [L. *Bacillus*]
bacillus

BACA bronchioalveolar carcinoma

bact bacterium

BAD biologic aerosol detection

BADGE Békésy Ascending-Descending Gap Evaluation

BAE
bone-anchored epithesis
bronchial artery embolization

BaE, BaEn barium enema

BAEP brainstem auditory evoked potential

BAER brainstem auditory evoked response

BAG buccoaxiogingival

BAHA bone-anchored hearing aid

25

BAI
    basilar artery insufficiency
    breath-actuated inhaler
BAL
    balance
    bioartificial liver
    blood alcohol level
    British anti-Lewisite
    bronchoalveolar lavage
BALB binaural alternate
    loudness balance
BALF bronchoalveolar lavage
    fluid
B-ALL B-cell acute
    lymphoblastic leukemia
bals balsam
BALT bronchus-associated
    lymphoid tissue
BAM, BAm brachial artery mean
    (pressure)
BaM barium meal
BAMO behavioral, anxiety,
    mood, and other types of
    disorders
BAN British approved name
Ba-N basion-nasion
band, stab neutrophil
BANS back, arm, neck, and
    scalp
BAO
    basal acid output
    basilar artery occlusion
BAP
    Behavioral Assessment of
      Pain
    blood agar plate
    bone alkaline phosphatase
    brachial artery pressure
    brightness area product
BAPS Biomechanical Ankle
    Platform System
bAPV baseline average peak
    velocity
BAQ brain-age quotient
BAR
    bariatrics
    barometer
barb. barbiturate
BARSIT Barranquilla Rapid
    Survey Intelligence Test

BAS
    balloon atrial septostomy
    Barnes Akathisia Scale
    behavioral activation system
    boric acid solution
BaS barium swallow
bas basilar
BASA Boston Assessment of
    Severe Aphasia
BASE Brief Aphasia Screening
    Examination
baso basophil
BaSO4 barium sulfate
BAT
    bilateral advancement
      transposition
    Brightness Acuity Test
    brown adipose tissue
batt battery
BAUP Bovie-assisted
    uvulopalatoplasty
BAV
    balloon aortic valvotomy
    bicuspid aortic valve
BAW bronchoalveolar washing
BB
    baby boy
    backboard
    beta blocker
    blood buffer (base)
    blow bottle
    both bones (fractures)
B/B backward bending
B&B bowel and bladder
Bb *Borrelia burgdorferi*
bb Bolton point
BBA born before arrival
BBB
    blood-brain barrier
    blood buffer base
    bundle branch block
BBC
    biceps, brachialis,
      coracobrachialis
    Brown-Buerger cystoscope
BBD
    baby born dead
    benign breast disease
BBE *Bacteroides* bile esculin
    (agar)

BBI Bowman-Birk inhibitor
BBM
  banked breast milk
  brush border membrane
BB to MM belly button to
  medial malleolus
BBN broadband noise
BBOW bulging bag of waters
BBPRL big big prolactin
BBR
  bibasilar rale
  bundle branch reentry
BBR-VT bundle branch reentry
  ventricular tachycardia
BBS
  bashful bladder syndrome
  benign breast syndrome
  BES buffered saline
  bilateral breath sounds
  brown bowel syndrome
BBT basal body temperature
BBTB blood-brain-tumor barrier
BBTOP Bankson-Bernthal Test
  of Phonology
BC
  backcross
  background count
  bactericidal concentration
  basal cell
  basket cell
  battle casualty
  beta carotene
  biliary colic
  birth control
  bladder cancer
  blast crisis
  blood cardioplegia
  blood count
  blood culture
  board certified
  bone conduction
  Bowman capsule
  brachiocephalic
  bronchial carcinoma
  buccal cartilage
  buccocervical
  buffy coat
  bulbus cordis

B&C
  bed and chair
  biopsy and curettage
  board and care
  breathed and cried
BCA
  balloon catheter angioplasty
  Barrett adenocarcinoma
  bell-clapper anomaly
  blood color analyzer
  brachiocephalic artery
  branchial cleft anomaly
  breast cancer antigen
BCAA branched-chain amino
  acid
BCB
  blood-cerebrospinal fluid
    barrier
  brilliant cresyl blue (stain)
BCC
  basal cell carcinoma
  benign cellular changes
  biliary cholesterol
    concentration
BCCa basal cell carcinoma
BCD
  bad conduct discharge
  basal cell dysplasia
  binary-coded decimal
  blepharocheilodontic
BCDDP Breast Cancer
  Detection Demonstration
  Project
BCDF B-cell differentiation
  factor
BCE
  basal cell epithelioma
  B-cell enriched
  benign childhood epilepsy
BCF
  basophil chemotactic factor
  bioconcentration factor
  breast cyst fluid
BCFA branched-chain fatty acid
BCG
  Bacille bilié de Calmette-
    Guérin
  Bacille Calmette-Guérin
    (vaccine)

27

BCG *(continued)*
ballistocardiogram
bicolor guaiac (test)
bilateral cystogram
bromcresol green

BCH
basal cell hyperplasia
benign cephalic histiocytosis
benign coital headache

BCHA bone conduction hearing
aid

bChl, Bchl bacterial chlorophyll

BCI
blunt cardiac injury
blunt carotid injury

BCKA branched-chain keto acid

BCL
basic cycle length
B-cell lymphoma
Békésy comfortable loudness

BCLL, B-CLL B-cell chronic
lymphocytic leukemia

BCLS basic cardiac life support

BCM
birth control medication
blood-clotting mechanism
(effects)
body cell mass

BCN
basal cell nevus
bilateral cortical necrosis

BCO
balloon coronary occlusion
biliary cholesterol output

BCOC bowel care of choice

BCP
biochemical profile
birth control pill
bromcresol purple

BCR
B-cell antigen receptor
B-cell reactivity
birth control regimen
breakpoint cluster region
bulbocavernosus reflex

BCRT Beast Cancer Risk tool

BCRx birth control drug

BCS
battered child syndrome
blood cell separator

BCSI breast cancer screening
indicator

BCSS Basic Clinical Scoring
System

BCT
benign cystic teratoma
brachiocephalic trunk
breast-conserving therapy

BCU burn care unit

BCVA best-corrected visual
acuity

BCW biologic and chemical
warfare

BCYE buffered charcoal yeast
extract

BD
base deficit
base-down prism
Becton Dickinson (catheter,
guidewire, spinal needle)
behavioral disorder
benzodiazepine
bile duct
birth date
birth defect
block design (test)
blood donor
blue diaper (syndrome)
board
borderline dull
bound
brain death
brain dysfunction
bronchial drainage
bronchodilator
buccodistal

B&D bondage and discipline

BDA
balloon dilation angioplasty
bile duct adenoma

BDAE Boston Diagnostic
Aphasia Examination

BDD
blistering distal dactylitis
body dysmorphic disorder

BDE bile duct epithelial (cells)

BDG buccal developmental
groove

BDGF bone-derived growth
factor

BDI
>Baseline Dyspnea Index
>Battelle Developmental Inventory
>Beck Depression Inventory
>burn depth indicator

BDIBS Boston Diagnostic Inventory of Basic Skills

BDIS Behavior Disorders Identification Scale

BDI SF Beck Depression Index Short Form

BDL
>below detectable levels
>bile duct ligation

BDM border detection method

BDMP Birth Defects Monitoring Program

bDNA, b-DNA branched chain deoxyribonucleic acid

BDNF brain-derived neurotrophic factor

BDRS Blessed Dementia Rating Scale

BDS biologic detection system

BDT bronchodilator

BDTVMI Beery Developmental Test of Visual-Motor Integration

BDV balloon dilation valvuloplasty

BDW buffered distilled water

BE
>bacillary emulsion (tuberculin)
>bacterial endocarditis
>barium enema
>Barrett esophagus
>base excess
>Baumé scale
>below elbow
>bile esculin (test)
>board eligible
>bovine enteritis
>brain edema
>bread equivalent
>breast examination
>bronchoesophagology

B↓E both lower extremities

B↑E both upper extremities

B&E brisk and equal

Be beryllium

BEA below-elbow amputation

BEAM brain electrical activity map

BEAP bronchiectasis, eosinophilia, asthma, pneumonia

BEB benign essential blepharospasm

BEC
>bacterial endocarditis
>biliary epithelial cell
>blood ethanol content

BECF blood extracellular fluid

BED binge eating disorder

BEEP both end-expiratoy pressures

BEF bronchoesophageal fistula

bef before

BEFV bovine ephemeral fever

BEH benign essential hypertension

beh behavior(al)

BEI
>back-scattered electron imaging
>Biological Exposure Indexes

BEIR biologic effects of ionizing radiation

BEL blood ethanol level

BEP brainstem evoked potential

BEPTI bionomics, environment, *Plasmodium*, treatment, immunity (malaria epidemiology)

BER
>basic electrical rhythm
>benign early repolarization

BERA brainstem electric response audiometry

BERG balloon-assisted, endoscopic, retroperitoneal, gasless

BES
>balanced electrolyte solution
>British Engineering System

BET
>benign epithelial tumor

BET *(continued)*
bleeding esophageal varix
Brunauer-Emmet-Teller
(method)
bet. between
beta-END beta endorphin
beta$_2$-GPI beta$_2$-glycoprotein I
BETS benign epileptiform
transients of sleep
BEV beam's eye view
BeV billion electron volts
Bex base excess
BF
bentonite flocculation (test)
bile flow
blastogenic factor
blister fluid
blocking factor
blood flow
body fat
Bolivian hemorrhagic fever
bone fragment
bouillon filtrate (tuberculin)
breast fed
breathing frequency
buccofacial
buffered
burning feet (syndrome)
butterfat
B:F bound to free (antigen
ratio)
BFA
baby for adoption
bifemoral arteriogram
BFB
biologic feedback
bronchial foreign body
BFC benign febrile convulsion
BFDT Békésy Functionality
Detection Test
BFL
bird fancier's lung
breast firm and lactating
BFM benign familial
macrocephaly
BFO
balanced forearm orthosis
ball-bearing forearm orthosis
blood-forming organ
buccofacial obturator

BFP biologic false-positive
BFR
blood filtration rate
blood flow rate
bone formation rate
buffered Ringer (solution)
BFS blood fasting sugar
BF-STS biological false-positive
serologic test for syphilis
BFT
bentonite flocculation test
biofeedback training
bladder flap tube
BFU burst-forming unit
BFV blood flow velocity
BFVW blood flow velocity
waveform
BG
baby girl
basal ganglion
basic gastrin
Bender-Gestalt
bicolor guaiac (test)
big gastrin
blood glucose
blood group (system)
bone graft
brilliant green
buccal groove
buccogingival
B-G Bordet-Gengou (agar,
bacillus, phenomenon)
BGA blue-green algae
BGAg blood group antigen
BGC
basal ganglion calcification
blood group class
BGCF buccal groove of central
fossa
BG-corr background corrected
BGD blood group degrading
(enzyme)
BGDR background diabetic
retinopathy
BGH bovine growth hormone
BGL blood glucose level
BGLB brilliant green lactose
broth
BGM blood glucose monitoring

BGP
> beta glycerophosphatase
> biliary glycoprotein
> bone Gla protein

BGS
> balance, gait, and station
> blood group substance

BGT
> basophil granulation test
> Bender-Gestalt test
> bungarotoxin

BH
> base hospital
> bill of health
> birth history
> Bishop-Harman (instrument)
> board of health
> Bolton-Hunter (reagent)
> borderline hypertensive
> both hands
> bowel habits
> brain hormone
> Braxton-Hicks (contraction)
> breath holding
> bronchial hyperreactivity
> Bryan high titer (strain of RSV)
> bundle of His

BHD bilateral hemisphere damage

BHF Bolivian hemorrhagic fever

BHI
> Battery for Health Improvement
> beef heart infusion (broth)
> biosynthetic human insulin
> bone healing index
> brain-heart infusion (broth)
> breath-holding index

BHL
> bilateral hilar lymphadenopathy
> biologic half-life

bHLH basic helix-loop-helix

BHN Brinell hardness number

BHP basic health profile

BHR
> basal heart rate

bronchial hyperreactivity
bronchial hyperresponsiveness

BHS
> Beck Hopelessness Scale
> beta-hemolytic streptococcus
> breath-holding spell

BHT
> borderline hypertension
> breath hydrogen test

BHU basic health unit

BH:VH (whole) body hematocrit to venous hematocrit ratio

BI
> background interval
> bactericidal index
> bacteriologic index
> Barthel index
> base (of prism) in
> basilar impression
> biologic indicator
> bodily injury
> bone injury
> bowel impaction
> brain infarct
> brain injury
> burn index

Bi bismuth

BIA bioelectrical impedance analysis

BIAD blind insertion airway device

BIB
> biliointestinal bypass
> brought in by

bib. drink [L. *bibe*]

biblio bibliography

BIC
> blood isotope clearance
> brain injury center

Bic biceps

BICAP bipolar circumactive probe

bicarb bicarbonate (*See also* CO_2, HCO_3)

BICROS, BiCROS bilateral contralateral routing of signals

BID
> bibliographic information and documentation

BID *(continued)*
    brought in dead
    twice a day [L. *bis in die*]
    (*See also* b.i.d.)
b.i.d. twice a day [L. *bis in die*] (*See also* BID)
BIDS
    bedtime insulin, daytime sulfonylurea (therapy)
    biological integrated detection system
    brittle hair, intellectual impairment, decreased fertility, short stature (syndrome)
BIE bayesian image estimation
BIEF bilateral inferior epigastric artery flap
bif bifocal
BIGGY bismuth glycine glucose yeast (agar)
BIH
    basal interhemispheric approach
    benign intracranial hypertension
bi isch between ischial tuberosities
BIL
    basal insulin level
    biceps interval lesion
    bilateral (*See also* bilat)
    brother-in-law
bilat bilateral (*See also* BIL)
bili bilirubin
BILI:ALB bilirubin to albumin ratio
bili-c conjugated bilirubin
BIMA bilateral internal mammary arteries
BINO binocular internuclear ophthalmoplegia
BINS Bayley Infant Neurodevelopmental Screener
biochem biochemistry
BIOD bony interorbital distance
biof biofeedback
biol biology
bioLH bioassay of luteinizing hormone

biophys biophysics
BIP
    Background Interference Procedure
    biparietal (diameter)
BiPAP bilevel positive airway pressure
BiPD biparietal diameter (fetal skull)
BIPP bismuth iodoform paraffin paste
BIR
    backward internal rotation
    basic incidence rate
BIRADS Breast Imaging Reporting and Data System
BIS
    behavioral inhibition system
    bone cement implantation syndrome
bis. twice [L.]
Bisp bispinous or interspinous (diameter)
BIU barrier isolation unit
BIVAD bilateral ventricular assist device
BIW biweekly
bi wk two times per week
BJ
    Bence Jones
    biceps jerk
B&J bones and joints
BJM bones, joints, and muscles
BJP Bence Jones protein
BK
    below knee
    bradykinin
    bullous keratopathy
Bk berkelium
BKA below-knee amputation
BKC blepharokeratoconjunctivitis
BKG, BKg background
bkly back lying
BKO below-knee orthosis
BKS beekeeper serum
BKTT below-knee-to-toe (cast)
BKWC below-knee walking cast
BKWP below-knee walking plaster

BL
  bacterial levan
  basal lamina
  baseline (fetal heart rate)
  bifurcation lesion
  black light
  blast (cell)
  blind loop
  blood
  blood lactate
  blood level
  blood loss
  bronchial lavage
  buccolingual
  Burkitt lymphoma
BLa buccolabial
BLADES Bristol Language
  Development Scale
BLAT Blind Learning Aptitude
  Test
BLB
  black light bulb
  Boothby, Lovelace, Bulbulian
   (mask)
  bulb (syringe)
BLD
  basal laminar deposit
  benign lymphoepithelial
   disease
Bld Bk blood bank
bld chem blood chemistry
bld tm bleeding time (*See also*
  BT)
BLE both lower extremities
BLEED (ongoing) bleeding, low
  (blood pressure), elevated
  (prothrombin time), erratic
  (mental status), (unstable
  comorbid) disease (risk
  factors for continued
  gastrointestinal bleeding
bleph blepharoplasty
BLES bovine lavage extract
  surfactant
BLESS bath, laxative, enema,
  shampoo, and shower
BLFD buccolinguofacial
  dyskinesia

BLFG bilateral firm (hand)
  grips
BLG beta-lactoglobulin
blk black
BLL
  below lower limit
  bilateral lower lobe
  blood lead level
  brows, lids, and lashes
  Burkitt-like lymphoma
BLM
  bilayer lipid membrane
  bimolecular liquid membrane
  borderline malignancy
  buccal-lingual-masticatory
BL PR blood pressure (*See also*
  BP)
BLQ both lower quadrants
BLS
  basic life support
  blind loop syndrome
  blood and lymphatic system
BLT
  bilateral lung transplant
  bladder tumor
  blood-clot lysis time
  blood test
  blood type
BLV
  blood viscosity
  blood volume (*See also* BV)
BM
  bacterial meningitis
  basal medium
  basal membrane
  basal metabolism
  basement membrane
  biomedical
  blind matching
  blood monocyte
  body mass
  bone marrow
  bowel movement
  breast milk
  buccal mass
  buccomesial
BMB
  biomedical belt
  bone marrow biopsy

BMC
balloon mitral
commissurotomy
bone marrow cell
bone marrow culture
bone mineral content

BMD
Becker muscular dystrophy
bone marrow depression
bone mineral densitometry
bovine mucosal disease

BME
basal medium, Eagle
biundulant meningoencephalitis
brief maximal effort

BMET basic metabolic panel

BMF bone marrow failure

BMG benign monoclonal
gammopathy

BMI body mass index

BMJ bones, muscles, joints

BMK birthmark

BMM bone mineral mass

BMNC blood mononuclear cell

BMOC Brinster medium for
ovum culture

Bmod behavior modification

B-mode brightness modulation
(ultrasonography)

BMP
basic metabolic profile
behavior management plan
bone morphogenetic protein

BMR
basal metabolic rate
best motor response
biologic response modifier

BMS
biomedical monitoring system
biometal surface
burning mouth syndrome

BMST Bruce maximal stress
test

BMT
behavioral marital therapy
bilateral myringotomy (and)
tubes
bone marrow transplantation
Buschke Memory Test

BMV
balloon mitral valvotomy
balloon mitral valvuloplasty

BMZ basement membrane zone

BN
bladder neck
brachial neuritis
bronchial node
bucconasal
bulimia nervosa

BNA bronchoscopic needle
aspiration

BNAS, BNBAS Brazelton
Neonatal Behavioral
Assessment Scale

BNB blood-nerve barrier

BNC
binasal cannula
bladder neck contracture

BND barely noticeable
difference

BNEG B negative (blood type)

BNMSE Brief
Neuropsychological Mental
Status Examination

BNO
bladder neck obstruction
bowels not open

BNP brain natriuretic peptide

BNPA binasal pharyngeal
airway

BNR bladder neck resection

BNS bladder neck suspension

BNT Boston Naming Test

BO
bacterial overgrowth
base (of prism) out
behavior objective
body odor
bowel obstruction
bowels open
bronchiolitis obliterans
buccoocclusal

B&O belladonna and opium

BOA
behavioral observation
audiometry
born on arrival
born out of asepsis

BOC
beat of clonus
blood oxygen capacity
BOD
bilateral orbital decompression
biochemical oxygen demand
braided occlusion device
burden of disease
Bod units Bodansky units (*See also* BU)
BOE bilateral otitis externa
BOF branchiooculofacial
bol bolus
BOLD blood oxygenation level-dependent
BOLT Basic Occupational Literacy Test
BOM
benign ovarian mass
bilateral otitis media
BOO
bladder outlet obstruction
buccinator-orbicularis oris
BOOP bronchiolitis obliterans-organizing pneumonia
BOR
basal optic root
before time of operation
branchiootorenal (syndrome)
BORD borderline
BOS
base of skull
Boix-Ochoa score
bronchiolitis obliterans syndrome
BOSS Becker orthopaedic spinal system
BOT
base of tongue
botulinum toxin
bot
botany
bottle
BOU burning on urination
BOW bag of waters
BOWI bag of waters intact
BOWR bag of waters ruptured
BOZR back optic zone radius

BP
bacillary peliosis
back pressure
barometric pressure
basic protein
bed pan
before present
behavior pattern
Bell palsy
bioequivalence problem
biotic potential
biparietal
bipolar
birthplace
bladder pressure
blood pressure (*See also* BL PR)
body part
body plethysmography
boiling point
borderline personality
bronchopleural
bronchopulmonary
buccopulpal
bullous pemphigus
bypass
Pharmacopoeia Britannica (British Pharmacopoeia) (*See also* PB)
bp base pair
BPA
bronchopulmonary aspergillosis
bullous pemphigoid antigen
burst-promoting activity
BPB
biliopancreatic bypass
black-pigmented bacteria
bone-patella-bone
brachial plexus block
bromphenol blue
BPC
Behavior Problem Checklist
British Pharmaceutical Codex
bronchial provocation challenge
BPCF bronchopleurocutaneous fistula
BPCS back pain classification scale

BPD
>biliopancreatic diversion
>biparietal diameter
>bipolar disorder (type 1, 2)
>borderline personality disorder
>bronchopulmonary dysplasia

BPE benign prostatic enlargement

BPEC bipolar electrocoagulation

BPF
>Brazilian purpuric fever
>bronchopleural fistula

BPG
>blood pressure gauge
>bypass graft

BPH benign prostatic hypertrophy

BPh buccopharyngeal

BPI
>Basic Personality Inventory
>beef-pork insulin
>bipolar illness
>Brief Pain Inventory

BPIG bacterial polysaccharide immune globulin

BPLB bone-patellar ligament-bone

B-PLL B-cell prolymphocytic leukemia

BPLN bilateral pelvic lymph node

BPM, bpm
>beat per minute
>birth per minute
>blood perfusion monitor
>blood pressure monitor
>breath per minute

BPN brachial plexus neuropathy

BPO benign prostatic obstruction

BPP
>biophysical profile
>Bloembergen, Purcell, and Pound (theory)

BP&P blood pressure and pulse

BP,P,R,T blood pressure, pulse, respiration, and temperature

BPPV benign paroxysmal positional vertigo

BPQ Berne pain questionnaire

BPR
>blood per rectum
>blood pressure recorder

BPRS Brief Psychiatric Rating Scale

BPRS-C Brief Psychiatric Rating Scale for Children

BPS
>beat per second
>biophysical profile score
>breath per second
>bronchopulmonary sequestration

BPSA bronchopulmonary segmental artery

BPTB bone-patellar tendon-bone

BPTI brachial plexus traction injury

BPV
>balloon pulmonary valvuloplasty
>benign paroxysmal vertigo
>benign positional vertigo
>bioprosthetic valve
>bovine papillomavirus

BP(VET) British Pharmacopoeia (Veterinary)

Bq becquerel (SI unit of radionuclide activity)

BR
>baseline recovery
>bathroom
>bedrest
>bedside rounds
>biologic response
>blink reflex
>bowel rest
>brachialis
>breathing rate
>breathing reserve
>bronchial responsiveness
>bronchitis
>brown
>buccal root

Br
>breech
>bregma
>bridge
>bromine
>brucellosis

br
boiling range
branch
breath
broiled
brother (*See also* BRO)

BRA
bone-resorbing activity
brain-reactive antibody

BRAC basic rest-activity cycle

brach brachial

brady bradycardia

brady-tachy bradycardia-tachycardia (syndrome) (*See also* BTS)

BRAFE brachial, radial, femoral

BrAP brachial artery pressure

BRAT bananas, rice cereal, applesauce, toast (diet)

BRATT bananas, rice, applesauce, tea, toast (diet)

BRB
blood-retinal barrier
bright red blood

BRBPR, BRBR bright red blood per rectum

br bx breast biopsy

BRCA1 breast cancer gene 1

BRCA2 breast cancer gene 2

BRD
baroreflex dysfunction
bladder retraining drill

BRDS Blessed-Roth Dementia Scale

Brit British

brkf breakfast

BRM biologic response modifier

BrM breast milk

BRMP Biological Response Modification Program

BRN Board of Registered Nursing

BRO brother (*See also* br)

BROM back range of motion

bron
bronchial
bronchus, bronchi

bronch bronchoscope

BRP-2 Behavior Rating Profile, Second Edition

Brph bronchophony

BRRS Bannayan-Riley-Ruvalcaba syndrome

BRS
baroreflex sensitivity
Behavior Rating Scale

BR S breath sounds

BRW-PB Brown-Roberts-Wells phantom base

BS
Bacillus subtilis
Bartter syndrome
bedside
before sleep
Behçet syndrome
Bennett seal
bilateral symmetric
bile salt
Binet-Simon (test)
blood sugar
bowel sounds
breaking strength
breath sounds
British Standard
buffered saline

BS 1–4 biosafety level 1–4

B&S
Bartholin and Skene (glands)
Brown and Sharp (suture)

BS=BL breath sounds equal bilaterally

BSA
bismuth-sulfite agar
body surface area
bovine serum albumin
bowel sounds active
broad-spectrum antibiotic

BSAP brief, small, abundant potential

BSAPP brief, small, abundant, polyphasic potential

BSB body surface burned

BSC
basosquamous carcinoma
bedside care
bedside commode
bench scale calorimeter

BSC *(continued)*
    bile salt concentrate
    Biological Stain Commission
    biosafety cabinet
    burn scar contracture
BSD
    baby soft diet
    bedside drainage
BSE
    Behavior Summarized Evaluation
    bilateral, symmetrical, equal
    bovine spongiform encephalopathy
    breast self-examination
BSEP brainstem evoked potential
BSER, BSERA brainstem evoked response (audiometry)
BSF
    backscatter factor
    basal skull fracture
    B-lymphocyte stimulatory factor
BSFR basal secretory flow rate
BSG brachioskeletogenital (syndrome)
BSGA beta-hemolytic streptococcus group A
BSH benign sexual headache
BSI
    Behavior Status Inventory
    bloodstream infection
    body substance isolation
    bound serum iron
    brainstem injury
    Brief Symptom Inventory
BSID-II Bayley Scales of Infant Development-II
BSK Barbour-Stoenner-Kelly (medium)
BSL
    biosafety level
    blood sugar level
BSLE bullous systemic lupus erythematosus
BSLM body surface laplacian mapping
BSM bile salt metabolism

BSM II Bilingual Syntax Measure II (Test)
BSN bowel sounds normal
BSNA bowel sounds normal and active
BSNT breasts soft and nontender
BSO
    bilateral sagittal osteotomy
    bilateral salpingo-oophorectomy
BSOM bilateral serous otitis media
BSP
    body segment parameter
    bone sialoprotein
    bromsulfophthalein (liver function test)
BSp bronchospasm
BSPA bowel sounds present and active
BSPM body surface potential mapping
BSPS Brief Social Phobia Scale
BSR
    basal skin resistance
    bowel sounds regular
    brain stimulation reinforcement
BSRI Bem Sex Role Inventory
BSS
    balanced salt solution
    bedside scale
    black silk suture
    buffered saline solution
    buffered single substrate
BSSI Basic School Skills Inventory
BSSO bilateral sagittal split osteotomy
BSSRO bilateral sagittal split ramus osteotomies
BST
    basic structural unit
    bedside testing
    biceps semitendinosus
    blood serologic test
    breast stimulation test
    brief stimulus therapy
BSV binocular single vision
BT
    Bacillus thuringiensis

base of tongue
bedtime
bitemporal (diameter of fetal head)
bitrochanteric
bituberous
bleeding time (*See also* bld tm)
blood transfusion
blood type
blue tongue
body temperature
brain tumor
breast tumor
bulbotruncal

BTA
biological terrain assessment
bladder tumor antigen
botulinum toxin A
brief tone audiometry

BTBV   beat-to-beat variability

BTC
basal temperature chart
by the clock

BTD   bolus thermodilution

BTE
Baltimore Therapeutic Equipment (work simulator)
behind-the-ear (hearing aid)
bovine thymus extract

BTEA   Boston Test for Examining Aphasia

BTF   blenderized tube feeding

BTg   bovine trypsinogen

BTHI   Brief Test of Head Injury

BTI   biliary tract infection

BTi   biomagnetometer

BTL   bilateral tubal ligation

BTLS   basic trauma life support

BTM
benign tertian malaria
bilateral tympanic membranes

BTO
balloon test occlusion
bilateral tubal occlusion

BTPD   body temperature, pressure, dry

BTPS   body temperature, ambient pressure, and saturated with water vapor (gas)

BTR
Bezold-type reflex
biceps tendon reflex
buccal triangular ridge

BTS
bioptic telescopic spectacle
Blalock-Taussig shunt
blood transfusion service
blue toe syndrome
bradycardia-tachycardia syndrome (*See also* brady-tachy)

BTU   British thermal unit

BTX
botulinum toxin
brevetoxin
bungarotoxin

BU
base (of prism) up
below the umbilicus
Bethesda unit
biologic unit
blood urea
Bodansky units (*See also* Bod units)
burn unit
butyl

BUA
blood uric acid
bone ultrasound attenuation

buc   buccal

BUE
both upper extremities
built-up edge

BUFA   baby up for adoption

BUG   buccal ganglion

BUI   brain uptake index

BULL   buccal of upper and lingual of lower

bull.
bulletin
let it boil [L. *bulliat*]

BUN   blood urea nitrogen

BUN:Cr   blood urea nitrogen to creatinine ratio

BUO
> bilateral ureteral obstruction
> bilirubin of undetermined origin
> bleeding of undetermined origin
> bruising of undetermined origin

BUQ both upper quadrants
BUR backup rate (ventilator)
Burd Burdick (suction)
BUS
> Bartholin, urethral, and Skene (glands)
> busulfan

BUSEG Bartholin, urethral, and Skene (glands), and external genitalia
BUSTOP Burke Stroke Time-Oriented profile
But butyric (acid)
BUV backup ventilation
BV
> bacterial vaginosis
> balloon valvuloplasty
> basilic vein
> billion volts
> biologic value
> blood vessel
> blood volume (*See also* BLV)
> bronchovesicular
> buccoversion
> bulboventricular

B&V binging and vomiting
BVA
> best-corrected visual acuity
> bioimpedance venous analysis

BVAD biventricular assist device
BVAS Birmingham Vasculitis Activity Score
BVAT Binocular Visual Acuity Test
BVC British Veterinary Codex
BVD bovine viral diarrhea
BVDT Brief Vestibular Disorientation Test
BVE
> binocular visual efficiency
> biventricular enlargement

> blood vessel endothelium
> blood volume expander

BVFI bilateral vocal fold (cord) immobility
BVFP bilateral vocal fold (cord) paralysis
BVH biventricular hypertrophy
BVI blood vessel invasion
BVL bilateral vas (deferens) ligation
BVM
> bag-valve-mask (ventilation)
> bronchovascular markings

BVMOT Bender Visual-Motor Gestalt Test
BVO branch vein occlusion
BVP
> back vertex power
> blood vessel prosthesis
> blood volume pulse

BVR
> balloon valvuloplasty registry
> basal vein of Rosenthal

BVRO bilateral vertical ramus osteotomy
BVRT-R Benton Visual Retention Test, Revised
BVS
> biventricular support
> blanked ventricular sense

BVT bilateral ventilation tubes
BW
> bacteriologic warfare
> bandwidth
> bed wetting
> below waist
> biologic warfare
> biologic weapon
> birth weight
> bite-wing (radiograph)
> bladder washout
> body water
> body weight

B&W black and white (milk of magnesia and cascara extract)
BWA bedwetter admission
BWD bacillary white diarrhea
BWFI bacteriostatic water for injection

BWGA birth weight for
gestational age
BWM Bad Wildungen Metz
(spinal instrumentation system)
BWS battered-woman syndrome
BWST black widow spider
toxin

BWSV black widow spider
venom
BWt birth weight
BX, Bx biopsy

B

C

ascorbic acid (vitamin C)
calorie (large) (*See also* Cal)
canine (tooth)(upper)
carbon
cathode
Celsius (temperature scale)
centigrade
cervical (nerve, vertebra)
Clostridium
coarse (bacterial colonies)
coefficient
colony count
convergence
cornea
cornu
cortex (*See also* cort)
costa (rib)
coulomb
cuspid (secondary dentition)
cylinder, cylindrical lens (*See also* cyl)
cytosine
hundred [L. *centum*]

°**C** degree Celsius

C_p constant pressure

-**C** convexoconcave

c

calorie (small) (*See also* cal)
canine (tooth)(lower)
capillary blood (subscript)
centi- (prefix)
circumference
culture [medium]
cuspid (primary dentition)

c̄ with [L. *cum*]

CI, CII, CIII, CIV, CV DEA
controlled substances
schedules I through V

CA

anterior commissure [L. *commissura anterior*]
calcium antagonist
cancer, carcinoma
cardiac-apnea (monitor)
cardiac arrest

cardiac arrhythmia
carotid artery
celiac artery
cerebral aqueduct
cerebral atrophy
chorioamnionitis
clotting assay
coagglutination (test)
coefficient of absorption
community acquired
conceptual age
coronary angioplasty
coronary arrest
coronary artery
corpus albicans
cricoid arch

CA125, CA-125 cancer antigen-125

CA19-9, CA 19-9 cancer antigen 19-9

C&A

Clinitest and Acetest
conscious and alert

Ca calcium

ca about [L. *circa*]

CAA

coloanal anastomosis
coronary artery aneurysm

CAB coronary artery bypass

CaBF carotid blood flow

CABG coronary artery bypass graft

CABGS coronary artery bypass graft surgery

CAC

cancer (malignant) cell
carotid artery canal
circulating anticoagulant
coronary artery calcification

CA:C convergence accommodation ratio

CACh cold air challenge

CaCO₃ calcium carbonate

CACx cancer of cervix

CAD

cadaver donor

43

CAD *(continued)*
   compressed-air disease
   computer assisted dialogue
   coronary artery disease
CADD Computerized
   Ambulatory Drug Delivery
   (pump)
CAE
   cellulose acetate
      electrophoresis
   contingent aftereffects
   coronary artery embolization
CaE calcium excretion
CAEP
   chronotropic exercise
      assessment protocol
   cortical auditory evoked
      potential
CAER
   community awareness and
      emergency response
   cortical auditory evoked
      response
CAF coronary artery fistula
caf caffeine
CAFAS Child and Adolescent
   Functional Assessment Scale
CAG
   cholangiogram
   continuous ambulatory gamma
      globulin (infusion)
   coronary angiogram
   coronary arteriography
CaG calcium gluconate
CAGE cut down (on drinking),
   annoyance, guilt (about
   drinking), (need for)
   eyeopener (alcohol screening)
CAH
   camber axis hinge
   chronic active hepatitis
   congenital adrenogenital
      hyperplasia
CAHD
   coronary arteriosclerotic heart
      disease
   coronary atherosclerotic heart
      disease
CAI
   Career Assessment Inventory

catheter-associated infection
complete androgen
   insensitivity
confused artificial insemination
cortical arousal index
Cultural Attitude Inventory
CAL
   café au lait
   calcium (test)
   calculated average life
   callus
   chronic airflow limitation
   coracoacromial ligament
Cal calorie (large) (*See also* C)
cal
   caliber
   calorie (small) (*See also* c)
Calb, C_{alb} albumin clearance
calc calculate
calcif calcification
cal ct calorie count
calib calibrated
cal/kg day calories per
   kilogram per day
cal/oz calories per ounce
CAM
   cell adhesion molecule
   child-adult mist
   chorioallantoic membrane
   controlled ankle motion
C_{am} amylase clearance
CAMC
   camera augmented mobile C-
      arm
   computer analysis of
      mammography phantom
      images
   computer application in
      medical care
CAMDEX Cambridge Mental
   Disorders in Elderly
   Examination
CAML Coarticulation
   Assessment in Meaningful
   Language
CAMP
   Childhood Asthma
      Management Program
   Christie-Atkins-Munch-Petersen
      (test)

CAMV congenital anomaly of mitral valve

CAN
continuous albuterol nebulization
cord (umbilical) around neck

CA/N child abuse and neglect

CANC cancelled

CANS
central auditory nervous system
computer-assisted neurosurgical navigational system

CANT LEAP cyclosporine, alcohol, nicotinic acid, thiazides, Lasix, ethambutanol, aspirin, pyrazinamide (substances causing hyperuricemia)

CAOD coronary artery occlusive disease

CAP
capacity
capillary
capillary blood
capsule
carcinoma of prostate
community-acquired pneumonia
compound action potential
continent anal cap
coupled atrial pacing

Ca:P calcium to phosphorus ratio

CAPA
caffeine, alcohol, pepper, and aspirin (diet free of)
Child and Adolescent Psychiatric Assessment

CAPB central auditory processing battery

CAPD
central auditory processing disorder
continuous ambulatory peritoneal dialysis

CAPE continuous anatomical passive exerciser

CAPR calcium pyrophosphate

CAPS
caffeine, alcohol, pepper, and spicy foods (diet free of)
Children of Aging Parents

CAQ Childhood Asthma Questionnaire

CAR
cancer-associated retinopathy
cardiac ambulation routine
conditioned avoidance response

CARB
carbohydrate (*See also* CHO)
carbonate

CARD
cardiac
cardiac automatic resuscitative device
cardiology
catalyzed reporter deposition

CARE Comprehensive AIDS Resources Emergency (ct)

CARIFS Canadian Acute Respiratory Illness and Flu Scale

CARS Childhood Autism Rating Scale

CART
cartilage
Classification and Regression Tree
combined antiretroviral therapy

CARTOS computer-assisted reconstruction by tracing of serial sections

CAS
calcarine sulcus
calcific aortic stenosis
cardiac adjustment scale
cardiac surgery
carotid angioplasty and stenting
carotid artery stenosis
casein
castrated
castration
cerebral arteriosclerosis
cerebral atherosclerosis
Chemical Abstracts Service

C

CAS *(continued)*
  computer-aided surgery
  congenital anterior staphyloma
  contralateral acoustic
    stimulation
  coronary artery scan
Cas casualty
CASA Child and Adolescent
  Services Assessment
CASH
  classic abdominal Semm
    hysterectomy
  comprehensive assessment of
    symptoms and history
  cruciform anterior spinal
    hyperextension (brace)
CASHD
  coronary arteriosclerotic heart
    disease
  coronary atherosclerotic heart
    disease
CASL-PI MRI continuous
  arterial spin-labeled perfusion
  magnetic resonance imaging
CASMD congenital atonic
  sclerotic muscular dystrophy
Ca-SP calcium urine spot (test)
CAS REGN Chemical Abstracts
  Service Registry Number
CASS computer-assisted
  stereotactic surgery
CAST Color Allergy Screening
  Test
CASTNO number of casts
  (urinalysis)
CAT
  California Achievement Test
  capillary agglutination test
  catalase (*See also* CAT'ase)
  catalyst
  cataract
  cellular atypia
  Children's Apperception Test
  Children's Articulation Test
  choline acetyltransferase
  classified anaphylatoxin
  computed axial tomography
    (*See also* CT)
CAT'ase catalase (*See also*
  CAT)

cat. c̄ IL, cat. ē IOL cataract
  with intraocular lens
cath catheter
CATT
  calcium tolerance test
  card agglutination
    trypanosomiasis test
caut cauterization
CAV
  cardiac allograft vasculopathy
  congenital absence of vagina
  congenital adrenal virilism
  constant angular velocity
cav cavity
CAVB complete atrioventricular
  block
CAVC common atrioventricular
  canal
CAVD
  cardiac allograft vascular
    disease
  complete atrioventricular
    dissociation
  completion, arithmetic
    problems, vocabulary,
    following directions (battery)
  congenital absence of vas
    deferens
CAVH continuous arteriovenous
  hemofiltration
CAVHD continuous
  arteriovenous hemodialysis
CAVHDF continuous
  arteriovenous hemodiafiltration
CAW
  carbonaceous activated water
  catalyst altered water
  central airways
C_{AW}, C_{aw} airway conductance
  (*See also* Gaw)
CAWO closing abductory
  wedge osteotomy
CB
  calcium blocker
  carotid body
  catheterized bladder
  ceased breathing
  centroblastic
  cesarean birth
  chest-back

chocolate blood (agar)
chondroblast
circumflex branch
color blind
compensated base
conjugated bilirubin
contrast bath
coracobrachial
cord blood

C&B
chair and bed
crown and bridge (*See also* Cr&Br)

Cb columbium

CBA
competitive-binding assay
congenital bronchial atresia
cost-benefit analysis
cutting balloon angioplasty
cytochemical bioassay

CBAT Coulter battery

CBB Coomassie brilliant blue R-250 (stain)

CBBB complete bundle branch block

CBC
child behavior characteristics
complete blood (cell) count

CBCL cutaneous B-cell lymphoma

CBCL/2-3 Child Behavior Checklist for ages 2-3

CBCME computer-based continuing medical education

CBD
carotid body denervation
closed bladder drainage
common bile duct

CBE clinical breast examination

CBF
capillary blood flow
cerebral blood flow
ciliary beat frequency
cochlear blood flow
coronary blood flow
cortical blood flow

CBFV
cerebral blood flow velocity

coronary blood flow velocity
cortical blood flow velocity

CBG
capillary blood gas
capillary blood glucose
cord blood gas
corticosteroid-binding globulin
cortisol-binding globulin

CBI
continuous bladder irrigation
convergent beam irradiation

CBL
chronic blood loss
circulating blood lymphocytes
(umbilical) cord blood leukocytes

CBM
capillary basement membrane
cryopreserved bone marrow

CBMC cord blood mononuclear cell

CBMT capillary basement membrane thickness

CBMW capillary basement membrane width

CBP
calcium-binding protein
carbohydrate-binding protein
cardiac bypass
casual blood pressure
cobalamin-binding protein
copper-binding protein

CBR
chemical, bacteriologic, and radiologic (warfare)
chemically bound residue
complete bedrest
cord blood registry

C_{BR} bilirubin clearance

CBRAM controlled partial rebreathing (anesthesia method)

CBRF child behavior rating form

CBRN chemical, biological, radiological or nuclear (weapons)

CBS
  capillary blood sugar
  child behavioral study
CBT
  carotid body tumor
  cognitive behavior therapy
  computed body tomography
  cord blood transplantation
  corticobulbar tract
CBV
  capillary blood (flow) velocity
  catheter balloon valvuloplasty
  cerebral blood volume
  circulating blood volume
  corrected blood volume
  cortical blood volume
CBV:CBF cerebral blood
  volume to cerebral blood
  flow ratio
CBVI computer based video
  instruction
CBW
  chemical and biological
    warfare
  critical bandwidth (range of
    frequencies)
CBWO closed base wedge
  osteotomy
CBX computer based
  examination
Cbx core biopsy
CC
  calcaneocuboid
  calcium cyclamate
  canal catheterization
  cardiac catheterization
  caval catheterization
  cerebral commissure
  cerebral concussion
  chest circumference
  chief complaint
  chronic complainer
  circulatory collapse
  clean catch (of urine)
  clinical course
  colorectal cancer
  commission-certified (stain)
  complications and
    comorbidities
  contrast cystogram

  coracoclavicular
  cord compression
  corpus callosum
  costochondral
  craniocaudal
  craniocervical
  crus cerebri
  crus communis
C-C convexoconcave
C1–C7 cervical vertebrae 1–7
C1–C8 cervical nerves 1–8
C1–C9 complement 1–9
C/C cholecystectomy and
  (operative) cholangiogram
C&C
  cold and clammy
  confirmed and compatible
Cc concave
cc
  carbon copy
  cubic centimeter (use mL)
    (*See also* cm³)
  with correction (with glasses)
c̄c̄ with meals
CCA
  calcium channel antagonist
  cholangiocarcinoma
  choriocarcinoma
  common carotid artery
  congential contractural
    arachnodactyly
CCAI Clinical Colitis Activity
  Index
CCAT Canadian Cognitive
  Abilities Test
CCB calcium channel blocker
CCBV central circulating blood
  volume
CCC
  central corneal clouding
    (grade 0+–4+)
  cholangiocellular carcinoma
  chronic calculous cholecystitis
  citrated calcium carbimide
  clear cell carcinoma
  craniocerebellocardiac
CC&C colony count and
  culture
CCCR closed-chest cardiac
  resuscitation

CCCS condom catheter collecting system
CCCT
clomiphene citrate challenge test
closed craniocerebral trauma
CCD
calibration curve data
central core disease
charge-coupled device
choriocapillaris degeneration
cortical collecting duct
countercurrent distribution
crossed cerebellar diaschisis
cumulative cardiotoxic dose
CCDA calcaneocuboid distraction arthrodesis
CCDS color-coded duplex sonography
CCE
cholesterol crystal embolization
clear-cell endothelioma
clubbing, cyanosis, and edema
countercurrent electrophoresis
CCEI Crown-Crisp Experimental Index
CCF
cardiolipin complement fixation
centrifuged culture fluid
cephalin-cholesterol flocculation
compound comminuted fracture
CCFA cycloserine-cefoxitin-fructose agar
CCG
cationic colloidal gold
cholecystogram
costochondral graft
CCGC capillary column gas chromatography
CCHD cyanotic congenital heart disease
cc/hr cubic centimeter per hour (use mL per hour)

CCI
chronic coronary insufficiency
Cronqvist cranial index
CCJ costochondral junction
CCK cholecystokinin
cc/kg day cubic centimeters per kilogram per day (use mL per kg day)
CCKNOW Crohn and Colitis Knowledge
CCL
carcinoma cell line
cardiac catheterization laboratory
centrocyte-like (cell)
certified cell line
critical condition list
ccl with contact lenses
CCLO child-centered literary orientation
CCM
congestive cardiomyopathy
contralateral competing message
craniocervical malformation
Crime Classification Manual
critical care medicine
CC/MCL centrocytic/mantle-cell lymphoma
CCMD-2 Chinese Classification of Mental Disorders, Second Edition
CCMSUA clean-catch midstream urinalysis
CCMT catechol methyltransferase
CCN
caudal central nucleus
cervical cord neurapraxia
coronary care nursing
critical care nursing
CCNS cell cycle nonspecific (agent)
CCO continuous cardiac output
C-collar cervical collar
CCP
ciliocytophthoria
colitis cystica profunda
crippled children's program

49

CCP *(continued)*
crystalloid cardioplegia
cytidine cyclic phosphate

CCPD
continuous cyclic peritoneal
dialysis
crystalline calcium
pyrophosphate dihydrate

CCPR
cerebral cortex perfusion rate
crypt cell production rate

CCR
chemokine receptor
continuous complete remission
cumulative conception rate
C_{cr} creatinine clearance (*See
also* CrCl)

CCRT, CC-RT concurrent
chemoradiotherapy

CCS
casualty clearing station
cell cycle specific (agent)
central cord syndrome
Children's Coma Score
cholecystosonography
Clinical Classification System
cloudy-cornea syndrome
concentration-camp syndrome
costoclavicular syndrome

CC&S cornea, conjunctivae, and
sclerae

CCSAS Canadian Cardiovascular
Society angina score

CCSC Canadian Cardiovascular
Society classification

CCSCS central cervical spinal
cord syndrome

CCT
carotid compression
tomography
chocolate coated tablet
closed cerebral trauma
coated compressed tablet
composite cyclic therapy
controlled cord traction
coronary care team
cranial computed tomography

cct circuit

CCTA coronal computed
tomographic arthrography

CCTET contact, control, test,
evaluate, treatment

CCTGA congenitally corrected
transposition of the great
arteries

CCU
Cherry-Crandall unit
coronary care unit
cricital care unit

CCUA clean-catch urinalysis

CCUP colpocystourethropexy

CCW counterclockwise

CD
cadaver donor
canine distemper
cardiac dullness
cardiac dysrhythmia
cardiovascular deconditioning
Carrel-Dakin (fluid)
caudad
celiac disease
cervical dystonia
cesarean delivery
character disorder
chemical dependency
childhood disease
circular dichroism
Clostridium difficile
cluster of differentiation
collecting duct
combination drug
common duct
communicable disease
communication disorder
completely denatured
complicated delivery
conduct disorder
conduction defect
conjunctiva diagonalis
consanguineous donor
contact dermatitis
contagious disease
continuous drainage
convulsive disorder
convulsive dose
corneal dystrophy
cutdown
cystic duct
Czapek-Dox (agar)

diagonal conjugate diameter of the pelvis [L. *conjugata diagonalis*]

C:D cup to disk ratio

C&D
curettage and desiccation
cystoscopy and dilation

CD₅₀ median curative dose

Cd cadmium

cd
candela (candle power)
caudal
color denial
condylion
cord

CDA
ciliary dyskinesia activity
completely denatured alcohol
congenital dyserythropoietic anemia (types I–III)

CDAI Crohn Disease Activity Index

CDAK Cordis Dow artificial kidney

CDAP continuous distending airway pressure

CDB, C&DB cough and deep breath

CDC
calculated date of confinement
capillary diffusion capacity
Centers for Disease Control
chemical dependency counselor
choledochocholedochostomy
Clostridium difficile colitis
Crohn disease of colon

CDCR conjunctivodacryocystorhinostomy

CDD
childhood disintegrative disorder
critical degree of deformation

CDE
canine distemper encephalitis
color Doppler energy
common duct exploration

CDEIS Crohn Disease Endoscopic Index of Severity

CDF
chondrodystrophia fetalis
color flow Doppler (*See also* CFD)

CDG central developmental groove

CDGA constitutional delay in growth and adolescence

CDGD constitutional delay in growth and development

CDH
congenital diaphragmatic hernia
congenital dislocation of hip
congenital dysplasia of hip

CDI
Children's Depression Inventory
color Doppler imaging
communicative development inventory

CDJ choledochojejunostomy

CDK climatic droplet keratopathy

CDM
chemically defined medium
childhood dermatomyositis
clinical decision making

cDNA complementary deoxyribonucleic acid

CDO
controlled depth osteotomy cutter
Cotrel-Dubousset Orthopaedic (instrumentation)

CDP
certified distinct part
collagenase-digestible protein
complete decongestive physiotherapy
continuous distending pressure

CDQ corrected development quotient

CDR
chronologic drinking record
Clinical Dementia Rating
complementarity-determining region

51

CDR *(continued)*
computed digital radiography
continuing disability review
CDR(H) cup to disk ratio horizontal
CDR(V) cup to disk ratio vertical
CDS
Chemical Data System
color Doppler sonography
cul-de-sac
cumulative duration of survival
CDSPIES congestive heart failure, drugs, spasm, pneumothorax, infection, embolism, drugs (mnemonic for differential diagnosis)
cd-sr candela-steradian
CDSS (computer assisted) clinical decision support system
CDT
carbon dioxide therapy
combined diphtheria tetanus
CDU
color Doppler ultrasonography
cumulative dose unit
CDV canine distemper virus
CDY cystoduodenostomy
CDYN, C_{dyn}, Cdyn dynamic compliance (of lung in pulmonary function test)
CE
California encephalitis
capillary zone electrophoresis
capital epiphysis
cardioesophageal (junction) (*See also* CEJ)
cataract extraction
central episiotomy
chloroform-ether
chromatoelectrophoresis
conjugated estrogens
constant estrus
continuing education
contrast echocardiology
crude extract
cytopathic effect

C&E
consultation and examination
cough and exercise
curettage and electrodesiccation
Ce cerium
CEA carotid endarterectomy
CEA-125, CEA 125 carcinoembryonic antigen-125
CEAP clinical manifestations, etiologic factors, anatomic involvement, pathophysiologic features
CECT contrast-enhanced computed tomography
CED
chondroectodermal dysplasia
convection-enhanced delivery
cranioectodermal dysplasia
cultural/ethnic diversity
cystoscopy-endoscopy dilation
CEE
central European encephalitis
conjugated equine estrogens
CEEA circular end-to-end anastomosis
CE-EUS contrast-enhanced endoscopic ultrasonography
CEF
centrifugation extractable fluid
constant electric field
CEFA continuous epidural fentanyl anesthesia
CE/FA capillary electrophoresis/frontal analysis
CE-FAST contrast-enhanced Fourier-acquired steady state
CEI
character education inquiry
converting enzyme inhibitor
corneal epithelial involvement
CEID crossed electroimmunodiffusion
CEJ
cardioesophageal junction (*See also* CE)
cementoenamel junction
CEM
central extensor mechanism

conventional transmission
electron microscope
CE-MRA contrast enhanced
magnetic resonance
angiography
CE-MRI contrast enhanced
magnetic resonance imaging
cen
central
centromere
CENMR capillary electrophoresis
nuclear magnetic resonance
CEP
continuing education program
cortical evoked potential
counterelectrophoresis
CEPH cephalic
CEPH FLOC cephalin
flocculation (test)
CER
conditioned emotional
response
cortical evoked response
CE&R central episiotomy and
repair
CERA cardiac-evoked response
audiometry
CEREC ceramic reconstruction
cert
certificate
certified
cerv cervix
CES
cardioembolic stroke
cauda equina syndrome
cranial electrical stimulation
CES-D Centers for
Epidemiologic Studies
Depression scale
CESI cervical epidural steroid
injection
CET
cerebral electrotherapy
congenital eyelid tetrad
controlled environment
treatment
CEU
congenital ectropion uveae
continuing education unit

CF
carbol-fuchsin (stain)
carotid foramen
Caucasian female
central fossa
choroid fissure
Christmas factor
circumflex (*See also* Cx)
clavicular fracture
clotting factor
clubfoot
colony-forming
color and form
complement fixation
computed fluoroscopy
contractile force
count fingers (visual acuity
test)
cystic fibrosis
C&F
cell and flare
curettage and fulguration
Cf californium
cf centrifugal force
cf. compare [L. *confer*]
CFA
common femoral artery
complete Freund adjuvant
CFA-SFA common femoral
artery-superficial femoral
artery
CFC
colony-forming cells
continuous-flow centrifugation
CFCL continuous-flow
centrifugation leukapheresis
CFD
cephalofacial deformity
color flow Doppler (*See also*
CDF)
craniofacial dysostosis
CFE colony-forming efficiency
CFF critical flicker fusion (test)
CFI
cardiac function index
color flow imaging
complement fixation inhibition
confrontation fields intact
contour-facilitating instrument

53

CFM
  cerebral function monitor
  close-fitting mask
cfm cubic feet per minute
CFMV constant flow
  mechanical ventilation
CFND
  craniofrontonasal dysostosis
  craniofrontonasal dysplasia
CFNS chills, fever, and night
  sweats
CFOS constrained fast
  orthogonal search
CFP
  chronic false-positive
  cystic fibrosis protein
CFPD critical frequency of
  photic driving
CFR
  case atality ratio
  complement-fixation reaction
  coronary flow reserve
CFS
  contoured femoral stem
  craniofacial stenosis
cfs cubic feet per second
CFT
  cardiolipin flocculation test
  complement-fixation test
  crystal field theory
CFU colony-forming unit
CFUC, CFU-C colony-forming
  unit-culture
CFU-E colony-forming unit-
  erythrocyte
CFU-EOS colony-forming unit-
  eosinophil
CFU-F colony-forming unit-
  fibroblast
CFU-GEMM colony-forming
  unit-granulocyte, erythrocyte,
  megakaryocyte, macrophage
CFU-GM colony-forming unit-
  granulocyte-macrophage
CFU-L colony-forming unit-
  lymphoid
CFU-Meg colony-forming unit-
  megakaryocyte
CFU/mL colony-forming units
  per milliliter

CFU-NM colony-forming unit-
  neutrophil-monocyte
CFU-S
  colony-forming unit-spleen
  colony-forming unit-stem (cell)
CFVR coronary flow velocity
  reserve
CFW
  calcofluor white stain
  cancer-free white (mouse)
CFZ capillary-free zone
CG
  calcium gluconate
  cardiography
  center of gravity
  choking gas (phosgene)
  cholecystogram
  chorionic gonadotropin
  cingulate gyrus
  colloidal gold
  control group
  cryoglobulin
  phosgene (choking gas)
cg centigram
CGA comprehensive geriatric
  assessment
CGAS Children's Global
  Assessment Scale
CGCF central groove of central
  fossa
CGI Clinical Global Impression
  (Scale)
CGIC Clinical Global
  Impression of Change
CGI-S Clinical Global
  Impression-Severity of Illness
  Scale
c gl correction with glasses
CGM
  central gray matter (spinal
  cord)
  coffee-grounds material
cgm centigram
cGMP cyclic guanosine
  monophosphate
CGMS continuous glucose
  monitoring system
CGS
  cardiogenic shock

centimeter-gram-second (system, unit)
CGTT cortisone-glucose tolerance test
CGY cystogastrostomy
cGy centigray
CH
case history
cervicogenic headache
Chinese hamster
chloral hydrate
Christchurch chromosome
cluster headache
common hepatic (duct)
communicating hydrocele
convalescent hospital
coracohumeral
crown-heel (infant length)
C-H carbon-hydrogen
C&H
coarse and harsh (breathing)
cocaine and heroin
CH$_{50}$ (total serum) hemolytic complement
C$_H$ constant domain of H chain
Ch
chest
child
cholesterol (*See also* CHOL)
choline
chromosome (*See also* chr)
C$_{H2O}$ clear water
CHA
common hepatic artery
compound hypermetropic astigmatism
congenital hypoplasia of adrenal glands
congenital hypoplastic anemia
continuous heated aerosols
CHAMPUS Civilian Health and Medical Programs of Uniformed Services
CHAMPVA
Civilian Health and Medical Program of Veterans' Administration

CHAR continuous hyperfractionated accelerated radiotherapy
CHASE cut holes and sink 'em (chemical weapons disposal operation)
CHAT conversational hypertext access technology
CHATH chemically hardened air transportable hospital
CHB
complete heart block
congenital heart block
CHC Canadian Heart Classification
CHD
center hemodialysis
childhood disease
chronic hemodialysis
common hepatic duct
congenital heart defect
congenital heart disease
congenital hip dislocation
congenital hip dysplasia
constitutional hepatic dysfunction
coronary heart disease
CHE cholinesterase
CHEDDAR chief complaint, history (present illness, social, and family), examination, details (of problems and complaints), drugs and dosage, assessment, return (medical history documentation)
CHEF contour-clamped homogeneous electric field (electrophoresis)
chem chemistry
CHEMLINE Chemical Dictionary On-Line
chemo chemotherapy
chem panel blood chemistry profile
chemrad chemotherapy and radiotherapy
CHF congestive heart failure

55

CHI
closed head injury
creatinine-height index

chi$_2$ chi-squared (distribution, test)

chi$_e$ electric susceptibility

chi$_m$ magnetic susceptibility

CHL
conductive hearing loss
crown-heel length

chlor chloroform

CHN
carbon, hydrogen, and nitrogen
child neurology
community health network

CHO
carbohydrate (*See also* CARB)
chorea

choc chocolate

CHOL cholesterol (*See also* Ch)

chold withhold

chole cholecystectomy

chol est cholesterol ester

CHPX chickenpox

CHQ child health questionnaire

chr chromosome (*See also* Ch)

CHROMINFO chromosome information (database)

chron
chronic
chronological

CHT
closed head trauma
contralateral head turning

CHTN Cooperative Human Tissue Network

CHVF chemically viewed functionally

CHVS chemically viewed structurally

CI
cardiac index
cardiac insufficiency
cephalic index
cerebral infarction
cervical incompetence
cesium implant
chemoimmunotherapy
chemotherapeutic index

cochlear implant
colony inhibition
complete iridectomy
constraint-induced
continuous imaging
continuous infusion
convergence insufficiency
cord insertion
coronary insufficiency
crystalline insulin
cumulative injury

C.I. Colour Index

Ci curie

CIA
chemiluminescent immunoassay
collagen-induced arthritis
colony-inhibiting activity
congenital intestinal aganglionosis

CIB
crying-induced bronchospasm
cytomegalic inclusion bodies

CIC
carbachol inhalation challenge
cardioinhibitor center
circulating immune complex
clean intermittent catheterization
completely in the canal (hearing aid)
constant initial concentration
crisis intervention center

CICA cervical internal carotid artery

CICE combined intracapsular cataract extraction

CICU cardiac intensive care unit

CID
cervical immobilization device
chick infective dose
combined immunodeficiency (disease)
cytomegalic inclusion disease

CIDEP chemically induced dynamic electron polarization

CIDI composite international diagnostic interview

CIE
chemotherapy-induced emesis

counbtercurrent (crossed) immunoelectrophoresis

CIF
claims inquiry form
cloning inhibiting factor

CIG
cardiointegram
cold-insoluble globulin

CIH
carbohydrate-induced hyperglyceridemia
children in hospital

Ci-hr curie-hour

CIIA common internal iliac artery

CIM
constraint-induced movement
cortically induced movement
Cumulated Index Medicus

Ci/mL curie per milliliter

CIMS chemical ionization mass spectrometry

CIN
cefsulodin-Irgasan-novobiocin (agar)
cerebriform intradermal nevus
cervical intraepithelial neoplasia
chemotherapy-induced neutropenia
conjunctival intraepithelial neoplasia

C_{IN}, C_{in} inulin clearance

CINE
chemotherapy-induced nausea and emesis
cineangiogram

cine MRI, cine-MRI cine magnetic resonance imaging

CIOP chromosomally incompetent ovarian failure

CIP cellular immunocompetence profile

CIPD chronic intermittent peritoneal dialysis

circ
circulation
circumcision
circumference

circ & sen circulation and sensation

CIRF cocaine-induced respiratory failure

CIRR cirrhosis

CI-S Simplified Calculus Index

CIS
carcinoma in situ
central inhibitory state
continuous interleaved sampling

CiS cingulate sulcus

CIT
citrate
cold ischemia time
combined intermittent therapy
conjugated-immunoglobulin technique
conventional immunosuppressive therapy
conventional insulin therapy
corneal impression test

CIV
common iliac vein
continuous interleaved sampling
continuous intravenous (infusion)

CJ conjunctivitis

CJD Creutzfeldt-Jakob disease

CJR centric jaw relationship

CK
cholecystokinin
color kinesis
contralateral knee
creatine kinase
cytokeratin

ck check(ed)

CK-BB creatine kinase (fraction brain)

CKC
closed kinetic chain
cold-knife conization

CKG cardiokymograph

c/kg coulomb per kilogram

CK-ISO creatine kinase isoenzyme

CK-MB creatine kinase fraction myocardial band

CK-MM creatine kinase fraction muscle (skeletal)
CKPT combined kidney and pancreas transplant
CK-PZ cholecystokinin-pancreozymin
CL
 capacity of lung
 cardinal ligament
 cardiolipin
 cell line
 center line
 centralis lateralis
 cervical line
 chemiluminescence
 cholelithiasis
 cholesterol-lecithin
 chronic leukemia
 cirrhosis of liver
 clear liquid
 cleft lip
 compliance of the lung (*See also* C$_L$)
 contact lens (*See also* ctl)
 corpus luteum
 cricoid lamina
 criterion level
 critical list
 cutaneous leishmaniasis
 cutis laxa
 cycle length
 cytotoxic lymphocyte
C$_L$
 compliance of the lung (*See also* CL)
 constant domain of L chain
Cl chloride
cL centiliter
CLA
 cervicolinguoaxial
 cleft lip and alveolus
 community living arrangements
 contralateral local anesthesia
 (X-linked) cerebral ataxia
C lam cervical laminectomy
CLAV clavicle
CLBP chronic low back pain
CLC Charcot-Leyden crystal

CLCS Comprehensive Level of Consciousness Scale
CLD
 central language disorder
 congenital limb deficiency
cldy cloudy
CLE
 columnar-lined esophagus
 continuous lumbar epidural (anesthesia)
CLED cystine-lactose electrolyte-deficient (agar)
CLIA
 chemiluminescent immunoassay
 Clinical Laboratory Improvement Act
 Clinical Laboratory Improvement Amendments
CLIF *Crithidia luciliae* immunofluorescence
CLIFT *Crithidia luciliae* indirect immunofluorescence test
clin clinic
CLINHAQ Clinical Health Assessment Questionnaire
clin path clinical pathology
clin proc clinical procedure
CLL
 cholesterol-lowering lipid
 chronic lymphatic leukemia
 chronic lymphocytic leukemia
 cow lung lavage
cl liq clear liquid
clmp clump(ed)
CLND complete lymph node dissection
CLO cod liver oil
C-loop anatomical position (shape) of duodenum
CLOtest *Campylobacter*-like organism test (for *H. pylori*)
CLOT R clot retraction
CLP
 cecal ligation and puncture
 cycle length, paced
CL&P cleft lip and palate
ClP clinical pathology
CLQ cognitive laterality quotient

CLSE calf lung surfactant extract
CLSH corpus luteum stimulating hormone
CLSL chronic lymphosarcoma (cell) leukemia
CLSM confocal laser scanning microscopy
CLT clot lysis time
CLV constant linear velocity
CL VOID clean voided specimen (urine)
CM
　California mastitis (test)
　cardiac monitor
　cardiomyopathy
　carpometacarpal
　cell membrane
　center of mass
　centrum medianum
　cerebral malaria
　cervical mucus
　chemotactic migration
　Chick-Martin (coefficient)
　chondromalacia
　chopped meat (medium)
　chylomicron
　cochlear microphonic
　congenital malformation
　congestive myocardiopathy
　contrast medium
　costal margin
　cow's milk
　culture medium
　cytometry
C&M cocaine and morphine
C$_m$ maximal clearance
Cm curium
cM centimorgan
cm centimeter
cm^2 square centimeter
cm^3 cubic centimeter (*See also* cc)
CMA
　cerebral microangiopathy
　complete maturation arrest
　compound myopic astigmatism
　cow's milk allergy

CMAP
　compound motor action potential
　compound muscle action potential
C$_{max}$ maximal drug concentration
CMB carbolic methylene blue
CMC
　care management continuity
　carpometacarpal (joint)
　cell-mediated cytotoxicity
　complement-mediated cytotoxicity
　corticomedullary contrast
　critical micelle concentration
CMD
　cerebromacular degeneration
　congenital muscular dystrophy
　corticomedullary differentiation
　count median diameter (of particles)
　craniomandibular dysfunction
　cystoid macular degeneration
　cytomegalic disease
CME
　cervical mucous extract
　continuing medical education
　cystoid macular edema
CMER current medical evidence of record
CMF
　calcium-magnesium free
　craniofacial microsomia
　craniomandibulofacial
CMG
　chopped-meat glucose (medium)
　congenital myasthenia gravis
　cyanmethemoglobin
　cystometrogram
CMGS chopped meat-glucose-starch (medium)
cm H$_2$O centimeter of water
CMI
　carbohydrate metabolism index
　cell-mediated immunity
　cell multiplication inhibition
　chronically mentally ill

c/min cycle per minute (*See also* cpm)

CMIR cell-mediated immune response

CMJ carpometacarpal joint

CML
cell-mediated lysis
chronic myelocytic leukemia
chronic myelogenous leukemia
count median length

cm/m² centimeter per square meter

CMML chronic myelomonocytic leukemia

CMN
congenital melanocytic nevus
congenital mesoblastic nephroma
cranial motor nuclei

CMO
calculated mean organisms
cardiac minute output
comfort measures only

CMoL chronic monocytic leukemia

CMOR craniomandibular orthopedic repositioning device

CMP
cardiomyopathy
cervical mucus penetration
colorimetric microtiter plate
cow's milk protein
cross-modal priming
cytidine monophosphate

CMP-FX complement fixation

CMR
cardiomodulorespirography
cerebral metabolic rate
common mode rejection
congenital mitral regurgitation
crude mortality ratio

CMRR common mode rejection ratio (of amplifiers)

CMS
cardiomediastinal silhouette
cervical mucous solution
chromosome modification site
circulation, motion, sensation
clean, midstream (urine)

cm/s centimeter per second

CMSS circulation, motor (ability), sensation, and swelling

CMSUA clean, midstream urinalysis

CMT
cervical motion tenderness
chemotherapy (*See also* CT, chemo)
circus-movement tachycardia
combined modality therapy
continuous memory test

CMU
cardiac monitoring unit
complex motor unit

CMV
continuous mechanical ventilation
cool mist vaporizer
cytomegalovirus

CMVIg cytomegalovirus immunoglobulin

CMVS culture midvoid specimen

CN
calcaneonavicular
calcineurin
caudate nucleus
cellulose nitrate
charge nurse
clinical nursing
cochlear nucleus
congenital nystagmus
cranial nerve
cyanogen
cyanosis neonatorum

C:N
carbon to nitrogen ratio
carrier to noise ratio
contrast to noise ratio

CN I–XII cranial nerves I–XII

CN I first cranial nerve (olfactory)

CN II second cranial nerve (optic)

CN III third cranial nerve (oculomotor)

CN IV fourth cranial nerve (trochlear)

CN V fifth cranial nerve (trigeminal)
CN VI sixth cranial nerve (abducent)
CN VII seventh cranial nerve (facial)
CN VIII eighth cranial nerve (vestibulocochlear)
CN IX ninth cranial nerve (glossopharyngeal)
CN X tenth cranial nerve (vagus)
CN XI eleventh cranial nerve (accessory)
CN XII twelfth cranial nerve (hypoglossal)
CNA calcium nutrient agar
CNAG chronic narrow angle glaucoma
CNAP
  compound nerve action potential
  continuous negative airway pressure
CNB
  core needle biopsy
  cutting needle biopsy
CNC clear, no creamy (layer)
CND
  canned
  cannot determine
CNE
  concentric needle electrode
  could not establish
CNEMG concentric needle electromyography
CNEP continuous negative extrathoracic pressure
CNL chronic neutrophilic leukemia
CNP
  continuous negative pressure
  cranial nerve palsy
  C-type natriuretic peptide
  cyclic nucleotide phosphodiesterase
CNPV continuous negative-pressure ventilation
CNS central nervous system

CNT
  continuous nebulization therapy
  could not test
CNV
  choroidal neovascularization
  cutaneous necrotizing vasculitis
CO
  calcium oxalate
  carbon monoxide
  cardiac output
  centric occlusion
  cervical orthosis
  coenzyme
  control
  corneal opacity
  crossover
C/O
  check out
  complains of
  in (under) care of
Co
  cobalt
  coenzyme
CO$_2$
  bicarbonate (*See also* bicarb, HCO$_3$)
  carbon dioxide
CO$_3^{2-}$ carbonate
COA
  calculated opening area
  coagglutination
  condition on admission
CoA
  coarctation of the aorta
  coenzyme A
COAG
  chronic open angle glaucoma
  coagulation (study, panel)
coarc coarctation (of aorta)
COAT chronic opioid analgesic therapy
COB coordination of benefits
COBRA Consolidated Omnibus Budget Reconciliation Act
COC
  calcifying odotogenic cyst
  cement-on-crown

COC *(continued)*
  coccygeal
  combined oral contraceptive
CO/CI cardiac output/cardiac
  index
Co-Cr-Mo cobalt-chromium-
  molybdenum
Co-Cr-W-Ni cobalt-chromium-
  tungsten-nickel (alloy metal
  implant)
COD
  cause of death
  cementoosseous dysplasia
  cerebroocular dysgenesis
  chemical oxygen demand
  computerized optical
    densitometry
  condition on discharge
CODA
  cadaveric organ donor act
  Canadian organ donors
    association
COE court-ordered examination
coeff coefficient
COF
  cementoossifying fibroma
  cutoff frequency
CoF cofactor
COG
  center of gravity
  cognitive (function tests)
CoHB carboxyhemoglobin
COI
  Central Obesity Index
  combination of isotonics
COL
  colony
  color
  column
  cost of living
COLD A, cold agg cold
  agglutinin (titer)
COLDER character, onset,
  location, duration,
  exacerbation, remission
COLL
  collect
  colloidal
collat collateral

collut. mouthwash [L. *colluere*
  to wash]
coll vol collective volume
COLLYR, collyr. eyewash [G.
  kollyrion]
col/mL colony per milliliter
color
  colorimetry, including
    spectrophotometry and
    photometry
  let it be colored [L.
    coloretur]
colp, colpo
  colporrhaphy
  colposcopy
COM chronic otitis media
COMA congenital ocular motor
  apraxia (type Cogan)
comb. combine
COMBIMAN Computerized
  Biomechanical Man
COMF comfortable
comm
  commission
  committee
  communicable
commun dis communicable
  disease
comp
  comparable
  compensate
  complaint
  composition
  compound
  compress
  compression
compd compounded
compet competition
compl
  complete
  complication
CON certificate of need
con. against [L. *contra*] (*See
  also* cont.)
conc, concentr concentrate(d)
cond
  condense(d)
  condition(ed)
cond ref conditioned reflex
cond resp conditioned response

conf conference
congen, cong congenital
congr congruent
coniz conization (of cervix)
conj conjunctiva
conjug conjugate(d)
CONS consultation
cons conserve
const constant
constit constituent
cont.
  against [L. *contra*] (*See also* con.)
  bruised [L. *contusus*]
contag contagious
contra contraindicated
contralat contralateral
contrib contributory
contrx contraction (*See also* CTXN, CX)
conv
  convalescent
  convergence
conv hosp convalescent hospital
conv strab convergent strabismus
coord coordinate(d)
CO-oximetry carbon monoxide oximetry
COP
  capillary osmotic pressure
  change of plaster
  cicatricial ocular pemphigoid
  circumoval precipitin
  coefficient of performance
  colloid oncotic pressure
  colloid osmotic pressure
COPD chronic obstructive pulmonary disease
COPRO coproporphyria
CoQ₁₀ coenzyme Q10
COR
  body [L. *corpus*]
  cardiac output recorder
  cervicoocular reflex
  conditioned orientation reflex (audiometry)
  coronary
  coroner

  corrosive
  heart
CoR corepressor
cor coronary (heart)
CORA conditioned orientation reflex audiometry
corr
  correct(ed)
  correspondence
cort
  cortex (*See also* C)
  cortical
CORTIS cortisol
COS
  childhood-onset schizophrenia
  clinically observed seizure
Cosm osmolar clearance
COSY correlated spectroscopy
COT
  colony overlay test
  continuous oxygen therapy
  contralateral optic tectum
  critical off-time
CO₂T total carbon dioxide content
COTX cast off, to x-ray (*See also* CRTX)
COV crossover value
COWAT Controlled Oral Word Association Test
COWS cold-opposite, warm-same (Hallpike caloric stimulation response)
COX
  cyclooxygenase
  cytochrome c oxidase
  uncoxsackievirus
COZ cranioorbitozygomatic osteotomy
CP
  capillary pressure
  cardiopulmonary
  Carr-Purcell (sequence)
  centric position
  cerebellopontine
  cerebral palsy
  chemically pure
  child psychiatry
  child psychology

CP *(continued)*
  chondromalacia patellae
  chronic pain
  cleft palate
  closing pressure
  cochlear potential
  cold pressor
  color perception
  constant pressure
  coracoid process
  cor pulmonale
  cortical plate

C:P cholesterol to phospholipid ratio

C&P
  compensation and pension
  complete and pain-free (range of motion)
  cystoscopy and pyelography

Cp
  ceruloplasmin
  peak concentration
  phosphate clearance

cP centipoise

CPA
  calcaneal pitch angle
  cardiophrenic angle
  cardiopulmonary arrest
  carotid phonoangiography
  cerebellopontine angle
  circulating platelet aggregate
  condylar plateau angle
  costophrenic angle

C-PACG chronic primary angle-closure glaucoma

CPA/OPG carotid phonoangiography/oculoplethysmography

CPAP continuous positive airway pressure

CPB cardiopulmonary bypass

CPBA competitive protein-binding assay

cPCR competitive polymerase chain reaction

CPCS circumferential pneumatic compression suit

CPD
  calcium pyrophosphate deposition

cephalopelvic disproportion
childhood polycystic disease
chorioretinopathy and pituitary dysfunction
chronic peritoneal dialysis
congenital penile deviation
congenital polycystic disease
contact potential difference
contagious pustular dermatitis
continuous peritoneal dialysis
critical point drying

CPE
  cardiogenic pulmonary edema
  Clostridium perfringens enterotoxin
  complex partial epilepsy
  corona-penetrating enzyme
  cytopathogenic effect

CPET cardiopulmonary exercise test

CP-EUS catheter probe-assisted endoluminal ultrasonography

CPF
  clot-promoting factor
  contraction peak force

CP&FD cephalopelvic disproportion and fetal distress

CPG
  capillary blood gas
  cardiopneumographic (recording)
  carotid phonoangiogram
  clinical practice guidelines

CPI
  congenital palatopharyngeal incompetence
  conventional planar imaging
  coronary prognostic index
  cysteine proteinase inhibitor

CPITN community periodontal index of treatment needs

CPK creatine phosphokinase

CPK-BB brain isoenzyme of creatine phosphokinase

CPKI, CPKISO creatine phosphokinase isoenzyme(s)

CPK-MB myocardial band enzyme of creatine phosphokinase

CPK-MM muscle fraction enzyme of creatine phosphokinase

CPL conditioned pitch level

CPLM cysteine-peptone-liver (infusion) medium

CPM
cognitive-perceptual-motor
Colored Progressive Matrices
confined placental mosaicism
continuous passive motion (device)

cpm cycle per minute (*See also* c/min)

CPmax (peak) maximum serum concentration

CPMG Carr-Purcell-Meiboom-Gill (sequence, spin-echo technique)

CPMI central principal moments of inertia

CPmin (trough) minimum serum concentration

CPN celiac plexus neurolysis

CPP
cerebral perfusion pressure
choroid plexus papilloma

CPPB continuous positive-pressure breathing

CPPD calcium pyrophosphate dihydrate deposition (disease)

CP&PD chest percussion and postural drainage

CPPV continuous positive-pressure ventilation

CPR cardiopulmonary resuscitation

CPRAM controlled partial rebreathing anesthesia method

CPS
Children's Protective Service
complex partial seizure
cycle per second (*See also* c/sec)

CPT
carotid pulse tracing
chest physical therapy (physiotherapy)
Current Procedural Terminology

CPTN culture-positive toxin-negative

CPTP culture-positive toxin-positive

CPU caudate putamen

CPV canine parvovirus

CPX
calciphylaxis
cardiopulmonary exercise
complete physical examination

CR
calorie restricted
cardiac rhythm
cardiorespiratory
cardiorrhexis
caries resistant
cathode ray
center of rotation
central ray
centric relation
chest roentgenogram
closed reduction
clot retraction
colorectal
computed radiology
congenital rubella
Congo red
controlled release
controlled respiration
controlled response
conversion rate
creatinine
cremaster ratio
cresyl red
critical ratio
crown-rump (length) (*See also* CRL)
cycloplegic refraction

CR0–10 category ratio 0–10

C&R
cardiac and respiratory
convalescence and rehabilitation

Cr chromium

CRA
central retinal artery

C

65

CRA *(continued)*
chemotherapy-related
amenorrhea
Chinese restaurant asthma
chronic rheumatoid arthritis
cis-retinoic acid
colorectal adenocarcinoma
colorectal anastomosis
coronary rotational
atherectomy
CR 1, 2, 3, 3a, 3b, 4, 5, 5a
complement receptor 1, 2, 3,
3a, 3b, 4, 5, 5a
CRAMS circulation, respiration,
abdomen, motor, and speech
CRB
chemical, radiological, and
biological
congenital retinitis blindness
Cr&Br crown and bridge (*See
also* C&B)
CRC
cardiovascular reflex
conditioning
cerebrovascular reserve
capacity
child-resistant container
colorectal cancer
concentrated red (blood) cell
CR&C closed reduction and
cast
CrCl, Crcl creatinine clearance
(*See also* C_{cr})
CR/CO centric relation-centric
occlusion
CRD
childhood rheumatic disease
child-restraint device
chorioretinal degeneration
chronic renal disease
chronic respiratory disease
cone-rod dystrophy
congenital rubella deafness
CRE
cardiorespiratory endurance
cumulative radiation effect
crep. crepitation [L. *crepitus*]
CRF
cardiac risk factor
chronic renal failure

chronic respiratory failure
coronary reserve flow
corticotropin-releasing factor
CRG, CR-gram cardiorespirogram
CRH corticotropin-releasing
hormone
CRI
Cardiac Risk Index
chronic renal insufficiency
chronic respiratory
insufficiency
CRIES crying (high pitched),
requires (oxygen), increased
(vital signs), expression
(grimace), sleepless (last
hour) (neonatal pain
assessment)
crit hematocrit (*See also* h'crit,
HCT)
CRL crown-rump length (*See
also* CR)
CRM Certified Reference
Materials
cr nn cranial nerves
CRO
cathode ray oscilloscope
centric relation occlusion
CROM cervical range of
motion
CROP compliance, rate,
oxygenation, and pressure
CROS contralateral routing of
signals
CRP C-reactive protein
CrP phosphocreatine
CRPS complex regional pain
syndrome
CRQ Chronic Respiratory
Questionnaire
CRS
Clinical Rating Scale
colorectal surgery
congenital rubella syndrome
CRSM cherry-red spot
myoclonus
CrSp craniospinal
CRT
cadaver renal transplant
cardiac resuscitation team
cathode-ray tube

chemoradiation therapy
circuit resistance training
computed renal tomography
conformal radiation therapy
Critical Reasoning Test

CRTX cast removed, take x-ray
(*See also* COTX)

CRV central retinal vein

CRW Cosman-Roberts-Wells
(stereotactic frame)

cryo
cryoglobulin
cryoprecipitate
cryosurgery
cryotherapy

crys, cryst crystal

crystal meth methamphetamine
(*See also* meth)

CS
cardiogenic shock
caries susceptible
carotid sinus
cavernous sinus
celiac sprue
cerebrospinal
chemical sympathectomy
clinical stage
completed suicide
concentrated strength (of
solution)
conditioned stimulus
congenital syphilis
conjunctivae-sclerae
conscious(ness)
contact sensitivity
coronary sinus
corpus striatum
crush syndrome

C&S
conjunctivae and sclerae
cough and sneeze

C$_s$ standard clearance

Cs cesium

CSA Controlled Substance Act

CSAP cryosurgical ablation of
the prostate

CSB Cheyne-Stokes breathing

CSC
administration of small doses
of drugs at short intervals
[Fr. blow on blow, *coup
sur coup*]
collagen sponge contraceptive
cornea, sclera, and
conjunctiva

C/S & CC culture and
sensitivity and colony count

CSD
cat-scratch disease
craniospinal defect

CS&D cleaned, sutured, and
dressed

CSE combined spinal/epidural
(anesthesia)

c/sec cycle per second (*See also*
CPS)

C-section cesarean section

CSEP cortical somatosensory
evoked potential

CSER
contoured femoral stem
coronary sinus flow
cortical somatosensory evoked
response

CSF-IFE cerebrospinal fluid
immunofixation electrophoresis

CSFP cerebrospinal fluid
pressure

CSFV cerebrospinal fluid
volume

CSF-WR cerebrospinal
fluid–Wassermann reaction

CSI
Calculus Surface Index
Caregiver Strain Index
cholesterol saturation index

CSL computerized speech lab

CSLM confocal scanning
microscopy

CSLR crossed straight leg
raising

CSM
circulation, sensation, mobility
Consolidated Standards
Manual

CSMT capillary refill, sensation, motor function, temperature
CSN
  cardiac sympathetic nerve
  carotid sinus nerve
CSNB congenital stationary night blindness
CSO
  common source outbreak
  crescentic shelf osteotomy
CSP
  Cancer Surveillance Program
  carotid sinus pressure
  cavum septum pellucidum
  chemistry screening profile
  criminal sexual psychopath
CSPAMM complementary spatial modulation of magnetization (imaging)
C-spine cervical spine
CSR
  Cheyne-Stokes respiration
  complete subtalar release
  corrective septorhinoplasty
CSRA cementless surface replacement arthroplasty
CSS
  Cancer Surveillance System
  chewing, sucking, swallowing
CSSEP cortical somatosensory evoked potential
CST
  cardiac stress test
  cavernous sinus thrombosis
  Compton scatter tomography
  convulsive shock therapy
  corticospinal tract
  static (lung) compliance (*See also* C_s)
cSt centistoke
CSU catheter specimen of urine
CSUF continuous slow ultrafiltration (for renal failure)
CT
  calcitonin
  cardiac tamponade
  carpal tunnel
  chemotherapy (*See also* CMT, chemo)
  chest tube
  Chlamydia trachomatis
  chordae tendineae
  circulation time
  closed thoracotomy
  coagulation time
  cobra toxin
  computed (axial) tomography (*See also* CAT)
  contraction time
  Coombs test
  corneal transplant
  coronary thrombosis
  corrected transposition
  corrective therapy
  crutch training
C3T clomiphene citrate challenge test
C:T
  compression to traction ratio
  crossmatch to transfusion ratio
C&T color and temperature
CTA
  clear to auscultation
  computed tomography angiography
  cytoplasmic aggregate
  cytotoxic assay
  menses [L. *catamenia*]
CTAP computed tomography arterial portography
CTB ceased to breathe
CTCL cutaneous T-cell lymphoma
ctCO$_2$ concentration of total carbon dioxide
CTD
  carpal tunnel decompression
  chest tube drainage
  clitoral therapy device
  connective tissue disease
  cumulative trauma disorder
CT&DB cough, turn, and deep breathe
CTF
  certificate
  Colorado tick fever

CTG
  cardiotocography
  cervicothoracic ganglion
C:TG cholesterol to triglyceride
  ratio
CTGA complete transposition of
  great arteries
CTGF connective tissue growth
  factor
CTH
  clot to hold
  computerized tomographic
    holography
CTHA computed tomographic
  hepatic angiography
CTI coffee table injury
CTL
  cervical, thoracic, and lumbar
  cytotoxic T lymphocyte
ctl contact lens (*See also* CL)
CTLSO cervicothoracolumbosacral
  orthosis
CTLV cross-table lateral view
CTM
  cardiotachometer
  computed tomographic
    myelography
  cricothyroid muscle
cTnI cardiac troponin I
cTNM clinical staging of
  tumor, node, and metastasis
cTnT cardiac troponin T
CTO cervicothoracic orthosis
CTR
  cardiothoracic ratio (*See also*
    CT)
  carpal tunnel release
  cricotracheal resection
ctr center
CT-RT chemo- and radiotherapy
CTS
  cardiothoracic surgery
  carpal tunnel syndrome
  clitoris tourniquet syndrome
  computed tomographic scan
  corneal topography system
CTSIB Clinical Test of Sensory
  Interaction & Balance

CTV cervical and thoracic
  vertebrae
CTVF Comprehensive Test of
  Visual Functioning
CTx cardiac transplantation
CTXN contraction (*See also*
  contrx, CX)
CU
  color unit
  control unit
  cusp
Cu copper [L. *cuprum*]
cu ft cubic foot
CUG cystourethrogram
cu in cubic inch (*See also* in^3)
cult. culture
cu mm cubic millimeter (*See
  also* mm^3)
CUP
  cancer of unknown primary
  carcinoma of unknown
    primary
CUR
  curettage
  cystourethrorectal
cur.
  curative
  cure
  current
CUS carotid ultrasound
cusp. cuspid
CuTS cubital tunnel syndrome
cu yd cubic yard
Cu/Zn copper-zinc
CV
  cardiovascular
  cerebrovascular
  cervical vertebra
  closed vitrectomy
  color vision
  conduction velocity
  consonant vowel (syllable)
  costovertebral
  cresyl violet
  curriculum vitae
  true conjugate (diameter of
    pelvic inlet) [L. *conjugata
    vera*]

C/V
 cervical/vaginal
 coulomb per volt
CVA
 cerebrovascular accident
 costovertebral angle
CVAD central venous access device
CVAT costovertebral angle tenderness
CVB chorionic villus biopsy
CVC
 central venous catheter
 consonant vowel consonant (syllable)
CVD
 cardiovascular disease
 cerebrovascular disease
 collagen vascular disease
 color vision deviant
cvd curved
CVF central visual field
CVG
 composite valve graft
 contrast ventriculography
CVI
 Children's Vaccine Initiative
 continuous venous infusion
 cortical visual impairment
CVIR Cardiovascular Information Registry
CVK computerized videokeratography
CVL central venous line
CVM congenital vascular malformation
CVN cochleovestibular neurectomy
CVO obstetric conjugate (of pelvic inlet) [L. *conjugata vera obstetrica*]
C$_v$O$_2$ mixed venous oxygen content
CVP
 cardiac valve procedure
 central venous pressure
 cerebrovascular profile
CVRI cardiovascular resistance index

CVS
 cardiovascular system
 chorionic villus sampling
 clean-voided specimen
 computer vision syndrome
CVT
 cerebral venous thrombosis
 congenital vertical talus
CVUG cystoscopy and voiding urethrogram
CW
 chemical warfare (weapon)
 chest wall
 circle of Willis
 clustered waves
 crutch walking
C/W
 compatible with
 consistent with
CWD continuous-wave Doppler
CWDF cell wall-deficient form (bacteria)
CWE cotton-wool exudate
CWH cardiomyopathy and wooly-hair coat (veterinary syndrome)
CWI cardiac work index
CWMS color, warmth, movement sensation
CWOP childbirth without pain
CWP coal worker's pneumoconiosis
CWS cotton-wool spots
Cwt, cwt hundredweight
CX
 contraction (*See also* contrx, CTXN)
 cylinder axis
Cx
 cervix
 circumflex (*See also* CF)
 convex
CxBx cervical biopsy
CXR chest x-ray
CXTX cervical traction
Cy cyst
cyc
 cycle
 cyclotron

cyl cylinder, cylindrical lens
  (*See also* C)
Cys cysteine
CYSTO
  cystogram
  cystoscopy

Cyt cytosine
cyt cytoplasm
cytol cytology
Cz central (electrode placement
  in electroencephalography)

C

D

central auditory processing
  disorder
cholecalciferol (vitamin D)
  (*See also* D_3)
debye (unit)
deciduous (upper teeth) (*See
  also* DEC)
deuterium
dorsal
dose [L. *dosis*]

D1

day one (first day of
  treatment)
first diagonal branch
  (coronary artery)

D2 second diagonal branch
  (coronary artery)

1D one-dimensional

2D two-dimensional

3D

delayed double diffusion (test)
three-dimensional

4D

four-dimensional
4 prism diopters

D5 dextrose 5% injection

°D mean dose

D_3 cholecalciferol (vitamin D_3)
  (*See also* D)

D- stereochemical structure

d

atomic orbital with angular
  momentum quantum number
  2
deci-
deciduous (lower teeth) (*See
  also* dec)
deuteron
dextro- (right, clockwise)
dyne
relative to rotation of a
  beam of polarized light

d- dextrorotatory

1/D diffusion resistance

D/3 distal third

D10W 10% dextrose in water

D15 Farnsworth panel D15
  color vision test

D20W 20% dextrose in water

D50 50% dextrose injection

D50W 50% dextrose in water

D5 1/2NS dextrose 5% in
  0.45% sodium chloride
  injection

D5-1/2S 5% dextrose in 0.45%
  sodium chloride (saline)
  injection

D5/45 dextrose 5% in 0.45%
  sodium chloride injection

D 5% DW 5% dextrose in
  distilled water

D-5-HS dextrose 5% in
  Hartmann solution

D5RL 5% dextrose in Ringer
  lactate (solution)

D5S dextrose 5% in saline
  (solution)

D5W 5% dextrose in water

D70W 70% dextrose in water

DA

dark adaptation (test)
decubitus angina
degenerative arthritis
delayed action
developmental age
diabetic acidosis
direct agglutination
disaggregated
donor-acceptor
drug addict(ion)
ductus arteriosus
give [L. *da*]

D&A dilatation and aspiration

D/A

date of accident
date of admission
digital to analog converter
  (*See also* DAC)
discharge and advise

Da dalton

da deca-

DAA
dead after arrival
digital auditory aerobics
dissecting aortic aneurysm
double aortic arch

DA/A drug/alcohol addiction

DAAF deoxyribonucleic acid
amplification fingerprinting

DAB day after birth

DAC
day activity center
Depressive Adjective Checklist
digital to analog converter
(*See also* D/A)
disabled adult child
disaster assistance center

dac dacryon

DACA Drug Abuse Control
Amendments

DAD
delayed afterdepolarization
diode array detector
dispense as directed
drug administration device

DAE diving air embolism

DAF
decay-accelerating factor
delayed auditory feedback
DNA amplification
fingerprinting
dynamic axial fixator

DAH disordered action of heart

daL decaliter

DALY disability-adjusted life
year(s)

dam decameter

DAMP deficits in attention,
motor control, perception

dAMP
deoxyadenosine monophosphate
deoxyadenylic acid

DAN diabetic autonomic
neuropathy

DAo descending aorta

DAOM depressor anguli oris
muscle

DAP
delayed after-polarization
depolarizing afterpotential
diastolic arterial pressure
direct (latex) agglutination
pregnancy (test) (*See also*
DAPT)
dose area product
Draw-A-Person (test)

DAPS dark-adapted pupil size

DAPST Denver Auditory
Phoneme Sequencing Test

DAPT direct (latex)
agglutination pregnancy test
(*See also* DAP)

DAQ Diagnostic Assessment
Questionnaire

DAR
daily affective rhythm
data, action, response

DARE
data, action, response, and
evaluation
Drug Abuse Resistance
Education

DAS
day of admission surgery
dead air space
dead at scene
death anxiety scale
developmental apraxia of
speech

DASE dobutamine-atropine stress
echocardiography

DASH
Dietary Approaches to Stop
Hypertension (diet)
disabilities of the arm,
shoulder, and hand

DASI Duke Activity Status
Index

DASP double antibody solid
phase (immunoassay)

DAT
dementia of Alzheimer type
dental aptitude test
Developmental Articulation
Test
diet as tolerated
differential agglutination test
diphtheria antitoxin
direct agglutination test
direct amplification test

direct antiglobulin (Coombs)
test
Disaster Action Team (of
Red Cross)
dau daughter
DAVM dural arteriovenous
malformation
DAW dispense as written
DB
Baudelocque diameter
(external conjugate diameter)
database
deep breath
demineralized bone
demonstration bath
dense body
dermabrasion
dextran blue
diabetes
diagonal band
diaphragmatic breathing
disability
distobuccal
double-blind (study)
dry bulb
duodenal bulb
D$_\beta$ total body bone mineral
density
dB decibel
DBA Diamond-Blackfan anemia
DBC
distance between centers
distobuccal cusp
dye-binding capacity
DB&C deep breathing and
coughing
DBCL dilute blood clot lysis
(method)
DBCR distobuccal cusp ridge
DBDG distobuccal developmental
groove
DBE deep breathing exercise
dBEMCL decibel effective
masking contralateral
D5BES dextrose 5% in
balanced electrolyte solution
DBF disturbed bowel function
dBHL decibel hearing level

DBI
development-at-birth index
diffuse brain injury
D bili direct bilirubin
dBk decibel above 1 kilowatt
DBL distance between nasal
lines
dbl double
DBM
demineralized bone matrix
diabetic management
dBm decibel above 1 milliwatt
dBnHL decibel normal hearing
level
DBO distobuccoocclusal
DBP
D-binding protein
demineralized bone powder
diastolic blood pressure
distobuccopulpal
Döhle body panmyelopathy
DBR
disordered breathing rate
distobuccal root
DBS
deep bonding system
Denis Browne splint
despeciated bovine serum
diminished breath sounds
direct bonding system
direct brain stimulation
dBSL decibel sensation level
dBSPL decibel sound pressure
level
DBT
disordered breathing time
dry bulb temperature
DBW
desirable body weight
dry body weight
dBW decibel above 1 watt
DC
deep compartment
descending colon
dextran charcoal
dextrocardia
diagonal conjugate (diameter)
direct Coombs (test)
direct current

DC *(continued)*
  discharge *(See also* disch)
  discomfort
  discontinue
  distal colon
  distal cusp
  distocervical
  donor cell
  dorsal column
  dual chamber
  Dupuytren contracture
D/C
  diarrhea/constipation
  disconnect
D&C
  dilation and curettage
  direct and consensual
DCA
  deoxycholate-citrate agar
  dicarboxylic acid
  directional color angiography
  directional coronary
    angioplasty
  directional coronary
    atherectomy
  disk-condyle adhesion
  double cup arthroplasty
DCAP-BTLS deformities,
  contusions, abrasions,
  puncture/penetration, burns,
  tenderness, lacerations,
  swelling (EMT assessment
  mnemonic)
DCB distal communicating
  branch
DC&B dilation, curettage, and
  biopsy
DCC
  dextran-coated charcoal
  direct cardiac compression
  direct current cardioversion
  dorsal calcaneocuboid
  dorsal cell column
DCc double concave
DCD developmental coordination
  disorder
DCF direct centrifugal flotation
DCFM Doppler color flow
  mapping

DCG
  dacryocystography
  diagnostic cardiogram
  dynamic electrocardiogram
DCHS dysarthria-clumsy hand
  syndrome
DCI delayed cerebral ischemia
DCIA deep circumflex iliac
  artery
DCIS ductal carcinoma in situ
DCIV deep circumflex iliac
  vein
DCLS deoxycholate citrate
  lactose saccharose (agar)
DCM
  dilated cardiomyopathy
  dyssynergia cerebellaris
    myoclonica
DCML dorsal column medial
  lemniscus
DCN
  dorsal column nucleus
  dorsal cutaneous nerve
DCOM dilated cardiomyopathy
DCP
  dicalcium phosphate
  dynamic compression plate
DCPN direction-changing
  positional nystagmus
DCR
  dacryocystorhinostomy
  delayed cutaneous reaction
  digitorenocerebral syndrome
  direct cortical response
  distal cusp ridge
3DCRT three-dimensional
  conformal radiation therapy
DCS
  decompression sickness
  dorsal column stimulation
  dorsal cord stimulation
  dyskinetic cilia syndrome
1D-CSI one-dimensional
  chemical-shift imaging
DCT
  deep chest therapy
  distal convoluted tubule
  diurnal cortisol test
  dynamic computed
    tomography

3D-CTA three-dimensional
  computed tomographic
  angiography
3D-CTP three-dimensional
  computed tomography
  pancreatography
DCUS duplex color
  ultrasonography
DCx double convex
DD
  daily [L. *de die*]
  dangerous drug
  Darier disease
  day of delivery
  degenerative disease
  delivery date
  delusional disorder
  dependent drainage
  Descemet (membrane)
    detachment
  detrusor dyssynergia
  developmentally delayed
  developmentally disabled
  development disorder
  dialysis dementia
  diaper dermatitis
  died of the disease
  disc diameter
  disc diffusion
  discharged dead
  discharge diagnosis
  Distortion of Dots
  double dose (contrast)
  drug dependence
  dry dressing
  due date
D1–D12 first through twelfth
  dorsal vertebrae (*See also*
  T1–T12)
D&D
  debridement and dressing
  diarrhea and dehydration
  drilling and drainage
DDA
  dideoxyadenosine
  dorsal digital artery
dDAVP deamino-8-ᴅ-arginine
  vasopressin
DDC dangerous drug cabinet

DDD
  defined daily dose
  degenerative disc disease
  dense deposit disease
  double-dose delay
  dual-mode, dual-pacing, dual-
    sensing (pacemaker)
DDDR pacemaker code: D,
  dual pace; D dual sense; D
  dual response; R,
  programmability rate
DDGE denaturing density
  gradient electrophoresis
DDH
  developmental dysplasia of
    hip
  dissociated double hypertropia
DDI
  dressing dry and intact
  drug dose intensity
D-Di D-dimer
ddI dideoxyinosine
DDIs drug-drug interactions
dDNA denatured
  deoxyribonucleic acid
DDNOS dissociative disorder
  not otherwise specified
DDP
  density-dependent
    phosphoprotein
  difficult-denture patient
DDR
  diastolic descent rate
  direct digital radiography
DDRA dead despite resuscitation
  attempt
DDS
  damaged disc syndrome
  dendrodendritic synaptosome
  dental distress syndrome
  Denys-Drash syndrome
  depressed DNA synthesis
  dialysis disequilibrium
    syndrome
  directional Doppler
    sonography
  disease disability scale
  double decidual sac

D

DDST Denver Developmental Screening Test

DDT
ductus deferens tumor
dye disappearance test

DDU dermodistortive urticaria

DDW double distilled water

D/DW dextrose in distilled water

DDx differential diagnosis (*See also* diff diag)

DE
deprived eye
dermal-epidermal (junction)
diagnostic error
dialysis encephalopathy
digestive energy
digitalis effect
dobutamine echocardiogram
dose equivalent

2DE two-dimensional echocardiography

3DE three-dimensional echocardiography

D5E75 5% dextrose and electrolyte 75% (solution)

D&E dilation and evacuation

DEA # Drug Enforcement Administration number (physicians' federal narcotic number)

DEB dystrophic epidermolysis bullosa

deb debridement

debil debility

DEC
decant
deciduous (upper teeth) (*See also* D)
decimal
pour off [L. *decanta*]

dec deciduous (lower teeth) (*See also* d)

decd, dec'd deceased

DECEL deceleration

decoct decoction

decomp decompose

decon decontamination

DECR decrease

dec (R) decrease, relative

DECUB
decubitus position
lying down [L. *decubitus*]
pressure ulcer

DED
date of expected delivery
defined exposure dose
delayed erythema dose
diabetic eye disease
died in emergency department

DEEDS drugs, exercise, education, diet, and self-monitoring

DEEG depth electroencephalogram

DEF
decayed, extracted, filled (permanent teeth)
defecation
deficiency
definite

2-DEF two-dimensional echo-derived ejection fraction

def decayed, extracted, filled (deciduous teeth)

defib defibrillate

DEFT driven equilibrium Fourier transform

DEG
degeneration
degree

dehyd dehydrated

DEI Disease Extent Index

DEJ, dej
dentinoenamel junction
dermal-epidermal junction

DEL deltoid

del
deletion
delivery
delusion

DELFIA dissociation-enhanced lanthanide fluoroimmunoassay

deliq deliquescence

DELTA Descriptive Language for Taxonomy

DEN dermatitis exfoliativa neonatorum

denat denatured

denom denominator

DENS direct electrical nerve stimulation
DENT Dental Exposure Normalization Technique
dent
dental
dentition
DEP dilution end point
dep
dependent
deposit
depr
depressed
depression
dept department
DEQ digital echo quantification
DER dual-energy radiograph
der derivative chromosome
DERM dermatology
DES
dermal-epidermal separation
diethylstilbestrol
DESAT desaturated
desc
descending
descent
DESD detrusor external sphincter dyssynergia
DEST
Denver Eye Screening Test
dichotic environmental sounds test
DET dipyridamole echocardiography test
determ
determination
determine
detn detention
detox detoxification
DEUC direct electronic urethrocystometry
DEV duck embryo vaccine
dev
deviate
deviation
devel development
DevPd developmental pediatrics
DEVR dominant exudative vitreoretinopathy

DEXA dual-energy x-ray absorptiometry (scan)
DF
day frequency (of voiding)
decapacitation factor (sperm)
decayed and filled (permanent teeth)
decontamination factor
deficiency factor
defined flora (of an animal)
degree of freedom
dengue (hemorrhagic) fever (*See also* DHF)
dermatofibrosis
diabetic father
diabetic fetopathy
diaphragmatic function
diastolic filling
dietary fiber
digital fluoroscopy
disseminated foci
distal fossa
dorsiflexion
dry (gas) fractional (concentration)
dye free
df
decayed and filled (deciduous teeth)
degree of freedom
DFA
delayed feedback audiometry
diet for age
difficulty falling asleep
direct fluorescence assay
direct fluorescent antibody (test)
direct fluorescent antigen (test)
distal forearm
dorsiflexion angle
dorsiflexion assist
DFC deletion of final consonants
DFD
defined formula diet
degenerative facet disease
DFDB demineralized freeze-dried bone

DFDBA
decalcified freeze-dried bone allograft
demineralized freeze-dried bone allograft

DFDCB decalcified freeze-dried cortical bone

DFE
dilated fundus examination
distal femoral epiphysis

d_{FF} density of the fat mass

d_{FFM} density of the fat-free mass

DFG direct forward gaze

DFI
deterioration following improvement
disease-free interval
dye fluorescence index

D-FISH double-fusion fluorescent in situ hybridization

DFLE disability-free life expectancy

DFM
decreased fetal movement
deep friction massage

DFMC daily fetal movement count

DFNA3 autosomal dominant nonsyndromic hearing loss

DFNB1 autosomal recessive nonsyndromic hearing loss

DFNX3 X-linked progressive mixed deafness with perilymphatic gusher

DFP diastolic filling period

DFPP double filtration plasmapheresis

DFR
designated family respondent
dialysate filtration rate

2DFr two-dimensional Fourier imaging

3DFr three-dimensional Fourier imaging

DFS
disease-free survival
Doppler flow study

DFT
defibrillation threshold
discrete Fourier transform
Doppler flow test

2DFT two-dimensional Fourier transform

3DFT three-dimensional Fourier transform

DFU dead fetus in utero

DFV
dengue fever vaccine
diarrhea with fever and vomiting

DFWO dorsiflexory wedge osteotomy

DG
dark ground
dentate gyrus
diastolic gallop
distogingival
downward gaze

dg decigram

DGA DiGeorge anomaly

DGCI delayed gamma camera image

DGE
delayed gastric emptying
density gradient electrophoresis

DGF
delayed graft function
digoxin-like factor

DGGE denaturing gradient gel electrophoresis

DG-L deep gastric-longitudinal

DGL deglycyrrhizinated licorice

DGS diabetic glomerulosclerosis

DGSX X-linked dysplasia-gigantism syndrome

DGV dextrose, gelatin, Veronal (solution)

DGVB dextrose-gelatin-Veronal buffer

DH
dehydrogenase
delayed hypersensitivity
dental habits
dermatitis herpetiformis
developmental history
diaphragmatic hernia

disseminated histoplasmosis
dominant hand
dorsal horn
drug hypersensitivity
ductal hyperplasia
D-H Dimon-Hughston (intertrochanteric osteotomy)
D:H deuterium to hydrogen ratio
D+H delusions and hallucinations
DHCP dental health care provider
DHD dissociated horizontal deviation
DHDA directed heteroduplex analysis
DHF
dengue hemorrhagic fever (*See also* DF)
dorsihyperflexion
DHFS dengue hemorrhagic fever shock (syndrome)
DHFT developmental hand-function test
DHIC detrusor hyperactivity with impaired contractility
DHO deuterium hydrogen oxide
DHPc dorsal hippocampus
DHPLC denaturing high-performance liquid chromatography
DHR delayed hypersensitivity reaction
DHS
delayed hypersensitivity
duration of hospital stay
dynamic hip screw
DHT
dissociated hypertropia
Dobhoff tube
domino heart transplantation
DI
date of injury
degradation index
dental index
dentinogenesis imperfecta
desorption ionization
detrusor instability

diabetes insipidus
diagnostic imaging
dispensing information
distal intestine
distoincisal
DNA index
donor insemination
dorsal interosseous
dorsoiliacus
dose intensity
drug information
drug interaction
dyskaryosis index
dyspnea index
D&I dry and intact
Di
didymium
Diego (blood group)
DIA
depolarization-induced automaticity
diabetes
dot immunobinding assay
drug-induced agranulocytosis
drug-induced amenorrhea
DiA Diego antigen
diag
diagonal
diagram
diam diameter
diaph diaphragm (*See also* DPH)
DIAPPERS delirium, infection, atrophic urethritis and vaginitis, pharmaceuticals, psychological disorders, excessive output, restricted mobility, stool impaction
dias diastole
DIAS BP diastolic blood pressure
diath diathermy
DIB dot immunobinding
DIBC drug-induced blood cytopenias
DIBS dead-in-bed syndrome
DIC
diagnostic imaging center

81

DIC *(continued)*
  differential interference contrast (microscopy)
  disseminated intravascular coagulation
  drip-infusion cholangiogram
dic dicentric
DICA-R Diagnostic Interview for Children and Adolescents-Revised
DICP demyelinated inflammatory chronic polyneuropathy
DICT dose-intensive chemotherapy
DID
  dead of intercurrent disease
  delayed ischemic deficit
  dissociative identity disorder
  double immunodiffusion (technique)
  drug-induced disease
  dystonia-improvement-dystonia
di-di dichorionic-diamniotic (twins)
DIDS Dermatology Index of Disease Severity
DIE drug-induced esophagitis
DIEA deep inferior epigastric artery
DIF
  differentiation-inducing factor
  diffuse interstitial fibrosis
  direct immunofluorescence (test)
DIFF
  different
  differential (blood count)
  diffusion
diff diag
  differential diagnosis (*See also* DDx)
DIG
  digitalis
  digoxin
DIGS Diagnostic Interview for Genetic Study
dig. tox digitalis toxicity
DIH died in hospital
DIL
  daughter-in-law

dilute
dilution (*See also* diln)
drug-induced lupus
dilat dilation
DILC dose-intensity limiting criterion
diln dilution (*See also* DIL)
DIM
  diminish
  divalent ion metabolism
dim. one-half [L. *dimidus*]
DIMS disorders of initiating and maintaining sleep
diopt diopter
DIP
  desquamative interstitial pneumonia
  digital imaging processing
  diphtheria toxoid vaccine
  diploid
  diplopia
  distal interphalangeal (joint)
  drip-infusion pyelogram
  drug-induced parkinsonism
DIPC dynamic infusion pharmacocavernosometry
diph diphtheria
DIPI direct intraperitoneal insemination
DIR
  direct
  disturbed interpersonal relationships
  double isomorphous replacement
DI-S Debris Index-Simplified
DIS digital imaging spectrophotometer
DISA-SPECT dual-isotope simultaneous acquisition single-photon emission computed tomography
DISC
  death-inducing signaling complex
  dynamic integrated stabilization chair
disch discharge (*See also* DC)
DISC-R Diagnostic Interview Schedule for Children-Revised

DISCUS Dyskinesia Identification System: Condensed User Scale
DISH diffuse idiopathic skeletal hyperostosis
DISI
  dorsal intercalated segment instability
  dorsiflexed intercalated segment instability
disloc dislocate
disod disodium
DISP disposition
disp dispense
DISS Diameter Index Safety system
diss dissolve(d)
dissem disseminate
dist
  distal
  distill(ed)
  distribute
  distribution
  district
dist fr distinguished from
DIT
  diet-induced thermogenesis
  drug-induced thrombocytopenia
DIU death in utero
DIV double-inlet ventricle
div
  divergence
  divergent
  divide
  division
DIVA digital intravenous angiography
div ex divergence excess
DJD degenerative joint disease
DJJ duodenojejunal junction
DK
  dark
  decay
DKA diabetic ketoacidosis
DKB deep knee bend
DKC
  double knee to chest
  dyskeratosis congenita

DKP
  dibasic potassium phosphate
  dikalium phosphate
DKS Damus-Kaye-Stansel (procedure)
DL
  developmental level
  diagnostic laparoscopy
  difference limen (threshold)
  diffusing capacity of lung
  directed listening
  direct laryngoscopy
  distolingual
  double lumen
  drug level
  lethal dose [L. *dosis letalis*]
DL- equal quantities of D and L enantiomorphs (formerly dl-)
dL deciliter
DLA, DLa distolabial
DLAI, DLaI distolabioincisal
DLAP, DLaP distolabiopulpal
DLB dementia with Lewy bodies
DL&B direct laryngoscopy and bronchoscopy
DLC
  differential leukocyte count
  distolingual cusp
  double-lumen catheter
DLCO diffusing capacity of lung for carbon monoxide
DLCO$_2$ diffusing capacity of the lungs for carbon dioxide
DLCR distolingual cusp ridge
DLD
  date of last drink
  developmental language disorder
DLE
  delayed light emission
  discoid lupus erythematosus
DLF
  distolingual fossa
  dorsolateral funiculus
  ductal lavage fluid
DLG distolingual groove

DLI
Digital Libraries Initiative
distolinguoincisal
donor leukocyte infusion
donor lymphocyte infusion
double label index

DLK deep lamellar keratoplasty

DLLI dulcitol lysine lactose iron (agar)

DLO distolinguoocclusal

DLO₂ diffusing capacity of lungs for oxygen

DLP
developmental learning problems
dislocation of patella
distolinguopulpal
dysharmonic luteal phase
dyslipoproteinemia

DLPFC dorsolateral prefrontal cortex

D₅LR dextrose 5% in lactated Ringer (solution)

DLS
digitalis-like substances
ductlike structure
dynamic light scattering

DLSC double lumen subclavian catheter

DLT
diode laser trabeculoplasty
dorsolateral tract
dose-limiting toxicity
double lung transplant

DLU diffused lung uptake

DLW doubly labeled water

DM
dehydrated and malnourished
dermatology
dermatomyositis
Descemet membrane
dextromaltose
diabetes mellitus (type 1, 2)
diabetic mother
diastolic murmur
distant metastases
dorsomedial
dose modification
double membrane
double minute (chromosome)

dry matter
membrane diffusing capacity
myotonic dystrophy

D_M membrane component of diffusion

dM decimorgan

dm decimeter

dm² square decimeter

dm³ cubic decimeter

DMAB, DMABA dimethylaminobenzaldehyde (Ehrlich reagent)

DMARD disease-modifying antirheumatic drug

DMAS deep muscular aponeurotic system

DMAT disaster medical assistance team

D_max
maximum density
maximum depth

DMB demineralized bone

DMC direct microscopic count

DMCC direct microscopic clump count

DMD
disciform macular degeneration
disease-modifying drug
drowsiness monitoring device
Duchenne (de Boulogne) muscular dystrophy
dystonia musculorum deformans

DME
degenerative myoclonus epilepsy
diabetic macular edema
drug-metabolizing enzyme
Dulbecco modified Eagle (medium)
durable medical equipment

DMF decayed, missing, filled (permanent teeth)

dmf decayed, missing, filled (deciduous teeth)

DMFS decayed, missing, filled surfaces (permanent teeth)

dmfs decayed, missing, filled surfaces (deciduous teeth)

DMI
    diaphragmatic myocardial
      infarct
    direct migration inhibition
DML distal motor latency
DMM
    diffuse malignant
      mesothelioma
    disproportionate micromelia
D0(mm/dd/yy) Day zero
    (treatment start date)
DMN
    dorsal motor nucleus (of
      vagus)
    dorsomedial nucleus
DMOOC diabetes mellitus out
    of control
DMORT
    disaster mortuary operational
      response team
    Disaster Mortuary Team
DMP
    diffuse mesangial proliferation
    dura mater prosthesis
DMPH dysgenetic male
    pseudohermaphroditism
DMQ developmental motor
    quotient
DMR
    direct myocardial
      revascularization
    distal marginal ridge
D-MRI dynamic magnetic
    resonance imaging
DMS
    delayed muscle soreness
    demarcation membrane system
    dense microsphere
    dermatomyositis
    diagnostic medical sonography
    diffuse mesangial sclerosis
    dysmyelopoietic syndrome
DMSLT daytime multiple sleep
    latency test
DMT dermatophytosis
D,M,V,P disk, macula, vessels,
    periphery
DMWP distal mean wave
    pressure

DMX diathermy, massage, and
    exercise
DN
    Deiters nucleus
    diabetic nephropathy
    diabetic neuropathy
    dicrotic notch
    dysplastic nevus
D&N distance and near (vision)
DNA
    deoxyribonucleic acid
    did not answer
    did not attend
    does not apply
DNAse, DNase deoxyribonuclease
DND died a natural death
DNFB dinitrofluorobenzene
    (Sanger reagent)
DNFC does not follow
    commands
DNH do not hospitalize
DNI do not intubate
DNKA did not keep
    appointment
DNLL dorsal nucleus of lateral
    lemniscus
DNN did not nurse
DNOA diabetic neuropathic
    osteoarthropathy
DNP
    Dendroaspis natriuretic peptide
    did not pay
    do not publish
Dnp deoxyribonucleoprotein
DNR
    do not resuscitate
    dorsal nerve root
DNS
    de novo synthesis
    deviated nasal septum
    diaphragmatic nerve
      stimulation
    do not substitute
    dysplastic nevus syndrome
D$_5$NS, D$_5$NSS dextrose 5% in
    normal saline solution
DNT did not test
DNV dorsal nucleus of vagus

DO
  distal-occlusal
  distraction osteogenesis
  doctor's orders
  drugs only
D/O
  died of
  disorder
DO2 oxygen delivery
DO2I oxygen delivery index
DOA
  date of admission
  dead on arrival
  diagnostic and operative
    arthroscopy
  dominant optic atrophy
  driver of automobile
  duration of action
DOB
  dangle out of bed
  date of birth
  delta over baseline
  doctor's order book
DOC
  date of conception
  death of other cause
  diet of choice
  drug of choice
  dynamic orthotic cranioplasty
DOCLINE Documents On-Line
DOD
  date of death
  date of discharge
  dementia (syndrome) of
    depression
  died of disease
  dissolved oxygen deficit
  drug overdose
DOE
  date of examination
  direct observation evaluation
  disease-oriented evidence
  dyspnea on exertion
DOES disorders of excessive
  somnolence (sleepiness)
DOG distal oblique groove
DOHb Döhle bodies
DOI
  date of implant (pacemaker)
  date of injury

  depth of insertion
  died of injuries
DOL day of life (followed by
  number)
dol dolorimetric unit (of pain
  intensity)
DOLLS (Lee) double-loop
  locking suture
DOLV double-outlet left
  ventricle
DOM
  dissolved organic matter
  dominant
DOMS delayed-onset muscle
  soreness
DOOC diabetes out of control
DOR date of release
dors dorsal
DORV double-outlet right
  ventricle
DoRx date of treatment
DOS
  day of surgery
  doctor's order sheet
  dysosteosclerosis
DOSA day of surgery
  admission
DOSC Dubois oleic serum
  complex
DOST direct oocyte sperm
  transfer
DOT
  date of transcription
  date of transfer
  died on (operating) table
  directly observed therapy
  direct oocyte transfer
  Doppler ophthalmic test
DOTS directly observed therapy,
  short course
DOU direct observation unit
DOV
  date of visit
  distribution of ventilation
doz dozen (*See also* dz)
DP
  debonding pliers
  deep pulse
  degradation product
  degree of polymerization

deltopectoral
dementia praecox
dementia pugilistica
dental prosthesis
diastolic pressure
diffuse precipitation
diffusion pressure
digestible protein
discharge planning
discriminating power
displaced person
distal pancreatectomy
distal phalanx
distal pit
distopulpal
dorsalis pedis
driving pressure
D:P dialysis to plasma (urea ratio)
DPA
descending palatine artery
dextroposition of aorta
dual-photon absorptiometry (*See also* DPX)
dynamic physical activity
DPAP diastolic pulmonary artery pressure
D-PAS, dPAS diastase-periodic acid-Schiff
DPB
days postburn
dynamic pedobarography
DPBS Dulbecco phosphate-buffered saline
DPC
delayed primary closure
distal palmar crease
dpc days post coitus
DPCRT double-blind placebo-controlled randomized clinical trial
DPD
diffuse pulmonary disease
dual-photon densitometry
dysgenetic polycystic disease
D-2PD dynamic two-point discrimination
dP/dt upstroke pattern on apex cardiogram

DPEG dual percutaneous endoscopic gastrostomy
DPF Dental Practitioners' Formulary
DPFR diastolic pressure-flow relationship
DPG displacement placentogram
DPH diaphragm (*See also* diaph)
DPI
daily protein intake
days postinoculation
dietary protein intake
diphtheria-pertussis immunization
Doppler perfusion index
drug-prescribing index
dry powder inhaler
dynamic pulmonary imaging
DPJ
dementia paralytica juvenilis
direct percutaneous jejunostomy
DPL
diagnostic peritoneal lavage
distopulpolingual
DPLa distopulpolabial
DPM
digital phase mapping
disabling pansclerotic morphea
disintegrations per minute
drop per minute
DPN
deep penetrating nevus
dermatosis papulosa nigra
diabetic peripheral neuropathy
diabetic polyneuropathy
DPNB dorsal penile nerve block
DPOA durable power of attorney
DPOAE distortion-product otoacoustic emission
DPOAHC durable power of attorney for health care
DPOC placebo-controlled oral challenge testing
DPP
Diabetes Prevention Program
dorsalis pedis pulse
duration of positive pressure

D

DPR
    diagnostic procedure room
    doctor to population ratio
    dynamic planar reconstructor
DPRHP duodenum-preserving
pancreatic head resection
DPS
    disintegrations per second
    distal perfusion system
DPST, dpst double-pole single-
throw (switch)
DPT
    dehydration, poisoning, trauma
      department
    dichotic pitch (discrimination)
      test
    diphtheria, pertussis, and
      tetanus (vaccine)
    diphtheric pseudotabes
    dumping provocation test
DPTI diastolic pressure-time
index
DPTP diphtheria, pertussis,
tetanus, and poliomyelitis
(vaccine)
DPTPM diphtheria, pertussis,
tetanus, poliomyelitis, and
measles (vaccine)
DPUD duodenal peptic ulcer
disease
DPV disabling positional vertigo
DPVS dilated perivascular space
DPW distal phalangeal width
DPX dual-photon absorptiometry
(*See also* DPA)
DQ developmental quotient
DQE detective quantum
efficiency
DQOL diabetes quality of life
DR
    diabetic retinopathy
    diagnostic radiology
    digital radiography
    disposable/reusable
    distal root
    diurnal rhythm
    donor-related
    dorsal raphe
    dorsal root
    dose ratio

    drug receptor
    drug resistant
    dual-chamber rate-responsive
      (pacemaker)
    reaction of degeneration
      (muscle fibers)
dr
    drain
    dram (drachm)
DRA
    despite resuscitation attempts
    dialysis-related amyloidosis
    digital rotational angiography
    distal reference axis
    drug-related admission
DRAM
    de-epithelialized rectus
      abdominis muscle (graft)
    Distress Risk Assessment
      Method
DRAT differential rheumatoid
agglutination test
DRBC denatured red blood cell
DRC
    damage risk criteria
    dendritic reticulum cell
    digitorenocerebral (syndrome)
    dorsal radiocarpal ligament
    dorsal root, cervical
    dose-response curve
DRD
    dopa-responsive dystonia
    dorsal root dilator
    dystrophia retinae pigmentosa-
      dysostosis syndrome
DRE digital rectal examination
DREAM downstream regulatory
element antagonistic modulator
(gene)
DREF dose reduction
effectiveness factor
DRESS depth-resolved surface
(coil) spectroscopy
DREZ dorsal root entry zone
DRF
    digestive-respiratory fistula
    dose-reduction factor
DRFS distant recurrence-free
survival

DRG
  diagnosis-related group
  dorsal respiratory group
    (neurons)
  dorsal root ganglion
  duodenal-gastric reflux
    gastropathy
DRI
  defibrillation response interval
  Dietary Reference Intakes
  Discharge Readiness Inventory
  Doppler Resistive Index
DRID
  double radial immunodiffusion
  double radioisotope derivative
DRIFT drainage, irrigation,
  fibrinolytic therapy
DRIP delirium and drugs,
  restricted mobility and
  retention, infection and
  inflammation and impaction,
  polyuria (causes of urinary
  incontinence)
DRL
  differential reinforcement of
    low (response rates)
  dorsal root, lumbar
  dorsoradial ligament
  drug-related lupus
DRM drug-related morbidity
DRMS drug reaction monitoring
  system
DRN
  dorsal raphe nucleus
  drug-related neutropenia
drng
  drainage
  draining
DRnt diagnostic roentgenology
DRP
  dorsal root potential
  drug-related problem
DRQ discomfort relief quotient
DRR
  digitally reconstructed
    radiograph
  dorsal root reflex
  drug regimen review

DRS
  descending rectal septum
  diffuse reflectance
    spectroscopy
  Disability Rating Scale
  disease-related symptoms
  dorsal root, sacral
  drowsiness
  Duane retraction syndrome
  dynamic renal scintigraphy
  Dyskinesia Rating Scale
DRSG dressing
DRSI disease-related symptom
  improvement
DRSP drug-resistant
  Streptococcus pneumoniae
DRT
  dorsal root, thoracic
  drug-related thrombocytopenia
dRTA distal renal tubular
  acidosis
DRUJ distal radioulnar joint
DRVV dilute Russell's viper
  venom
DRVVT dilute Russell's viper
  venom time
DS
  dead (air) space
  deep sedative
  deep sleep
  defined substrate
  delayed sensitivity
  dendritic spine
  density (optical) standard
  dental surgery
  deprivation syndrome
  desynchronized sleep
  diaphragm stimulation
  diastolic murmur
  diencephalic syndrome
  difference spectroscopy
  digit span
  digit symbol
  dilute strength
  diopter sphere
  dioptric strength
  discharge summary
  discrimination score
  discriminative stimulus

DS *(continued)*
    disseminated sclerosis
    dissolved solids
    donor's serum
    Doppler sonography
    double strength
    double subordinance
    driving signal
    drug store
    dry swallow
    dumping syndrome
    duration of systole
D-S Doerfler-Stewart (test)
D&S dilation and suction
ds double-stranded (DNA, RNA)
DSA
    density spectral array
    digital subtraction angiography
    digital subtraction
      arteriography
DSACT direct sinoatrial
    conduction time
DSAP disseminated superficial
    actinic porokeratosis
DSB
    detachable silicone balloon
    drug-seeking behavior
Dsb single-breath diffusing
    (capacity)
DSBT donor-specific blood
    transfusion
DSC
    differential scanning
      colorimeter
    dobutamine stress
      echocardiography
    dynamic susceptibility contrast
DSCF Doppler-shifted constant
    frequency
DSCT dorsal spinocerebellar
    tract
DSD
    degenerative spinal disease
    digital selenium drum
      (radiology)
    dry sterile dressing
DSDDT double-sampling dye
    dilution technique
dsDNA double-stranded
    deoxyribonucleic acid

DSE
    digital subtraction
      echocardiogram
    dobutamine stress
      echocardiography
DSEA deep superior epigastric
    artery
DSF dry sterile fluff
DSG dry sterile gauze
Dsg desmoglein
DSH dexamethasone-suppressible
    hyperaldosteronism
DSHR delayed skin
    hypersensitivity reaction
DSI
    deep shock insulin
    digital subtraction imaging
DSIAR double-stapled ileoanal
    reservoir
DS-ICGA digital subtraction
    indocyanine green angiography
DSL distal sensory latency
dslv dissolve
DSM
    degradable starch microsphere
    Diagnostic and Statistical
      Manual of Mental Disorders
DSM-IV-TR Diagnostic and
    Statistical Manual of Mental
    Disorders, 4th Edition, Text
    Revision
DSO
    diffuse sclerosing osteomyelitis
    distal subungual
      onychomycosis
DSP
    delayed sleep phase
    diarrheic shellfish poisoning
    dibasic sodium phosphate
    digital signal processing
    digital sound processing
    digital subtraction
      phlebography
DSp digit span
D spine dorsal spine
DSPN
    distal sensory polyneuropathy
    distal symmetrical
      polyneuropathy

DSPS delayed sleep phase syndrome

DSR
dental stain remover
direct suicide risk
distal splenorenal
double simultaneous recording
dynamic spatial reconstructor

dsRNA double-stranded ribonucleic acid

DSRS distal splenorenal shunt

DSS
disease-specific survival
distal splenorenal shunt
double simultaneous stimulation

DSSEP dermatomal somatosensory-evoked potential

DSSLR double seated straight leg raise

DSSN distal symmetric sensory neuropathy

DSST digit symbol substitutional test

DST
daylight saving time
desensitization test
dexamethasone suppression test
digit substitution test
donor-specific transfusion
double stapling technique
duodenal secretin test

D-stix Dextrostix

DSU
day surgery unit
double setup

DSV digital subtraction ventriculography

DSVNI Distress Scale for Ventilated Newborn Infants

DSVP downstream venous pressure

DT
diphtheria-tetanus (immunization)
diphtheria toxin
diplöe thickness
dipole tracing

distal tubule
distance test (hearing)
double tachycardia
doubling time (of tumor size)
dye test

D/T
date/time
date of treatment
due to

D&T diagnosis and treatment

Dt duration of tetany

dT diphtheria-tetanus toxoid

DTA
descending thoracic aorta
differential thermoanalysis

2D-TCCS two-dimensional transcranial color-coded sonography

DTD
delivered total dose
diastrophic dystrophia

DTE desiccated thyroid extract

2D TEE two-dimensional transesophageal echocardiography

DTF
deep temporal fascia
desmoid-type fibromatosis
distal triangular fossa

D-TGA dextro-transposition of great arteries

DTH delayed-type hypersensitivity (reaction)

DTI
diffusion-tensor imaging
Doppler tissue imaging

DTICH delayed traumatic intracerebral hematoma

DTM
deep tissue massage
dermatophyte test media

DTMVmax diastolic transmembrane voltage, maximum

DTO deodorized tincture of opium

2D TOF two-dimensional time-of-flight

D

DTP
> differential time to positivity
> distal tingling on percussion
> (Tinel sign)

DTR deep tendon reflex

DTRTT digital temperature recovery time test

DTS
> danger to self
> dense tubular system
> differential temperature sensor
> diphtheria toxin sensitivity
> discrete time sample
> donor transfusion, specific

DTs delirium tremens

3D TSE three-dimensional turbo-spin echo (images)

DTT
> device for transverse traction
> diphtheria-tetanus toxoid
> direct transverse reaction

DTUS diathermy, traction, and ultrasound

DTV due to void

DTVMI Developmental Test of Visual Motor Integration

DTVP Developmental Test of Visual Perception

DTX detoxification

DU
> decubitus ulcer
> density (optical) unknown
> dermal ulcer
> developmental unit
> diabetic urine
> diagnosis undetermined
> dialytic ultrafiltration
> diffuse and undifferentiated
> dose unit
> duodenal ulcer

D$_U$ urea dialysance

DUA dorsal uterine artery

DUB
> Dubowitz (score)
> dysfunctional uterine bleeding

DUE drug use evaluation

DUF Doppler ultrasonic flowmeter

DUG dynamic urinary graciloplasty

DUI driving under the influence

DUL diffuse undifferentiated lymphoma

DUM
> dorsal unpaired median (axon, neuron)
> drug use monitoring

DUN dialysate urea nitrogen

duod
> duodenal
> duodenum

DUP duodenal ulcer perforation

dup
> duplicate
> duplication

DUR
> Drug Usage Review
> duration
> hard [L. *durus*]

DUS
> digital ultrasound
> distal urethral stenosis
> Doppler ultrasound stethoscope

3DUS three-dimensional ultrasound

DUSN diffuse unilateral subacute neuroretinitis ("wipe-out" syndrome)

DUV
> damaging ultraviolet
> degree of voicelessness

DV
> dependent variable
> dilute volume (of solution)
> distance vision
> domestic violence
> domiciliary visit
> dorsoventral
> double vision

D&V
> diarrhea and vomiting
> discs and vessels (ophthalmology)
> ductions and versions

dv double vibrations (unit of frequency of sound waves)

DVA
> developmental venous anomaly
> directional vacuum-assisted (biopsy)

distance visual acuity
duration of voluntary apnea (test)
dynamic visual acuity
D/VA diffusion per unit of alveolar volume
DVC
direct visualization of vocal cords
dorsal vein complex
DVD
dissociated vertical deviation
double-vessel disease
DVG double vein graft
DVH dose-volume histogram
DVI
atrioventricular sequential pacing
deep venous insufficiency
device-independent
digital vascular imaging
Doppler (systolic) velocity index
DVL deep vastus lateralis
DVM digital voltmeter
DVMI Developmental Test of Visual Motor Integration
DVN dorsal vagal nucleus
DVR
derotational varus osteotomy
digital vascular reactivity
double valve replacement
double vein graft
double ventricular response
DVS direct vesicoureteral scintigraphy
DVSA digital venous subtraction angiography
DVSS dysfunctional voiding scoring system
DVT deep vein thrombosis
DVTS deep venous thromboscintigram
D-W Danis-Weber ankle fracture (type A, B, C)
DW
deionized water
dextrose in water
diffusion-weighted (imaging)

distilled water
doing well
double wrap
dry weight
D/W
dextrose in water
discussed with
dry to wet
DWA died from wounds in action (by enemy)
DWCL daily-wear contact lens
DWD died with disease
DWDL diffuse well-differentiated lymphocytic (lymphoma)
DWI
diffusion-weighted (magnetic resonance) imaging
driving while impaired
driving while intoxicated
DWI/PI diffusion-weighted imaging/perfusion imaging
DWMHI deep white matter hyperintensity
DWMI deep white matter infarct
DWML deep white matter lesion
DWRT delayed work recall test
DWS
Dandy-Walker syndrome
Disaster Warning System
dorsal wrist syndrome
DWSCL daily-wear soft contact lens
DWT Dichotic Word Test
dwt pennyweight
DWW dynamic wall walk
Dx diagnosis
Dxd diagnosed
DxLS diagnosis responsible for length of stay
DXR
deep x-ray
delayed xenograft rejection
DXRT deep x-ray therapy
DY dense parenchyma
Dy dysprosium
dyn
dynamics

D

dyn *(continued)*
   dynamometer
   dyne
dysp dyspnea
DYTRO dynamic tone-reducing
   orthosis

DZ
   dizygous
   dizziness
Dz disease
dz dozen (*See also* doz)
DZT dizygotic twins

E

cortisone (compound E)
East
einstein (unit of energy)
Enterococcus
Escherichia
exa-
extraction (fraction, ratio)
glutamate (*See also* Glu)
methylenedioxy-
  methamphetamine (MDMA;
  Ecstasy)
opposite (stereo descriptor to
  indicate configuration at a
  double bond) [Ger.
  entgegen]
vectorcardiography electrode
  (midsternal)

E° standard electrode potential

E′ esophoria (for near)

E$_o$ skin (epidermis) dose
  (radiation)

E$_o$+, E° oxidation-reduction
  potential

e

erg
from [L. *ex*]

e− negative electron

e+ positron (positive electron)

EA

early antigen
educational age
electroanesthesia
embryonic (antibody, antigen)
enteral alimentation
enteroanastomosis
epidural anesthesia
episodic ataxia
erythrocyte (antibody, antisera)
estivoautumnal (malaria)

E&A evaluate and advise

E→A E to A changes

ea each

EAA

electrothermal atomic
  absorption
essential amino acid

EAAS electrothermal atomic
  absorption spectrophotometry

EAB extraanatomic bypass

EAC

Ehrlich ascites carcinoma
electroacupuncture (analgesia)
erythema action (spectrum)
erythema annulare centrifugum
erythrocyte, antibody, and
  complement
expandable access catheter
external auditory canal

EACD eczematous allergic
  contact dermatitis

EAD

early afterdepolarization
effective airspace dimension
extracranial arterial disease

EAG

electroantennogram
electroatriogram
endovascular aortic graft

EAHF eczema, asthma, and hay
  fever (complex)

EAI

electronically assisted
  instruction
erythema ab igne
erythrocyte antibody inhibition

EAL

electronic apex locator
electronic artificial larynx
endoscopic aspiration
  lumpectomy

EAM

endoscopic aspiration
  mucosectomy
external auditory meatus

EAP

endoscopic access port
evoked action potential

e-aq aqueous electron

E

95

EAR
electroencephalographic
audiometry
(expired air) resuscitation

ear ox ear oximetry

EAS
endoskeletal alignment system
external anal sphincter

EASI
Eczema Area and Severity
Index
extraamniotic saline infusion

EAST
elevated-arm stress test
enzyme allergosorbent test
external rotation-abduction
stress test

EAT
Eating Attitudes Test
ectopic atrial tachycardia
Edinburgh Articulation Test
Ehrlich ascites tumor
electroaerosol therapy
equine assistance therapy

EAUS endoanal ultrasound

EB
elbow bearing
elementary body
endometrial biopsy
epidermolysis bullosa
esophageal body
Evans blue (dye)

EBB electron beam boosts

EBC
early (stage) breast cancer
esophageal balloon catheter

EBCT electron beam computed
tomography

EBD
emotional and behavioral
difficulties
endoscopic balloon dilation
epidermolysis bullosa
dystrophica
evidence-based decision
(making)

EBE equal bilateral expansion

EBEA Epstein-Barr (virus) early
antigen

EBER Epstein-Barr early region
(protein)

EBF erythroblastosis fetalis

EBG electroblepharogram

EBGS electrical bone-growth
stimulator

EBIORT, EB-IORT electron-
beam intraoperative radiation
therapy

EBL
endoscopic band ligation
erythroblastic leukemia
estimated blood loss

EBM
electrophysiologic behavior
modification
evidence-based medicine
expressed breast milk

EBNA Epstein-Barr (virus)
nuclear antigen

EBNS endoscopic bladder neck
suspension

EBP epidural blood patch

EBR embolus-to-blood ratio

EBRT external beam radiation
therapy

EBS electrical brain stimulation

EBSB equal breath sounds
bilaterally

EBSD endoscopic balloon
sphincter dilation

EBSS Earle balanced salt
solution

EBT
electron beam tomography
external beam (photon)
therapy

EBV
effective blood volume
Epstein-Barr virus

EB-VCA Epstein-Barr viral
capsid antigen

EC
effect of closing (of eyes in
electroencephalography)
effective concentration
ejection click
electrochemical
electron capture
endocervical

endometrial carcinoma
endothelial cell
enteric-coated (tablet)
enterochromaffin cell
entorhinal cortex
Enzyme Commission
enzyme-treated cell
epidermal cell
epithelial cell
equalization-cancellation
ether-chloroform (mixture)
Euro-Collins (solution)
excitation-contraction
experimental control
external carotid
external conjugate (pelvis)
extracellular
extracranial
eye care

EC50, EC$_{50}$ median effective concentration

E/C endoscopy/cystoscopy

ECA
electric control activity
electrocardioanalyzer
epidemiologic catchment area
external carotid artery

E-CABG endoscopic coronary artery bypass grafting

ECAD extracranial carotid arterial disease

ECBD exploration of common bile duct

ECBV effective circulating blood volume

ECC
early childhood caries
edema, clubbing, and cyanosis
electrocorticogram
emergency cardiac care
Emergency Communications Center
endocervical cone
endocervical curettage
enterochromaffin cell
estimated creatinine clearance
external cardiac compression
extracorporeal circulation

ECCE extracapsular cataract extraction (*See also* XCCE)

ECCO$_2$R extracorporeal carbon dioxide removal

ECD
electrochemical detection
electron capture detector
endocardial cushion defect
equivalent current dipole
excision, curettage, and drilling
extended criteria donor
external cardioverter-defibrillator
extracellular domain
extracranial carotid disease
extracranial Doppler sonography

ECE
early childhood education
endocervical ecchymosis
extracapsular extension

ECEMG evoked compound electromyography

ECF
eosinophil chemotactic factor
erythroid colony formation
Escherichia coli filtrate
executive cognitive function(ing)
extended care facility
extracellular fluid

ECG electrocardiogram (*See also* EKG)

ECGE extracorporeal gas exchange

echino echinocyte

ECHO
echocardiogram
echoencephalography
enterocytopathogenic human orphan (virus)

ECHOG electrocochleography (*See also* ECoG)

ECHO-RV echocardiography-radionuclide ventriculography

ECHO-VM echoventriculometry

ECI
electrocerebral inactivity

ECI *(continued)*
    extracorporeal irradiation (of blood)
ECIC
    external carotid and internal carotid
    extracranial-intracranial
ECIS endometrial carcinoma in situ
ECL
    electrochemiluminescence
    emitter-coupled logic
    enhanced chemiluminescence
ECLA
    excimer laser coronary angioplasty
    extracorporeal lung assist
ECliPS encoded combinatorial libraries in polymeric support
ECLP extracorporeal liver perfusion
ECLRS electronic clinical laboratory reporting system
ECLS extracorporeal life support
ECLT euglobulin clot lysis time
ECM
    endoscope-controlled microsurgery
    erythema chronicum migrans
    external cardiac massage
    extracellular material
    extracellular matrix
ECM:BCM extracellular mass to body cell mass ratio
ECMO extracorporeal membrane oxygenation
ECN extended-care nursery
EC No. Enzyme Commission Number
ecNOS endothelial constitutive nitric oxide synthetase
ECoG
    electrocochleography *(See also* ECHOG)
    electrocorticogram
E. coli *Escherichia coli*
ECOR extracorporeal carbon dioxide removal

ECP
    effective conduction period
    emergency care provider
    emergency contraceptive pill
    endocardial potential
    erythropoietic coproporphyria
    external cardiac pressure
    external counterpulsation
    extracorporeal photochemotherapy
    extracorporeal photopheresis
ECPOG electrochemical potential gradient
ECPR external cardiopulmonary resuscitation
ECR
    electrocardiographic response
    emergency chemical restraint
    endocervical resection
    evoked cortical response
    extensor carpi radialis
ECRB extensor carpi radialis brevis
ECRL extensor carpi radialis longus
ECS
    elective cosmetic surgery
    electrocerebral silence
    electroconvulsive shock
    epileptic confusional state
    extracapsular spread
    extracellular-like, calcium-free solution
    extracellular space
ECT
    electrochemotherapy
    electroconvulsive therapy
    emission computed tomography
    euglobulin clot test
    European compression technique (bone screw and internal fixation)
    extracellular tissue
ECTR endoscopic carpal tunnel release
ECU
    extensor carpi ulnaris
    extracorporeal ultrafiltration

ECV
esophageal collateral vein
external cephalic version
extracellular (fluid) volume
extracorporeal volume

ECVD extracellular volume of distribution

ECVE extracellular volume expansion

ECW extracellular water

ED
early differentiation
eating disorder(s)
ectodermal dysplasia
ectopic depolarization
education
effective dose
elbow disarticulation
electrodialysis
electron diffraction
elemental diet
embryonic death
emergency department
emotional disorder
emotionally disturbed
end diastole
Entner-Doudoroff (metabolic pathway)
epidural
epileptiform discharge
equilibrium dialysis
equivalent dose
erectile dysfunction
erythema dose
evidence of disease
extensor digitorum
external diameter
extra-low dispersion

ED$_{50}$ median effective dose

E$_d$ depth dose

EDA
elbow disarticulation
electrodermal activity
electrodermal audiometry
electrolyte-deficient agar
electron donor-acceptor (interaction)
end-diastolic area

EDAM electron-dense amorphous material

EDAMS encephaloduroarteriomyosynangiosis

EDAS encephaloduroarteriosynangiosis

EDAX energy-dispersive x-ray analysis

EDB extensor digitorum brevis

EDBP erect diastolic blood pressure

EDC
effective dynamic compliance
emergency decontamination center
end-diastolic count
expected date of confinement
extensor digitorum communis

ED&C electrodesiccation and curettage

EDCP eccentric dynamic compression plate(plating)

EDD
effective drug duration
end-diastolic diameter
end-diastolic dimension
expected date of delivery
extended daily dialysis

EDE eating disorders examination

EDe erosion depth

edent edentulous

ED-ES endolymphatic duct-endolymphatic sac

EDF
elongation, derotation and lateral flexion
end-diastolic flow
erythroid differentiation factor
extradural fluid

EDG
electrodermography
electrodynogram

EdGr Edmondson grade

EDH
epidural hematoma
extradural hematoma

E

EDI
Eating Disorders Inventory
electrodeionization
EDL
end-diastolic load
end-diastolic (segment) length
estimated date of labor
extensor digitorum longus
ED/LD emotionally disturbed
and learning disabled
EDM
esophageal Doppler monitor
extensor digiti minimi
EDMA euclidean distance
matrix analysis
EDN electrodesiccation
EDP
electron-dense particle
emergency department
physician
end-diastolic pressure
endoscopic digital
pancreatography
EDQ extensor digiti quinti
EDR
early diastolic relaxation
effective direct radiation
electrodermal response
(biofeedback)
electrodialysis with reversed
(polarity)
extreme drug resistance
EDRA electrodermal response
audiometry
EDRF endothelial derived
relaxant factor
EDS
Ego Development Scale
energy-dispersive spectrometer
excessive daytime sleepiness
extended data stream
extradimensional shift
EDSS Expanded Disability
Status Scale (Score)
EDT
end-diastolic (cardiac wall)
thickness
exposure duration threshold
EDTA ethylenediaminetetraacetic
acid (edathamil, edetic acid)

EdU eating disorder unit
EDV
end-diastolic velocity
end-diastolic volume
EDVA Erhardt Developmental
Vision Assessment
EDW estimated dry weight
EDx electrodiagnosis (*See also*
EI Dx)
EDXA energy-dispersed x-ray
analysis
EDXRF energy-dispersive x-ray
fluorescence
E_{dyn} respiratory system elastance
EE
electrosurgical excision
emetic episodes
end-expiration
end-to-end (bite, occlusion)
energy expenditure
equine encephalitis
esophageal endoscopy
exercise echocardiogram
external ear
E&E eyes and ears
EEA
electroencephalic audiometry
energy expended with activity
EEC
endogenous erythroid colony
enteropathogenic *Escherichia
coli*
EECD endothelial-epithelial
corneal dystrophy
EEE
Eastern equine encephalitis
edema, erythema, and exudate
external eye examination
EEEP end-expiratory esophageal
pressure
EEG electroencephalogram
EEGA electroencephalographic
audiometry
EEHS emergency evacuation
hyperbaric stretcher
EEJ electroejaculation
EELS electron energy loss
spectroscopy
EELV end-expiratory lung
volume

EEM
   erythema exudativum
     multiforme
   external elastic membrane
EEMG evoked electromyogram
EENT eyes, ears, nose, throat
EEO electroendoosmosis
EEP
   end-expiratory pressure
   equivalent effective photon
EER electroencephalographic
   response
EESG evoked electrospinogram
EEU environmental exposure
   unit
EEV
   elastic equilibrium volume
   encircling endocardial
     ventriculotomy
EF
   eccentric fixation
   ejection fraction
   electric field
   embryo fibroblast
   eosinophilic fasciitis
   erythroblastosis fetalis
   extended field (radiation
     therapy)
   extrinsic factor
EFA essential fatty acid
EFAS embryofetal alcohol
   syndrome
EFBW estimated fetal body
   weight
EFD episode free day
EFE endocardial fibroelastosis
EFF electromagnetic focusing
   field (probe)
eff
   effect(ive)
   efficient
   effusion
effer efferent
EFL effective focal length
EFM electronic fetal monitoring
EFMM external fetal-maternal
   monitor
EFMT electric field mediated
   transfer

EFP effective filtration pressure
EFPS epicardial fat pad sign
EFR
   effective filtration rate
   extended field radiation
E FRAG erythrocyte fragility
(test)
EFS
   electric field stimulation
   event-free survival
EFT Embedded Figures Test
EFV extracellular fluid volume
EFVC expiratory flow-volume
   curve
EFW estimated fetal weight
EF/WM ejection fraction/wall
   motion
EG
   esophagogastrectomy
   esophagogastric
   external genitalia
e.g. for example [L. *exempli
gratia*]
EGA estimated gestational age
EGBT esophagogastric balloon
   tamponade
EGBUS external genitalia,
   Bartholin, urethral, and Skene
   (glands)
EGD esophagogastroduodenos-
   copy
EGDF embryonic growth and
   development factor
EGF
   endothelial growth factor
   epidermal growth factor
eGFP enhanced green
   fluorescent protein
EGG
   electrogastrogram
   electroglottography
EGJ esophagogastric junction
EGLT euglobulin lysis time
EGM
   electrogram
   extraglandular manifestation
   extraglomerular mesangium

E

EGR
early growth response
erythema gyratum repens
EGRA equilibrium-gated
radionuclide angiography
EGS electrogalvanic stimulation
EGTA esophagogastric tube
airway
EH
eccentric hypertrophy
educationally handicapped
emotionally handicapped
endometrial hyperplasia
enlarged heart
enteral hyperalimentation
epidermolytic hyperkeratosis
E&H environment and heredity
EHB
elevate head of bed
extensor hallucis brevis
EHC
enterohepatic circulation
enterohepatic clearance
essential hypercholesterolemia
extrahepatic cholestasis
EH-CF *Entamoeba histolytica*-
complement fixation
EHD
electrohemodynamic
epizootic hemorrhagic disease
EHEC enterohemorrhagic
Escherichia coli
EHF
electrohydraulic fragmentation
epidemic hemorrhagic fever
exophthalmos hyperthyroid
factor
extremely high frequency
EHH esophageal hiatal hernia
EHI
Edinburgh Handedness
Inventory
exertional heat illness
EHL
effective half-life (of
radioactive substance)
electrohydraulic lithotripsy
endogenous hyperlipidemia
endoscopic hemorrhoid
ligation

Environmental Health
Laboratory
essential hyperlipidemia
extensor hallucis longus
EHM embryonic heart motion
EHMS electrohydrodynamic
ionization mass spectrometry
EHP
Environmental Health
Perspectives
excessive heat production
extra high potency
EHPH extrahepatic portal
hypertension
EHS
employee health service
exertional heat stroke
EHT electrohydrothermal
EHV
Edge Hill virus
equine herpesvirus
EI
electrolyte imbalance
electron ionization
emotionally impaired
endovascular irradiation
environmental illness
enzyme immunoassay
enzyme inhibitor
eosinophilic index
erythema infectiosum
excretory index
extensor indicis
external intervention
E:I expiration to inspiration
ratio
E&I endocrine and infertility
EIA
electroimmunoassay
enzymatic immunoassay
enzyme immunosorbent assay
equine infectious anemia
exercise-induced anaphylaxis
exercise-induced asthma
EIAB extracranial-intracranial
arterial bypass
EIB
electrophoretic immunoblotting
erythema induration of Bazin
exercise-induced bronchospasm

EIC
  elastase inhibition capacity
  electrical impedance
    cardiography
  endometrial intraepithelial
    carcinoma
  enzyme inhibition complex
  epidermal inclusion cyst
EID
  egg-infectious dose
  electroimmunodiffusion
  electronic induction desorption
  electronic infusion device
EIDCR endoscopic intranasal
  dacryocystorhinostomy
EIEE early infantile epileptic
  encephalopathy
eIF eukaryotic initiation factor
EIFT embryo intrafallopian
  transfer
EIL elective induction of labor
EILV end-inspiratory lung
  volume
EIMS electron ionization mass
  spectrometry
EI/MV endotracheal intubation
  and mechanical ventilation
EIP
  early intervention program
  elective interruption of
    pregnancy
  end-inspiratory pause
  extensor indicis proprius
EIS
  endoscopic injection
    sclerotherapy
  Environmental Impact
    Statement
  Epidemic Intelligence Service
EISA electroencephalogram
  interval spectrum analysis
EIT
  electrical impedance
    tomography
  erythroid iron turnover
EITB enzyme-linked
  immunotransfer blot
EIV external iliac vein
EJ elbow jerk

EJB ectopic junctional beat
EJP excitatory junction potential
EJV external jugular vein
EK electrophoretic karyotyping
EKC epidemic
  keratoconjunctivitis
EKG electrocardiogram (*See also*
  ECG)
EKO echoencephalogram
EKY electrokymogram
EL
  early latent
  electrolarynx
  electroluminescence
  elopement
  erythroleukemia
  exercise limit
  external lamina
E-L external lids
El elastase
ELA excimer laser-assisted
  angioplasty
ELAD extracorporeal liver assist
  device
E-LAM, ELAM endothelial-
  leukocyte adhesion molecule
ELAT enzyme-linked
  antiglobulin test
ELBNS extraperitoneal
  laparoscopic bladder neck
  suspension
ELBW extremely low birth
  weight
ELC earlobe crease
ELCA excimer laser coronary
  angioplasty
ELD egg lethal dose
ELDH extraforaminal lumbar
  disk herniation
El Dx electrodiagnosis (*See also*
  EDx)
ELEC
  elective
  electric
  electuary (confection)
elem elementary
elev elevate
ELF
  elective low forceps (delivery)

ELF *(continued)*
 endoscopic laser foraminotomy
 epithelial lining fluid
 extremely low frequency
ELFA enzyme-linked fluorescent
 immunoassay
ELG
 endoluminal gastroplication
 endoluminal graft
elgon electrogoniometer
ELH
 egg-laying hormone
 endolymphatic hydrops
ELI
 endomyocardial lymphocytic
 infiltrates
 exercise lability index
ELIA enzyme-labeled
 immunoassay
ELICT enzyme-linked
 immunocytochemical technique
ELIEDA enzyme-linked
 immunoelectrodiffusion assay
ELIFA enzyme-linked
 immunofiltration assay
ELIG eligible
ELISA enzyme-linked
 immunoabsorbent assay
ELISPOT enzyme-linked
 immunoSPOT
ELITT endometrial laser
 intrauterine thermal therapy
elix elixir
ELLIP elliptocyte
ELM
 epiluminescence microscopy
 external limiting membrane
ELND elective lymph node
 dissection
ELOP estimated length of
 program
ELOS estimated length of stay
ELP
 early labeled peak
 electrophoresis
 extracorporeal liver perfusion
ELS
 electron loss spectroscopy
 endolymphatic sac

 extracorporeal life support
 extralobar sequestration
ELSS emergency life support
 system
ELT
 endless loop tachycardia
 endoscopic laser therapy
 euglobulin lysis test (time)
ELUS endoluminal rectal
 ultrasonography
ELVIS Enzyme Linked Virus
 Inducible System
EM
 ejection murmur
 electromechanical
 electron micrograph
 electron microscope
 electrophoretic mobility
 emergency medicine
 emmetropia (normal vision)
 erythema migrans
 erythema multiforme
 erythrocyte mass
 esophageal manometry
 esophageal motility
 external monitor
E-M Embden-Meyerhof
 (glycolytic pathway)
E of M error of measurement
E&M endocrine and metabolic
e:m ratio of (electron) charge
 to mass
em electromagnetic
EMA
 early morning awakening
 electronic microanalyzer
 endomysial antibody
 epithelial membrane antigen
EMAP evoked muscle action
 potential
Emax maximum ventricular
 elastance
EMB
 endometrial biopsy
 endomyocardial biopsy
 engineering in medicine and
 biology
 eosin-methylene blue (Levine
 agar)

emb
  embolus
  embryo
EMC
  emergency medical care
  encephalomyocarditis
  endometrial curettage
E&M codes evaluation and management codes
EMC&R emergency medical care and rescue
EMD
  electromechanical dissociation
  esophageal motility disorder
EMDA electromotive drug administration
EMDR eye movement desensitization and reprocessing
EME
  epithelial-myoepithelial (carcinoma)
  extreme medical emergency
EMEG electromagnetoencephalograph
EMER electromagnetic molecular electronic resonance
emer, emerg emergency
EMF
  elective midforceps
  electromagnetic flowmeter
  electromotive force
  endomyocardial fibrosis
  erythrocyte maturation factor
  evaporated milk formula
emf electromagnetic field
EMG
  electromyelogram
  electromyogram
  eye movement gauge
EMH educationally mentally handicapped
EMI
  electromagnetic interference
  electromechanical impactor
EMIC emergency maternal and infant care

EMI/RFI electromagnetic interference/radiofrequency interference
EMIT enzyme-multiplied immunoassay technique (test)
EMJH Ellinghausen-McCullough-Johnson-Harris (medium)
EML
  effective mandibular length
  essential medicine lists (WHO)
EMLA eutectic mixture of local anesthetics
EMM erythema multiforme major
EMO Epstein-Macintosh-Oxford (inhaler)
emot emotion
EMP
  electrical membrane property
  electromagnetic pulse
  electromolecular propulsion
  external membrane protein
EMPEP
  electrophoretic pattern
  erythrocyte membrane protein
emph emphysema
EMR
  educable mentally retarded
  electrical muscle stimulation
  electromagnetic radiation
  electronic medical record
  emergency mechanical restraint
  empty, measure, and record
  endoscopic magnetic resonance
  endoscopic mucosal resection
  eye movement recording
E-MRI extremity magnetic resonance imaging
EMS
  early morning stiffness
  electrical muscle stimulation
  emergency medical services
  endometriosis
  eosinophilia-myalgia syndrome
  esophageal manometric sequence

EMSA electrophoretic mobility shift analysis (assay)
EMT
electronic medical textbook
emergency medical technician
EMTALA Emergency Medical Treatment and Active Labor Act
EMT-B emergency medical technician basic
EMT-D emergency medical technician providing basic life support or defibrillation
EMT-I emergency medical technician intermediate
EMT-W emergency medical technician wilderness
emu electromagnetic unit
emul emulsion
EMVC early mitral valve closure
EMW electromagnetic waves
EN
easy normal
electronarcosis
enteral nutrition
erythema nodosum
E 50% N extension 50% of normal
ENB esthesioneuroblastoma
END
early neonatal death
elective neck dissection
endocrinology
endorphin
ENDO
endocardium
endocrine
endodontia
endodontics
endoscopy
endo-ECG endocoronary electrocardiography
endos endosteal
enem enema
ENG
electronystagmogram
engorged
ENK enkephalin

ENL
easy normal left
erythema nodosum leprosum
enl enlarge
ENL-DCR endonasal laser dacryocystorhinostomy
ENMG electroneuromyography
ENNAS Einstein Neonatal Neurobehavioral Assessment Scale
ENNS Early Neonatal Neurobehavior Scale
Eno enolase
eNO exhaled nitric oxide
ENog electroneurogram
ENR easy normal right
ENS
enteric nervous system
exogenous natural surfactant
ENT ears, nose, and throat
ENTOM entomology
environ environment
enz enzyme
EO
effect of opening (eyes in electroencephalography)
elbow orthosis
embolic occlusion
eyes open
E&O evaluation and observation
EOA
effective orifice area
erosive osteoarthritis
esophageal obturator airway
examination, opinion, and advice
EOAE evoked otoacoustic emission
EOB
edge of bed
explanation of benefits
EOC
electrooptical characteristic
Emergency Operations Center
EOD
electrical organ discharge
end of day
end organ damage
every other day
extent of disease

EOG
  electrooculogram
  electroolfactogram
EOIT ego-oriented individual therapy
EOL end of life
EOM
  error of measurement
  external otitis media
  extraocular motion
  extraocular movement
  extraocular muscle
EOM F & Conj extraocular movements full and conjugate
EOMI
  extraocular movements intact
  extraocular muscles intact
EOP equivalent oxygen performance
EOR end of range
EOS
  early-onset schizophrenia
  eligibility on-site
  end of study
eos eosinophil
EOT effective oxygen transport
EP
  ectopic pregnancy
  electrophoresis
  electrophysiology
  electroprecipitin
  endorphin
  end point
  ependymal (cell)
  epicardial
  epithelium
  erythrophagocytosis
  esophageal pressure
  esophoria
  evoked potential
  excretory phase
EPA
  erect posterior-anterior (projection)
  extrinsic plasminogen activator
EPAP expiratory positive airway pressure

EPB extensor pollicis brevis
EPBD endoscopic papillary balloon dilation
EPBF effective pulmonary blood flow
EPC
  electronic pain control
  end-plate current
  epilepsia partialis continua
  extent of pleural carcinomatosis (score)
  external pneumatic compression
EPCA external pressure circulatory assistance
EPCG endoscopic pancreatocholangiography
EPCL Everyday Problem Checklist
EPD
  electrode placement device
  embolic placement device
  endoscopic papillary balloon dilation
  enzyme potentiated desensitization
  equilibrium peritoneal dialysis
  extramammary Paget disease
EPDML epidemiology
EpDRF epithelium-derived relaxation factor
EPDS Edinburgh Postnatal Depression Scale
EPE extrapyramidal effect
EPEA expense-per-equivalent admission
EPEC enteropathogenic *Escherichia coli*
EPEM Emory Pain Estimate Model
EPF
  endoscopic plantar fasciotomy
  exophthalmos producing factor
EPG
  eggs per gram
  electronic pupillography
  electropneumogram

EPH
 edema, proteinuria, hypertension
 extensor proprius hallucis
EpHM intraesophageal pH monitoring
EPI
 echo-planar imaging
 evoked-potential index
 exercise pressure index
 Expanded Program of Immunizations (WHO)
 extremely premature infant
EPIC evaluation, prediction, intervention, and control
EPID
 epidemic
 epidural
epig epigastric
epil epilepsy
EPIS
 epileptic postictal sleep
 episiotomy
 episode
 epistaxis
EPITH epithelium
EPL
 effective path length
 extensor pollicis longus
 extracorporeal piezoelectric lithotripsy
EPM
 electronic pacemaker
 electron-probe microanalysis
 energy-protein malnutrition
EPN
 emphysematous pyelonephritis
 estimated protein needs
EPO
 epoetin alfa
 erythropoietin
 evening primrose oil
EPP
 endplate potential
 equal-pressure point
 erythropoietic protoporphyria
 extrapleural pneumonectomy
EPPB end positive-pressure breathing

EPR
 early-phase reaction
 early progressive resistance
 electron paramagnetic resonance
 electrophrenic respiration
 emergency physical restraint
 estimated protein requirement
 evoked potential response
EPS
 elastosis perforans serpiginosa
 electrophysiologic study
 endoscopic pancreatic sphincterotomy
 endoscopic pancreatic stenting
 extrapyramidal syndrome
EPSA
 early postoperative suture adjustment
 evoked potential signal averaging
EPSD E-point to septal distance
EPSEM equal probability of selection method
EPSP excitatory postsynaptic potential
EPT
 early pregnancy test
 endoscopic papillotomy
EPTE existed prior to enlistment
EPTFE, E-PTFE, e-PTFE expanded polytetrafluoroethylene
EPTS existed prior to service
EPXMA electron probe x-ray microanalyzer
EQ
 education quotient
 encephalization quotient
 energy quotient
 equal to
 equation
 equilibrium
 equivalent
EQA external quality assessment
EQP extensor quinti proprius
equip. equipment
equiv
 equivalency
 equivocal

ER
early repolarization
ejection rate
electroresection
emergency room
endoplasmic reticulum
end range
epigastric region
equine rhinopneumonia
equivalent roentgen (unit)
estrogen receptor
evoked response
expiratory reserve
external reduction
external rotation
extraction ratio
ER− estrogen receptor-negative
ER+ estrogen receptor-positive
E&R
equal and reactive
examination and report
Er erbium
ERA
electrical response activity
electric response audiometry
endometrial resection and
ablation
estrogen receptor assay
evoked-response audiometry
%ERAD eradication rate
ERB ethnic relational behavior
ERBAC excimer laser, rotational
atherectomy, and balloon
angioplasty
ERBD endoscopic retrograde
biliary drainage
ERBF effective renal blood
flow
ERC endoscopic retrograde
cholangiogram
ERCCE endoscopic retrograde
cholecystoendoprosthesis
ERCP endoscopic retrograde
cholangiopancreatography
ERD
early retirement with
disability
evoked-response detector

ERE external rotation in
extension
ERF
edge response function
external rotation in flexion
erf error function
ERFC, E-RFC erythrocyte
rosette-forming cell
ERG
electrolyte replacement with
glucose
electron radiography
electroretinogram
erg energy unit
ERH egg-laying release
hormone
ERI erythrocyte rosette inhibitor
ERIA electroradioimmunoassay
ER/IR external rotation/internal
rotation
ERISA Employee Retirement
Income Security Act
ERL effective refractory length
ERM
electrochemical relaxation
method
epiretinal membrane
ERMS exacerbating-remitting
multiple sclerosis
ERNA equilibrium radionuclide
angiography
ERP
early receptor potential
effective refractory period
endocardial resection
procedure
endoscopic retrograde
pancreatogram
estrogen receptor protein
event-related (brain) potential
ERPC evacuation of retained
products of conception
ERPP endoscopic retrograde
parenchymography of pancreas
ER/PR estrogen
receptor/progesterone receptor
ERR error

ERS
  endoscopic retrograde sphincterotomy
  evacuation of retained secundines (afterbirth)
  extended, rotated, sidebent

ERSL extended, rotated, sidebent left

ERSP event-related slow-brain potential

ERSR extended, rotated, sidebent right

ERSS Edinburgh Rehabilitation Status Scale

ERT
  electronic textbook of radiology
  emergency room thoracotomy
  emergent resuscitative thoracotomy
  estrogen replacement therapy
  external radiation therapy
  (pancreatic) enzyme replacement therapy

ERUS endorectal ultrasound

ERV expiratory reserve volume

e-RX electronic prescription

Er:YAG erbium:yttrium-aluminum-garnet (laser)

eryth
  erythema
  erythrocyte

ES
  ejection sound
  electrical stimulation
  electroshock
  electrospray
  embryonic stem (cells)
  emission spectrometry
  endometritis-salpingitis
  endoscopic sclerotherapy
  endoscopic sphincterotomy
  end stage
  end systole
  environmental stimulation
  esophageal scintigraphy
  Ewing sarcoma
  excretory-secretory
  extracapsular spread
  extrasystole

Es einsteinium

ESA epididymal sperm aspiration

ESAP evoked sensory (nerve) action potential

ESAS Edmonton Symptom Assessment Scale

ESAT extrasystolic atrial tachycardia

ESB electric stimulation of the brain

ES/BS erosion surface per bone surface

ESC
  electromechanical slope computer
  end-systolic count

ESCC
  epidural spinal cord compression
  esophageal squamous cell carcinoma

ESCS electrical spinal cord stimulation

ESD
  emission spectrometric detector
  end-systolic diameter
  end-systolic dimension
  environmental sex determination
  esophagus, stomach, and duodenum

ESE electrostatic unit [Ger. *electrostatische Einheit*]

ESEP
  elbow sensory potential
  extreme somatosensory evoked potential

ESF
  electrosurgical filter
  erythropoiesis-stimulating factor
  external skeletal fixation

ESG electrospinogram

ESI
  enamel surface index
  enzyme substrate inhibitor
  epidural steroid injection

ESIMS electrospray ionization mass spectrometry

ES-IMV expiration-synchronized intermittent mandatory ventilation

ESL
end-systolic (segment) length
English as a second language

ESLD
end-stage liver disease
end-stage lung disease

ESLF end-stage liver failure

ESM endothelial specular microscope

ESN educationally subnormal

ESN(M) educationally subnormal-moderate

ESN(S) educationally subnormal-severe

ESO
electrospinal orthosis
esophagoscopy

esoph
esophagoscopy
esophagus

esoph steth esophageal stethoscope

ESP
electrosensitive point
electrosurgical pencil
endometritis-salpingitis-peritonitis
end-systolic pressure
evoked synaptic potential
extrasensory perception

esp especially

ESPA electrical stimulation-produced analgesia

ESPI electronic speckle pattern interferometry

ESR
electric skin resistance
electron spin resonance
erythrocyte sedimentation rate

ESRD end-stage renal disease

ESRRL extension, sidebent right, rotated left

ESRS extrapyramidal symptom rating scale

ESS
empty sella (turcica) syndrome
endoscopic sinus surgery
end-systolic stress
Epworth Sleepiness Scale (Score)
European Stroke Scale
euthyroid sick syndrome

ESSF external spinal skeletal fixator

ess neg essentially negative

EST
electroshock therapy
electrosleep therapy
electrostimulation therapy
endoscopic sphincterotomy
esterase
exercise stress test
expression sequence tagged

E_{st} static elastance

est
ester
estimate

esth esthetic

E-stim electrical stimulation

ESU
electrostatic unit
electrosurgical unit

ESV
end-systolic (ventricular) volume
esophageal valve

ESVS epiurethral suprapubic vaginal suspension

ESWI end-systolic wall index

ESWL
electrohydraulic shock wave lithotripsy
extracorporeal shock wave lithotripsy

ESWT
end-systolic wall thickness
extracorporeal shock wave therapy

ESY expressed sequence tag

ET
edge thickness
ejection time

E

ET *(continued)*
    embryo transfer
    endometrial thickness
    endotoxin
    endotracheal
    end-tidal
    endurance time
    enterostomal therapy
    esotropia
    essential tremor
    eustachian tube
    Ewing tumor
    exchange transfusion
    exercise treadmill
    expiration time
ET′, ET− near esotropia
ET@20' esotropia at 6 meters (infinity)
E:T effector to target ratio
E(T) intermittent esotropia
E(T') intermittent near esotropia
Et ethyl
et and [L.]
ETA
    electron-transfer agent
    endotracheal aspirate
    estimated time of arrival
ETAB extrathoracic-assisted breathing
ETAC electrothermally assisted capsulorrhaphy
et al. and others [L. *et alii*]
ETBD etiology to be determined
ETC
    esophagotracheal combination tube
    estimated time of conception
ETc corrected ejection time
etc. and so forth [L. *et cetera*]
ETCO$_2$ end-tidal carbon dioxide (concentration)
ETD
    estimated time of death
    eustachian tube dysfunction
    eye-tracking dysfunction
ETE end-to-end (anastomosis)
ETEC enterotoxigenic *Escherichia coli*

ETF
    eustachian tube function
    extension teardrop fracture
ETFVL exercise tidal flow-volume loop
ETG episodic treatment group
ETH ethmoid
ETI endotracheal intubation
ETKTM every test known to mankind
ETL
    echo-train length
    expiratory threshold load
ETO
    estimated time of ovulation
    eustachian tube obstruction
EtO ethylene oxide
Et$_2$O ether
E-TOF electron time-of-flight
EtOH ethanol
ETP
    elective termination of pregnancy
    electron transport particle
ETPS electrotherapeutic point stimulation
ETR epitympanic recess
ETS
    electrical transcranial stimulation
    elevated toilet seat
    endoscopic transthoracic sympathectomy
    endotracheal suction
    end-to-side (anastomosis)
ETT
    endotracheal tube
    esophageal transit time
    exercise tolerance test
    exercise treadmill test
EU
    Ehrlich unit
    equivalent unit
    esophageal ulcer
    etiology unknown
    European Union
    excretory urography
Eu
    europium
    euryon

EUA examination under anesthesia
EUD external urinary device
EUG extrauterine gestation
EUL
    expected upper limit
    extrauterine life
EUM external urethral meatus
EUP extrauterine pregnancy
EUS
    echoendoscopy
    endorectal ultrasonography
    endoscopic ultrasound
    esophageal ultrasound
    external urethral sphincter
EUS-FNA endoscopic ultrasound-guided fine-needle aspiration
eust eustachian
EUV extreme ultraviolet (laser)
EV
    esophageal varices
    evoked (response)
    expected value
    extravascular
eV electron volt
EVA ethyl violet azide (broth)
EVAC evacuate
eval evaluate
evap evaporate
EVB esophageal variceal bleeding
eve evening
ever.
    eversion
    everted
EVG
    electroventriculogram
    electrovomerogram
EVH esophageal variceal hemorrhage
EVL endoscopic variceal ligation
EVM
    electronic voltmeter
    eye, verbal, motor (Glasgow Coma Scale)
evol evolution

EVP
    episcleral venous pressure
    evoked visual potential
EVR evoked visual response
EVS esophageal variceal sclerotherapy
EVUS endovaginal ultrasound
EW
    Edinger-Westphal (nucleus)
    expiratory wheeze
EWB
    emotional well-being
    estrogen withdrawal bleeding
EWCL extended-wear contact lens
EWHO elbow-wrist-hand orthosis
EWL
    estimated weight loss
    evaporation water loss
EWT erupted wisdom teeth
EX
    exacerbation
    example
    exophthalmos
    exposure
    external movement
exag exaggerated
exam examine
exc
    except
    excision
exec executive
Ex-ECG exercise stress electrocardiography
Ex-Echo exercise stress echocardiography
ExEF ejection fraction during exercise
exer exercise
EXIT ex utero intrapartum tracheloplasty
ex lap exploratory laparotomy
EXO exophoria
EXOPH exophthalmos
EXP
    experience
    exploration
    expose

E

113

exp
expected
exponential (function)
expect. expectorant
exper experiment(al)
expir
expiration
expiratory
expired
expn expression
EXREM external radiation-emission-man (radiation dose)
EXT, ext
exchange transfusion
extension
extract
ext extensor
ext aud external auditory
extd
extended
extracted

ext FHR external fetal heart rate (monitoring)
ext mon external monitor
extr extremity
extrap extrapolate
extrav extravasation
ext rot external rotation
EXTUB extubation
EXU excretory urogram
EY epidemiology year
EYA egg yolk agar
EYES Early Years Easy Screen
EZ Edmonston-Zagreb (vaccine)
Ez eczema
EZ-HT Edmonston-Zagreb high-titer (vaccine)
EZW embedded zero tree wavelet (picture archiving and communication)

F

conjugative plasmid in F⁺ bacterial cells
Fahrenheit
faraday (constant)
father
female
fermentative
fermi (energy)
fertility (factor)
field of vision
filial generation
first degree of fineness of abrasive particles
fluorine
focus
force
fractional (composition of gas in gas phase) (*See also* FX)
French (catheter size)
frontal electrode placement in electroencephalography
Helmholtz free energy
hydrocortisone (compound F)
inbreeding coefficient
(luminous) flux
phenylalanine (*See also* Phe)
vectorcardiography electrode (left foot)
visual field (*See also* VF)

F0 fundamental frequency
F′ secondary focal point (of lens)
°F degree Fahrenheit
/F full lower denture (*See also* FLD)
F+ good form response
F/ full upper denture (*See also* FUD)
F⁺ bacterial cell with an F plasmid
F⁻

bacterial cell lacking an F plasmid
fluoride
poor form response

F$_t$ ferritin

f

atomic orbital with angular momentum quantum number 3
femto-
fission
focal
respiratory frequency

F$_1$ first filial generation
F$_2$ second filial generation
FI–FXIII factor I through XIII (blood)
F= firm and equal
FA

fatty acid
femoral artery
fetal age
fetus active
fibrinolytic activity
filterable agent
filtered air
first aid
fluorescein angiography
fluorescent antibody (stain)
fluorescent assay
folic acid
follicular area
forearm
fortified aqueous (solution)
Freund adjuvant
Friedreich ataxia
functional activities

FAAD fetal activity acceleration determination
FAAP family assessment adjustment pass
FAASOL formalin, acetic, and alcohol solution
FAB

French-American-British (leukemia classification system)
functional arm brace

115

Fab fragment (of immunoglobulin G involved in) antigen binding

FABER flexion, abduction, external rotation

FABERE flexion, abduction, external rotation, extension

FABF femoral artery blood flow

FAB L1 acute lymphoblastic leukemia, child type

FAB L2 acute lymphoblastic leukemia, adult type

FAB L3 lymphoma-like leukemia (Burkitt)

FAB M0
leukemia with large granular blasts and negative myeloperoxidase
undifferentiated leukemia

FAB M1 myeloblastic leukemia without maturation

FAB M2 myeloblastic leukemia with maturation

FAB M3 acute promyelocytic leukemia

FAB M4 combination myeloblastic-monoblastic leukemia, acute

FAB M5 monoblastic leukemia

FAB M6 erythroleukemia

FAB M7 megakaryocytic leukemia

FAB/MS fast atom bombardment mass spectrometry

FABP finger arterial blood pressure

FAC
femoral arterial cannulation
fetal abdominal circumference
fractional area change
fractional area concentration
functional aerobic capacity
Functional Ambulation Categories

FACH forceps to aftercoming head

FACO$_2$ fraction of alveolar carbon dioxide

FACS fluorescence-activated cell sorting

FACT
focused appendix computed tomography
Functional Acuity Contrast Test
Functional Assessment of Cancer Therapy

FACT-B Functional Assessment of Cancer Therapy-Breast

FACT-F Functional Assessment of Cancer Therapy-Fatigue

FACT-G Functional Assessment of Cancer Therapy-General

FACT-HN Functional Assessment of Cancer Therapy–Head and Neck

FACT-L Functional Assessment of Cancer Therapy-Lung

FACT-O Functional Assessment of Cancer Therapy-Ovarian

FACT-P Functional Assessment of Cancer Therapy-Prostate

FAD
familial autonomic dysfunction
fetal abdominal diameter
fetal activity acceleration determination

FADF fluorescent antibody dark-field

FADIR flexion, adduction, internal rotation

FADIRE flexion, adduction, internal rotation, and extension

FADS fetal akinesia deformation sequence

FAE
fetal alcohol effect
Fogarty arterial embolectomy

FAF
fatty acid free
fibroblast-activating factor

FAGA full-term appropriate for gestational age

FAHI functional assessment of human immunodeficiency

FAI
first aid instruction

functional aerobic impairment

functional assessment inventory

FAIDS feline AIDS

FAJ fused apophyseal joints

FAL

femoral arterial line

functional and anatomic loading

FALP fluoroscopic-assisted lumbar puncture

FALS familial amyotrophic lateral sclerosis

FAM functional assessment measure

FAMA fluorescent antimembrane antibody (test)

fam doc family doctor

FAME

fast acquisition multiple excitation

finger-assisted malar elevation

fam hist family history (*See also* FHx)

FAMM

facial artery musculomucosal

familial atypical multiple melanoma

FAMMM familial atypical multiple-mole melanoma (syndrome)

fam per par familial periodic paralysis

fam phys family physician

FANA fluorescent antinuclear antibody (assay)

FANCAP fluids, aeration, nutrition, communication, activity, and pain (nursing)

FANCAS fluids, aeration, nutrition, communication, activity, and stimulation (nursing)

FANG fluorescent angiography

FANSS&M fundus anterior, normal size and shape, and mobile

FAP

familial adenomatous polyposis

femoral artery pressure

fibrillating action potential

fixed action pattern

FAQ

Family Attitudes Questionnaire

frequently asked question(s)

FAR flight aptitude rating

FARS Fatal Accident Reporting System

FAS

femoral access stabilization

fetal alcohol syndrome

fluorescent actin staining

fasc

fascicle

fasciculation

fasciculus

FASE fast asymmetric spin echo

FASIAR follicle aspiration, sperm injection, and assisted rupture

FASS foot and ankle severity scale

FAST

fetal acoustic stimulation testing

Filtered Audiometer Speech Test

flow-assisted short-term (balloon catheter)

Flowers Auditory Screening Test

fluorescent allergosorbent test

fluorescent antibody staining technique

focused abdominal sonography for trauma

Fourier-acquired steady-state technique

Frenchay Aphasia Screening Test

Functional Assessment Staging

FAT

female athlete triad

Fetal Activity Test

F

FAT *(continued)*
  fluorescent antibody technique
  food awareness training
  function, appearance, time
FATS
  face and thigh squeeze
    (position for bag mask
    ventilation)
  fast adiabatic trajectory in
    steady state
FATSA Flowers Auditory Test
  of Selective Attention
FAV
  facioauriculovertebral
  floppy aortic valve
FAZ foveal avascular zone
FB
  factor B
  feedback
  fingerbreadth
  flexible bronchoscope
  foreign body
F/B
  followed by
  forward/backward
  forward bending
f-b face-bow
FBA fecal bile acid
FBC functional bactericidal
  concentration
FBCOD foreign body of the
  cornea, oculus dexter (right
  eye)
FBCOS foreign body of the
  cornea, oculus sinister (left
  eye)
FBD
  familial British dementia
  functional bowel disorder
FBDSI Functional Bowel
  Disorder Severity Index
FBEP Fort Bragg evaluation
  project
FBF forearm blood flow
FBG
  fasting blood glucose
  foreign body-type granuloma
FBH familial benign
  hypercalcemia

FBHH familial benign
  hypocalciuric hypercalcemia
FBI
  fat-blood interface
  flossing, brushing, and
    irrigation
  food-borne illness
  full bony impaction
FBL
  fecal blood loss
  follicular basal lamina
FBM
  fetal bone marrow
  fetal breathing movement
  foreign body, metallic
FBP
  femoral blood pressure
  fibrin/fibrinogen breakdown
    product
FBR fresh-blood reaction [Ger.
  Frischblut]
FBS
  failed back syndrome
  fasting blood glucose
  fasting blood sugar
  feedback signal
  feedback system
  foreign body sensation (eye)
FBU fingers below umbilicus
  (measurement) *(See also* F↓U)
FBV fiber bundle volume
FBW fasting blood work
FC
  family conference
  fasciculus cuneatus
  fast component (of neuron)
  febrile convulsion
  fecal coli (broth)
  feline conjunctivitis
  female child
  fever, chills
  fibrocyte
  finger clubbing
  finger counting
  flexion contracture
  flow compensation
  flow cytometry
  foam cuffed (tracheal or
    endotracheal tube)
  Foley catheter

follows commands
free cholesterol
frontal cortex
functional capacity
functional class

F/C
facilitated communication
fever and chills

F&C
flare and cell
foam and condom

Fc
centroid frequency
fragment, crystallizable (of immunoglobulin)

Fc′ fragment crystallized in minute quantities (immunoglobulin)

fc footcandle

FCA
Federal False Claims Act
fracture, complete, angulated
Freund complete adjuvant

FCBD fibrocystic breast disease

FCC
familial colon cancer
family centered care
femoral cerebral catheter
fracture complete and compound
fracture compound and comminuted

fcc face-centered-cubic

FCCC fracture complete, compound, and comminuted

FCCL follicular center cell lymphoma

FCCU family centered care unit

FCD
fecal containment device
feces collection device
fibrocystic disease
final consonant deletion
fracture complete and deviated

FCE functional capacity evaluation

FCF
fetal cardiac frequency
fibroblast chemotactic factor

FCG fifth cusp groove

FCH, FCHL
familial combined hyperlipidemia
fibrosing cholestatic hepatitis

FCI
fixed cell immunofluorescence
food-chemical intolerance

FCIS Flint Colon Injury Scale

FCL fibular collateral ligament

fcly face lying (position)

FCM
fetal cardiac motion
flow cytometry

FCMC family-centered maternity care

FCMD Fukuyama congenital muscular dystrophy

FCMN family-centered maternity nursing

F/C/N/V fever, cough, nausea, and vomiting

FCOD focal cementoosseous dysplasia

FCOU finger count, both eyes

FCP
fasting chemistry profile
final common pathway
flow cytometric platelet
formocresol pulpotomy
Functional Communication Profile (of aphasic adults)
functional conduction period

FCPD fibrocalculous pancreatic diabetes

FCR flexor carpi radialis (muscle)

FCRB flexor carpi radialis brevis (muscle)

FCRT
fetal cardiac reactivity test
focal cranial radiation therapy

FCS
faciocutaneoskeletal
fecal containment system
feedback control system

119

FCS *(continued)*
fever, chills, and sweating
fluorescence correlation spectroscopy
foot compartment syndrome
full cervical spine

FCSNVD fever, chills, sweating, nausea, vomiting, and diarrhea

FCSW female commercial sex worker

FCT
fluorescein clearance test
food composition table

FCU flexor carpi ulnaris (muscle)

FCVD fracture complete and varus deformity

FCx frontal cortex

FCXM flow cytometry crossmatch

FD
failure to descend
familial dysautonomia
fan douche
fatal dose
feeding disorder
fetal demise
fetal distress
fibrous dysplasia
field desorption
fixed and dilated
fluorescence depolarization
focal distance
Folin-Denis (assay)
foot drape
forceps delivery
freedom from distractibility
free drain
freeze-dried
frequency deviation
full denture
fully dilated

F&D fixed and dilated

F/D fracture-dislocation (*See also* Fx-dis)

FD$_{50}$ median fatal dose

Fd
animo-terminal portion of heavy chain of immunoglobulin
fundus

FDA
Frenchay Dysarthria Assessment
right frontal anterior (position of fetus) [L. *frontodextroanterior*]

FDB
first-degree burn
flexor digitorum brevis (muscle)

FDBL fecal daily blood loss

FDC
flexor digitorum communis (muscle)
follicular dendritic cell

FDCT Franck Drawing Completion Test

FDDB freeze-dried demineralized bone

FDE
female day equivalent
final drug evaluation
fixed drug eruption

FDF
fast death factor
further differentiated fibroblast

FDFG free dermal-fat graft

FDFQ Food/Drink Frequency Questionnaire

FDG
feeding
fluorodeoxyglucose

FDI
Facial Disability Index
first digital interosseous (muscle)
first dorsal interosseus
food-drug interaction
frequency domain imaging (ultrasound)
frequency-duration index
Functional Disability Index

FDICT frequency-difference interferential current therapy

FDIP Facial Disability Index Physical

FDIU fetal death in utero

FDL flexor digitorum longus (muscle)

FDLMP first day of last menstrual period

FDM
fetus of diabetic mother
fibrous dysplasia of the mandible
flexor digiti minimi (muscle)
flexor digiti quinti (muscle)

FDMA first dorsal metatarsal artery

FDP
factitious disorder by proxy
fibrin/fibrinogen degradation products
fixed-dose procedure
flexor digitorum profundus (muscle)
right frontal posterior (position of fetus) [L. *frontodextroposterior*]

FDPCA fixed-dose patient-controlled analgesia

FD-PET fluorodopa-positron emission tomography

FDQB flexor digiti quinti brevis (muscle)

FDR
first-dose reaction
fractional disappearance rate
frequency dependence of resistance

FDS
for duration of stay
fiberduodenoscope
flexor digitorum sublimis
flexor digitorum superficialis

FDT right frontal transverse (position of fetus) [L. *frontodextrotransversa*]

FDTVMP Frostig Developmental Test of Visual Motor Perception

FDTVP Frostig Developmental Test of Visual Perception

FDZ fetal danger zone

FE
fatty ester
fecal emesis
fetal erythroblastosis
fluid extract
fluorescing erythrocyte
forced expiratory

Fe iron [L. *ferrum*]

FEAST feeding education and support team

feb febrile

FEBP fetal estrogen-binding protein

FEC
forced expiratory capacity
free erythrocyte coproporphyrin
Friend erythroleukemia cell

FECO$_2$, F$_{ECO2}$ fractional concentration of carbon dioxide in expired gas

FECV functional extracellular (fluid) volume

FED fish eye disease

FeD, Fe def iron (ferrum) deficiency

FEE forced equilibrating expiration

FEEG fetal electroencephalogram

FEER field-echo sequence with even-echo rephasing

FEES
fiberoptic endoscopic evaluation of swallowing
flexible endoscopic evaluation of swallowing

FEF
Family Evaluation Form
forced expiratory flow
frontal eye field

FEFmax maximal forced expiratory flow

FEFV forced expiratory flow volume

FEKG fetal electrocardiogram

FEM
femoral
femur

121

FEM *(continued)*
    finite element method
    fluid-electrolyte malnutrition
fem feminine
FEM-FEM femoral-femoral
    (bypass)
FEM-POP femoral-popliteal
    (bypass)
FEM-TIB femoral-tibial (bypass)
FEN fluids, electrolytes,
    nutrition
FENa fractional excretion of
    sodium
FEN-PHEN fenfluramine and
    phentemine
FENS field-electrical neural
    stimulation
F_{EO2} fractional concentration of
    oxygen in expired gas
FEP
    free erythrocyte porphyrin
    free erythrocyte protoporphyrin
    functional exercise program
FEPB functional electronic
    peroneal brace
FER
    flexion, extension, and
      rotation
    fractional esterification rate
    frozen embryo replacement
FERG focal electroretinogram
fert
    fertility
    fertilize
FES
    fat embolism syndrome
    flame emission spectroscopy
    forced expiratory spirogram
    functional electrical
      stimulation
FESE flexible endoscopic
    swallowing examination
FESEM field emission scanning
    electron microscopy
$FeSO_4$ ferrous sulfate
FESS functional endoscopic
    sinus surgery
FET
    field-effect transistor
    finger extension test

    Fisher exact test
    fixed erythrocyte turnover
    forced expiratory time
FETE Far Eastern tick-borne
    encephalitis
FETENDO fetal endoscopic
FETI fluorescence energy
    transfer immunoassay
Fe/TIBC iron/total iron-binding
    capacity
FETs forced expiratory time in
    seconds
FEU fibrinogen equivalent unit
FEUO for external use only
Fe-UR iron in urine
FEV-1, FEV_1 forced expiratory
    volume at one second
FEV_1:FVC forced expiratory
    volume in one second to
    forced vital capacity ratio
FEV:FVC forced expiratory
    volume timed to forced vital
    capacity ratio
FEV_t forced expiratory volume
    timed
FF
    fat free
    father factor
    fear of failure
    fecal frequency
    femorofemoral
    fertility factor
    fibrillation-flutter
    fields of Forel
    filtration fraction
    fine fiber
    fine fraction
    finger flexion
    fixation fluid
    flatfoot
    fluorescent focus
    follicular fluid
    force fluids
    forward flexion
    free fraction
    fresh frozen
    fundus firm
    further flexion
    second finest degree of
      abrasive particles

F/F face to face
F&F
  filiform (bougie) and follower
  fixes and follows
fF
  ultrafine fiber
  ultrafine fraction
ff following
f→f finger-to-finger (*See also* FTF)
FFA
  free fatty acid
  fundus fluorescein angiogram
FFB
  fast feedback
  flexible fiberoptic bronchoscopy
FFC
  fixed flexion contracture
  free from chlorine
FFCS forearm flexion control strap
FFD
  fat-free diet
  focal film distance
FFDCA Federal Food, Drug, and Cosmetic Act
FFDM
  free from distant metastases
  full field digital mammography
FFDW fat-free dry weight
FFE
  fast-field echo
  fecal fat excretion
  flexible fiberoptic endoscope
  free flow electrophoresis
FFEM freeze fracture electron microscopy
FFF
  field-flow fractionation
  finest degree of abrasive particles
  flicker fusion frequency (test)
  fuzzy functional form (protein)
FFG free fat graft
FFI
  fatal familial insomnia

  Foot Function Index
  free from infection
  fundamental frequency indicator
FFIT fluorescent focus inhibition test
FFL fetal foot length
FFM
  fat-free (body) mass
  five-finger movement
  freedom from metastases
FFP
  freedom from progression
  fresh frozen plasma
FFPB flexible fiberoptic bronchoscopy with protected brush
FFPE formalin-fixed paraffin-embedded
FFR
  fixed frequency response
  fractional flow reserve
  freedom from relapse
  frequency-following response
FFROM full, free range of motion
FFr-TMS fast-frequency repetitive transcranial magnetic stimulation
FFS
  failure-free survival
  five-factor score
  flexible fiberoptic sigmoidoscopy
FFT
  flicker fusion test
  flicker fusion threshold
  free-floating thrombus
FFTP first full-term pregnancy
FFU
  femur-fibula-ulna (syndrome)
  focus-forming unit
FF1/U fundus firm 1 cm above umbilicus
FF2/U fundus firm 2 cm above umbilicus
FFU/1 fundus firm 1 cm below umbilicus

FFU/2 fundus firm 2 cm below umbilicus
FF@u fundus firm at umbilicus
FFW fat-free weight
FFWC fractional free-water clearance
FFWW fat-free wet weight
FG
    fasciculus gracilis
    fast-glycolytic (muscle fiber)
    fast green
    Feeley-Gorman (agar)
    fibrin glue
    field gain
fg femtogram
FGC
    familial gigantiform cementoma
    fibrinogen gel chromatography
    full gold crown
FGD
    familial glucocorticoid deficiency
    fatal granulomatous disease
FGF fibroblast growth factor
FGFR, FGF-R fibroblast growth factor receptor
FGG free gingival groove
FGL fasting gastrin level
FGLU fasting glucose
FGM
    female genital mutilation
    focal glomerulonephritis
FGR fetal growth restriction
FGS
    Facial Grading System
    focal glomerular sclerosis
FGT
    female genital tract
    fluorescent gonorrhea test
FH
    facial hemihyperplasia
    familial hypercholesterolemia
    fasting hyperbilirubinemia
    favorable histology
    femoral hypoplasia
    fetal head
    fetal heart
    Ficoll-Hypaque (technique)
    floating hospital

    follicular hyperplasia
    Frankfort horizontal (plane of skull)
    fundal height
FHA
    familial hypoplastic anemia
    filamentous hemagglutinin
    functional hypothalamic amenorrhea
FHB flexor hallucis brevis (muscle)
FHBL familial hypobetalipoproteinemia
FHC
    familial hypertrophic cardiomyopathy
    family health center
    Ficoll-Hypaque centrifugation
    Fuchs heterochromic cyclitis
FHD family history of diabetes
FHF
    familial Hibernian fever
    fetal heart frequency
    fulminant hepatic failure
FHH fetal heart heard
FHI frontal horn index
FHL
    familial hemophagocytic lymphohistiocytosis
    femoral head line
    flexor hallucis longus (muscle)
    focal hypoechoic lesion
    functional hearing loss
FHLDL familial hypercholesterolemia, low-density lipoprotein
FHM fetal heart motion
FHN family history negative
FHNH fetal heart not heard
FHP family history positive
FHR
    familial hypophosphatemic rickets
    fetal heart rate
    fetal heart rhythm
FHRB fetal heart rate baseline
FHR-NST fetal heart rate nonstress test

FHRV fetal heart rate variability

FHS

fetal heart sound

fetal hydantoin syndrome

Floating-Harbor syndrome

FHT fetal heart tone

FHx family history (*See also* fam hist)

FI

fasciculus interfascicularis

fixateur interne

fixed interval (schedule)

flame ionization

forced inspiration

frontoiliacus

functional inquiry

Functional Integration (test)

fundamental imaging

fungal infection

fusion inhibitor

FIA

feline infectious anemia

fluorescent immunoassay

Freund incomplete adjuvant

FIB

fibrillation

fibrin

fibrinogen

fibrositis

fibula

FIC

forced inspiratory capacity

fractional inhibitory concentration

functional inhibitory concentration

FICO$_2$, FiCO$_2$ fraction of inspired carbon dioxide

FID

father in delivery

flame ionization detector

free induction decay

fungal immunodiffusion

FIDD fetal iodine deficiency disorder

FIF

feedback inhibition factor

forced inspiratory flow

formaldehyde-induced fluorescence

Functional Intact Fibrinogen (test)

fig. figure

FIGE Field inversion gel electrophoresis

FIGLU formiminoglutamic acid (test)

FIGO International Federation of Gynecology and Obstetrics

FIGO I carcinoma of vaginal wall

FIGO II carcinoma of the subvaginal tissue without involving pelvic wall

FIGO III endometrial carcinoma extending outside the uterus but not outside the pelvis

FIGO IV endometrial carcinoma extending outside the true pelvis or involving bladder and rectum

FIGO IVa endometrial carcinoma spreading to adjacent organs

FIGO IVb endometrial carcinoma spreading to distant organs

FIH

familial isolated hypoparathyroidism

fat-induced hyperglycemia

FIM

field ion microscopy

functional independence measure

FIN

fine intestinal needle

flexible intramedullary nail

FIND follow up intervention for normal development

FIO$_2$, FI$_{O2}$, FiO2, FiO$_2$ fraction of inspired oxygen

FIPH full scan with interpolation projection

FIPT periarteriolar transudate

FIQ
Fibromyalgia Impact Questionnaire
full scale intelligence quotient

FIR
far infrared
fold increase in resistance

FIRDA frontal intermittent rhythmic delta activity

FIRI fasting insulin resistance index

FIS
fiberoptic injection sclerotherapy
forced inspiratory spirogram

FISC Facial Impairment Scales for Children

FISCA Functional Impairment Scale for Children and Adolescents

FISH fluorescent in situ hybridization

FISP fast imaging with steady-state precession

FISS Flint Infant Security Scale

FIT
Flanagan Industrial Test
Fracture Intervention Trial
fusion-inferred threshold (test)

FITT frequency, intensity, time, and type (exercise)

FIUO for internal use only

FIV forced inspiratory volume

FIV₁ forced inspiratory volume in one second

FIVC forced inspiratory vital capacity

F-J Fisher-John (melting point method)

FJB facet joint block

FJD facet joint disease

FJP familial juvenile polyposis

FJROM full joint range of motion

FJS finger joint size

FJV first jejunal vein

FK
feline kidney
functioning kasai (Belgian Congo anemia)

FKA formally known as

FKE full knee extension

FL
fatty liver
feline leukemia
femur length
fetal length
fibers of Luschka
flow limitation
fluorescein
follicular lymphoma
frontal lobe
full liquids (diet)
functional length

fL femtoliter

fl
flank
flexible
flutter

FLA
fluorescent-labeled antibody
free-living ameba
left frontal anterior (position of fetus) [L. *frontolaeva anterior*]

FL:AC femur length to abdominal circumference ratio

flac flaccid

FLACC face, legs, activity, cry, consolability

FLAIR fluid attenuated inversion recovery

FLASH fast low-angle shot

FLB
four-layer bandage
funny-looking beat (heart)

FLC Friend leukemia cell

FLCOD florid local cementoosseous dysplasia

FLD
fatty liver disease
fibrotic lung disease
fluid
full lower denture (*See also* /F)

fld field

fld ext fluid extract

fl dr fluid dram

fld rest. fluid restriction

fl drs fluff dressing

FLE frontal lobe epilepsy
flex.
  flexion
  flexor
flex sig flexible sigmoidoscopy
FLGA full-term, large for gestational age
FLIC Functional Living Index-Cancer
FLIE Functional Living Index-Emesis
FLM
  fasciculus longitudinalis medialis
  fetal lung maturity
floc flocculation
flor. flowers (mineral substance in powdery state after sublimation) [L. *flores*]
fl oz fluid ounce
FLP
  fasting lipid profile
  Functional Limitation Profile
  left frontal posterior (position of fetus) [L. *frontolaeva posterior*]
FLPD flashlamp pulsed dye laser
FLR funny-looking rash
FLS
  fatty liver syndrome
  flashing lights and/or scotoma
  flow-limiting segment
  Functional Life Scale
FLSP fluorescein-labeled serum protein
FLT left frontal transverse (position of fetus) [L. *frontolaeva transversa*]
FLTA Fullerton Language Test for Adolescents
FLTAC Fisher-Logemann Test of Articulation Competence
flu influenza
flu A influenza A
fluores fluorescence
fluoro fluoroscopy
FLUP front-loading ultrasound probe

fl up flareup
FM
  face mask
  feedback mechanism
  fetal movement
  fibromuscular
  fibromyalgia
  filtered mass
  fine motor
  flowmeter
  fluid movement
  fluorescent microscopy
  foramen magnum
  forensic medicine
  formerly married
  foster mother
  frequency modulation
  Friend-Moloney (antigen)
  functional movement
F&M firm and midline (uterus)
Fm fermium
fm femtometer
FMA Frankfort mandibular (plane) angle
FMAC fetal movement acceleration test
FMAIT fetomaternal alloimmune thrombocytopenia
FMAP feeding mean arterial pressure
FMB full maternal behavior
FMC
  fetal movement count
  focal macular choroidopathy
FMD
  family medical doctor (*See also* fam doc)
  fibromuscular dysplasia
  foot-and-mouth disease
  foramen magnum decompression
  frontometaphyseal dysplasia
FME full-mouth extraction
FMF
  familial Mediterranean fever
  fetal movement felt
  flow microfluorometry
  forced midexpiratory flow

127

FMG
    fibrin matrix gel
    fine mesh gauze
FMH
    familial hemiplegic migraine
    family medical history
    fetomaternal hemorrhage
    first metatarsal head
FMI
    fixed mandibular implant
    Foods and Moods Inventory
FMIA Frankfort mandibular
    incisor angle
FMIV forced mandatory
    intermittent ventilation
FML flail mitral leaflet
FMLA Family and Medical
    Leave Act of 1993
FMN frontomaxillonasal (suture)
fmol femtomole
fmol/mg femtomole per
    milligram
FMP
    fasting metabolic panel
    first menstrual period
    functional maintenance
    program
FMPA full-mouth periapicals
FMPSPGR fast multiplanar
    spoiled gradient-recalled
    (imaging)
FMR
    fetal movement record
    focused medical review
    Friend-Moloney-Rauscher
    (antigen)
fMRA functional magnetic
    resonance angiography
FMRD full-mouth restorative
    dentistry
fMRI functional magnetic
    resonance imaging
FMRP fragile X mental
    retardation protein
FMS
    fat-mobilizing substance
    fatty meal sonogram
    fibromyalgia syndrome
    full-mouth series (dental x-ray
    films)

FMSTB Frostig Movement
    Skills Test Battery
FMT
    floating mass transducer
    functional muscle test
FMU first morning urine
FMV
    floppy mitral valve
    flow-mediated vasodilation
FN
    facial nerve
    false negative (*See also* Fneg)
    fastigial nucleus
    febrile neutropenia
    femoral neck
    flight nurse
F→N finger-to-nose
    (coordination test) (*See also*
    FTN)
F/N fluids and nutrition
FNA
    fine-needle aspiration
    Functional Needs Assessment
FNAB fine-needle aspiration
    biopsy
FNAC fine-needle aspiration
    cytology
FNB femoral nerve block
FNCJ fine-needle catheter
    jejunostomy
FND
    focal neurological deficit
    frontonasal dysplasia
    functional neck dissection
Fneg false negative (*See also*
    FN)
FNF
    false-negative fraction
    femoral neck fracture
FNHL follicular non-Hodgkin
    lymphoma
FNI facial nerve injury
FNR false-negative rate
FNS functional neuromuscular
    stimulation
F/NS fever and night sweats
FNSD face near straight down
    (infant sleep position)
FNTC, FNTHC fine-needle
    transhepatic cholangiogram

FO
  fiberoptic
  focus out
  foot orthosis
  foramen ovale
  foreign object
  frontooccipital (fetal position)
Fo
  fomentation
  phonation
FOAM fluorescence overlay antigen mapping
FOAR faciooculoacousticorenal (syndrome)
FOAVF failure of all vital forces
FOB
  father of baby
  fecal occult blood
  feet out of bed
  fiberoptic bronchoscope
  foot of bed
  foreign object/body
FOBT fecal occult blood test
FOC
  father of child
  frequency of contact (scale)
  frontooccipital circumference
FOCALCROS focal contralateral routing of signals
FOD
  fixing right eye
  focus object distance
  free of disease
FOEB feet over edge of bed
FOG full-on gain
FOI flight of ideas
FOIA Freedom of Information Act
FOID fear of impending doom
FOL
  fiberoptic laryngoscopy
  fiberoptic light
fol following
FOM
  figure of merit (measure of diagnostic value per radionuclide radiation dose)
  floor of mouth

FONAR field focused nuclear magnetic resonance
FONSI finding of no significant impact
FOOB fell out of bed
FOOSH fall on outstretched hand
FOP
  fibrodysplasia ossificans progressiva
  forensic pathology
FOPS fiberoptic proctosigmoidoscopy
FO-PT fiberoptic phototherapy
FOR forensic
for. foreign
form. formula
FOS
  fiberoptic sigmoidoscope
  fissura orbitalis superior
  fixing left eye
  full of stool
FOSQ Functional Outcomes of Sleep Questionnaire
FOT
  Finger Oscillation Test
  forced oscillation technique
  form of thought
  frontal outflow tract
found. foundation
FOUR full outline of unresponsiveness (eye, motor, brainstem, respiratory functions in trauma)
four Rs remove, replace, reinoculate, repair
FOV field of view
FOVI field of vision intact
FOW fenestration of oval window
FOZR front optic zone radius
FP
  fall precautions
  false-positive
  familial porencephaly
  family planning
  filling pressure
  filter paper
  fixation protein

FP *(continued)*
  fluid pressure
  food poisoning
  foot process
  forearm pronated
  freezing point
  frontoparietal
  frontopolar
  frozen plasma
  full period
  fundal pressure
  fusion point
F:P
  fluid-plasma ratio
  fluorescein to protein ratio
Fp frontal polar electrode
  placement in
  electroencephalography
FPA
  filter paper activity
  foot-progression angle
  frontopolar artery
fpa far point of accommodation
FPAA female pattern
  androgenetic alopecia
FPAL full-term (deliveries),
  premature (deliveries),
  abortion(s), living (children)
FPB
  femoral-popliteal bypass
  flexor pollicis brevis (muscle)
FPC
  familial polyposis coli
  family planning clinic
  fish protein concentrate
  forced pair copulation
  frozen packed cells
FPD
  fetopelvic disproportion
  fixed partial denture
  flame photometric detector
FPDVP Frostig Program for the
  Development of Visual
  Perception
FPE first-pass effect
F-18-PET fluoride ion positron
  emission tomography
FPF false-positive fraction
FPG
  fasting plasma glucose

  fluorescence plus Giemsa
  (stain)
FPHx family psychiatric history
FPI femoral pulsatility index
FPIA
  fluorescence polarization
  immunoassay
  fluorescence-polarization
  immunoassay
FPL
  fasting plasma lipid
  flexor pollicis longus (muscle)
FPM
  filter paper microscopic (test)
  first-pass metabolism
  full passive movements
fpm foot per minute
FPMA first plantar metatarsal
  artery
FPN ferric chloride, perchloric
  acid, and nitric acid
  (solution)
FPNA first-pass nuclear
  angiocardiography
FPO
  faciopalatoosseous
  freezing point osmometer
FPOR follicle puncture for
  oocyte retrieval
FPP free portal pressure
FPR
  facilitated positional release
  fastigial pressor response
  fluorescence photobleaching
  recovery
  fractional proximal resorption
  Functional Performance
  Record
FPRA first-pass radionuclide
  angiogram
fps
  foot per second
  foot-pound-second (system,
  unit)
  frame per second
FPU
  family participation unit
  fetoplacental unit
FPVB femoral-popliteal vein
  bypass

FR
> failure rate (contraception)
> Federal Register
> feedback regulation
> first responder
> fixed ratio
> flocculation reaction
> flow rate
> fluid restriction
> fluid retention
> fractional reabsorption
> free radical
> frequency of respiration
> frequent relapses
> full range
> functional reach
> functional residual (capacity) reticular formation [L. *formatio reticularis*]

F&R force and rhythm (of pulse)
F/R fire/rescue
Fr
> francium
> franklin (unit charge)

FRA
> fall risk assessment
> fluorescent rabies antibody

fra
> fragile gene
> fragile site (chromosome in cytogenetics)

frag fragment
FRAP
> family risk assessment program
> fluorescence recovery after photobleaching

FRAST Free Running Asthma Test
FRAT free radical assay technique
FRAX, fra(X) fragile X (chromosome, gene, syndrome)
FRAXA X-linked first site of fragility
FRAXE X-linked second site of fragility
FRBS fast red B salt

FRC
> feedback reduction circuit
> functional residual capacity (of lungs)

FRD flexion-rotation-drawer (test)
frem. vocal fremitus [L. *fremitus vocalis*]
freq frequency (*See also* F)
FRF fasciculus retroflexus
FRG Functional Related Groups
FRHS fast-repeating high sequence
Fried Friedman (test for pregnancy)
FRN fully resonant nucleus
FRNT focus-reduction neutralization test
FROA full range of affect
FROM full range of motion
FROMAJE functioning, reasoning, orientation, memory, arithmetic, judgment, and emotion (mental status evaluation)
FROS front routing of signal
FRP
> follicle regulatory protein
> functional refractory period

FRPS functional resting position splint
FR r friction rub
FRS
> first rank symptom
> flexed, rotated, sidebent
> fluid retention syndrome

FRSL flexed, rotated, sidebent left
FRSR flexed, rotated, sidebent right
FRV functional residual volume
FS
> factor of safety
> fetoscope
> fibrosarcoma
> fibrous synovium
> field stimulation
> fine structure
> fingerstick

131

FS *(continued)*
  fire setter (psychology)
  flexible sigmoidoscopy
  food service
  forearm supination
  Fourier series
  fractional shortening
  fracture, simple
  fracture site
  Friesinger score
  frozen section
  full-scale (IQ test)
  full strength
  functional shortening
  functional status
  function study
  (human) foreskin (cells)
F/S female, spayed (animal)
F&S full and soft (diet)
FSA frozen section assay
FSAD female sexual arousal
  disorder
FSB
  fetal scalp blood
  full spine board
FSBG
  fingerstick blood gas
  fingerstick blood glucose
FSBM full-strength breast milk
FSBP finger systolic blood
  pressure
FSBS fingerstick blood sugar
FSBT Fowler single breath test
FSC
  Fatigue Symptom Checklist
  flexible sigmoidoscopy
  fracture simple and
  comminuted
  fracture simple and complete
FSCC fracture simple complete
  and comminuted
FSD
  face-straight-down (infant
  sleep position)
  female sexual dysfunction
  Fletcher-Suit-Delclos
  (applicator)
  focus-skin distance
  fracture simple and depressed
  full-scale deflection

FSE
  fast spin echo
  fetal scalp electrode
FSG
  fasting serum glucose
  focal segmental
  glomerulosclerosis
FSGA full-term, small for
  gestational age
FSGO floating spherical
  gaussian orbital
FSH
  facioscapulohumeral
  follicle-stimulating hormone
FSH/LR-RH follicle-stimulating
  hormone and luteinizing
  hormone-releasing hormone
FSHMD facioscapulohumeral
  muscular dystrophy
FSH-RF follicle-stimulating
  hormone-releasing factor
FSH-RH follicle-stimulating
  hormone-releasing hormone
FSI
  foam stability index
  Functional Status Index
FSIQ Full-Scale Intelligence
  Quotient
FSL
  fasting serum level
  fixed slit lamp
FSM functional status measure
F-SM/C fungus, smear, and
  culture
FSO for screws only (prosthetic
  cups)
FS$_p$O$_2$ fetal arterial oxygen
  saturation
FSP
  familial spastic paraplegia
  fibrinogen split product
  fine suspended particulate
F-SP special form (taxonomy)
  [L. *forma specialis*]
FSQ Functional Status
  Questionnaire
FSR
  film screen radiography

fractionated stereotactic
radiosurgery
fusiform skin revision

FSRRL flexion, sidebent right,
rotated left

FSRT fractionated stereotactic
radiotherapy

FSS

Familiar Sensory Stimulation
fetal scalp sampling
French steel sound
frequency-selective saturation
full-scale score
functional systems scale

FSSE fat-suppressed spin-echo

FSU

functional spinal unit
functional subunit

FSV forward stroke volume

fsw feet of sea water

FT

false transmitter
fast twitch
feeding tube
ferromagnetic tamponade
filling time
finger tapping
fingertip
flexor tendon
fluidotherapy
followthrough (after barium
meal)
Fourier transform
free testosterone
frontotemporal
full term
function test

FT₃ free triiodothyronine

FT₄ free (unbound) thyroxine

ft foot

FTA

femorotibial angle
fluorescent titer antibody

FTA-Abs fluorescent treponemal
antibody absorption (test)

FTBD

fit to be detained
full term, born dead

FTBI fractionated total body
irradiation

FTC

fibulotalocalcaneal
frames to come (optometry)
frequency threshold curve
full to confrontation

fTCD functional transcranial
Doppler sonography

FTD

failure to descend
frontotemporal dementia
full-term delivery

FTE

failure to engraft
full-time equivalent (resident)

FTF

finger-to-finger (test) (*See also*
f→f)
free thyroxine fraction

FTFTN finger-to-finger-to-nose
(test)

FTG full-thickness graft

FTI force-time integral

FT₃I free triiodothyronine index

FT₄I free thyroxine index

FTIR Fourier transform infrared
(spectroscopy)

FTIUP full-term intrauterine
pregnancy

FTJ femorotibial joint

FTLB full-term live birth

ft·lbf foot pound-force

FTLE full-thickness local
excision

FTLFC full-term living female
child

FTLMC full-term living male
child

FTN finger-to-nose (*See also*
F→N)

FTNB full-term newborn

FTND full-term normal delivery

FTNS functional transcutaneous
nerve stimulation

FTNSD full-term, normal,
spontaneous delivery

FTO fulltime occlusion (eye
patch)

F

133

FTP
   failure to progress (in labor)
   full-term pregnancy
F:T PSA free to total prostate-specific antigen
FTR
   failed to report
   failed to respond
   force translation
   fractional turnover rate
   for the record
FTS
   feminizing testis syndrome
   fetal tobacco syndrome
   fingertips
   fissured tongue syndrome
   serum thymic factor [Fr. *facteur thymique sérique*]
FTSD full-term spontaneous delivery
FTSG full-thickness skin graft
FTSP fallopian tube sperm perfusion
FTT
   failure to thrive
   fat tolerance test
   fetal tissue transplant
   Finger-Tapping Test
   fraternal twins raised together
   fructose tolerance test
FTU fingertip unit
FTUPLD full-term uncomplicated pregnancy, labor, and delivery
FTV fetal thrombotic vasculopathy
FTW failure to wean
FTX field training exercise
FU
   finsen unit
   followup
   fractional urinalysis
   fraction unbound
F↑U fingers above umbilicus (measurement)
F↓U fingers below umbilicus (measurement)
F/U fundus at umbilicus
FUB functional uterine bleeding

FU$_{CO}$ functional uptake of carbon monoxide
FUD
   fear, uncertainty, and doubt
   full upper denture (*See also* F/)
FUDS fluorourodynamic study
FUDT forensic urine drug testing
FU/FL full upper, full lower (denture)
FUL
   federal upper limit (price list)
   functional urethral length
fulg fulguration
FU/LP full upper denture, partial lower denture
FUM fumigation
funct function(al)
FUNG-C fungus culture
FUNG-S fungus smear
FUO fever of unknown origin
FUS
   feline urologic syndrome
   first-use syndrome
   fusion
FV
   femoral vein
   flow velocity
   flow volume
   fluid volume
F(v) velocity distribution function
f/V$_t$ frequency to tidal volume
FVA Friend virus anemia
FVC
   false vocal cord
   forced vital capacity
FVE forced volume, expiratory
FVFR filled voiding flow rate
FVH
   focal vascular headache
   fulminant viral hepatitis
FVL
   femoral vein ligation
   flexible video laparoscope
   flow-volume loop
   force, velocity, length
FVOP finger venous opening pressure

FVP   Friend virus polycythemia
FVR
    forearm vascular resistance
    fractional velocity reserve
FVS   fetal varicella syndrome
FVU   first-void urine
FVWs   flow-velocity waveforms
    (umbilical artery Doppler)
FW
    fetal weight
    Folin and Wu (method)
    forced whisper
    fragment wound
F/W   followed with
Fw   F wave (fibrillatory wave,
    flutter wave)
FWB
    full weightbearing
    functional well-being
FWCA   functional work capacity
    assessment
FWD   fairly well developed
FWHM   full width (of
    photopeak measured at) half
    maximal (count) (tomography)
FWR
    Felix-Weil reaction
    Folin-Wu reaction
FWS   fetal warfarin syndrome
FWW   front wheel walker

FX
    factor X
    fluoroscopy
    fornix
    fractional (composition of gas
      in gas phase) (*See also* F)
Fx   fracture
Fx BB   fracture of both bones
Fx-dis   fracture-dislocation (*See
    also* F/D)
FXN   function
FY
    fiscal year
    full year
FYA   Duffy antigen A positive
    phenotype
FYAN   Duffy antigen A
    negative phenotype
FYB   Duffy antigen B positive
    phenotype
FYBN   Duffy antigen B
    negative phenotype
FYC   facultative yeast carrier
FYI   for your information
FZ
    focal zone
    frontozygomatic
Fz   frontal midline placement of
    electrodes in
    electroencephalography

G

force (pull of gravity)
gap (in cell cycle)
gas
gauss
general factor (single variance common to different intelligence tests)
Giemsa (banding stain)
giga-
glabella
glycine (*See also* Gly)
gonidial (colony)
Grafenberg spot
Gram (stain)
gravida (pregnant)
gravitational (constant)
gravity (unit)
Greek
Gross (leukemia antigen)
guanine
Newtonian constant of gravitation

G1

first pregnancy
grid 1 (in electroencephalography)
presynthetic gap (phase of cells prior to DNA synthesis)
primigravida
well differentiated tumor (TNM classification)

G2

grid 2 (in electroencephalography)
moderately differentiated tumor (TNM classification)
postsynthetic gap (phase of cells following DNA synthesis)
second pregnancy
secundigravida

G3

poorly differentiated tumor (TNM classification

tertigravida
third pregnancy

G4 undifferentiated tumor (TNM classification)

G° standard free energy

G0

gap zero (quiescent phase of cells leaving the mitotic cycle)
gravida 0, never pregnant

G− guaiac negative

G+ guaiac positive

g

acceleration due to gravity, 9.80665 m/s^2
gram

g relative centrifugal force

g% gram percent

GΩ gigaohm (one billion ohms)

G1–G6 grade 1–6 (heart murmur)

G=G grips equal and good

GA

gastric antrum
general appearance
genetic algorithm
gestational age
gingivoaxial
Golgi apparatus
granulocyte agglutination
granuloma annulare
gut-associated
gyrate atrophy

G:A globulin to albumin ratio

Ga gallium

ga gauge (of needle)

GABA gamma-aminobutyric acid

GABHS group A beta hemolytic streptococcus

GAD generalized anxiety disorder

GADS

gas atomized dispersion strengthened
gonococcal arthritis/dermatitis syndrome

137

GAF global assessment of functioning

GAHS galactorrhea amenorrhea hyperprolactinemia syndrome

GAI guided affective imagery

Gal galactose

gal gallon

G-ALB globulin-albumin

gal/min gallon per minute

GALOP gait disorder, autoantibody, late-age onset, polyneuropathy

GALS gait, arms, legs, and spine

GALT gut-associated lymphoid tissue

galv
galvanic
galvanized

GAN giant axonal neuropathy

gangl ganglion

GAP
glans approximation procedure
growth-associated protein

GAPO growth retardation, alopecia, pseudoanodontia, and optic atrophy (syndrome)

GAR
genitoanorectal (syndrome)
gonococcal antibody reaction

GARF Global Assessment of Relational Functioning

garg gargle

GARS Gait Abnormality Rating Scale

GARS-M Gait Abnormality Rating Scale Modified

GAS
galactorrhea-amenorrhea syndrome
gastric acid secretion
gene-activating sequence
general adaptation syndrome
Glasgow Assessment Schedule
group A streptococcus

GASA growth-adjusted sonographic age

Gas Anal F&T gastric analysis, free and total

gastroc gastrocnemius (muscle)

GAT
gelatin agglutination test
Gerontological Apperception Test

gav gavage

Gaw airway conductance (*See also* C_{AW})

GB
gallbladder
goofball (barbiturate pill)

GBA gingivobuccoaxial

GBD
gallbladder disease
gender behavior disorder
glassblower's disease
granulomatous bowel disease

GBEF gallbladder ejection fraction

GBF gingival blood flow

GBI
gingival bleeding index
globulin-bound insulin

GBIA Guthrie bacterial inhibition assay

GBM
glioblastoma multiforme
glomerular basement membrane

GBO gastric bacterial overgrowth

GBP gated blood pool

GBq gigabecquerel

GBR
gamma band response (audiology)
good blood return
guided bone regeneration

GBS
gallbladder series
gastric bypass surgery
glycerine-buffered saline
group B (beta-hemolytic) streptococcus
Guillain-Barré syndrome

GBSS Grey balanced saline solution

GBT gastric bleeding time

GBW generalized body weakness

GC
- gas chromatography
- gel chromatography
- geriatric care
- germinal center
- gingival curettage
- goblet cell
- Golgi complex
- goniocurettage
- gonococcal (infection)
- gonorrhea culture
- granular cast
- granular cyst
- granule cell
- group-specific component

Gc
- gigacycle
- group-specific component

GCA giant cell arteritis
g-cal gram calorie (small calorie)
GCBP gated cardiac blood pool
GCDAS Gesell Child Development Age Scale
GCE general conditioning exercise
GCF
- gingival crevicular fluid
- greatest common factor

GCFT gonococcal complement-fixation test
G-CFU granulocyte colony-forming unit
GCI
- General Cognitive Index
- gestational carbohydrate intolerance

g-cm gram-centimeter
GC-MS, GC/MS gas chromatography-mass spectrometry
GCS
- Glasgow Coma Scale
- graduated compression stockings

Gc/s gigacycle per second
G-CSF granulocyte colony-stimulating factor
GCST Gibson-Cooke sweat test

GCU gonococcal urethritis
GCV great cardiac vein
GD
- gastroduodenal
- Gaucher disease
- general diagnostics
- gestational diabetes (mellitus)
- glare disability
- gonadal dysgenesis
- gravely disabled
- Graves disease

G&D growth and development
Gd gadolinium
GDA gastroduodenal artery
GDB
- gas-density balance
- Guide Dogs for the Blind

GDC Guglielmi detachable coil
GDD glaucoma drainage device
GDF growth differentiation factor
GDH
- gonadotropic hormone
- growth and differentiation hormone (in insects)

GDID genetically determined immunodeficiency disease
g/dL grams per deciliter
GDM gestational diabetes mellitus
Gd-MRI gadolinium-enhanced magnetic resonance imaging
GDP
- gastroduodenal pylorus
- gel diffusion precipitin

GDS
- Geriatric Depression Scale
- Gesell Developmental Schedules
- Global Deterioration Scale
- gradual dosage schedule

GDSS Glasgow Dyspepsia Severity Score
GDT gel development time
GDW glass-distilled water
GE
- gainfully employed
- gastric emptying
- gastroemotional

GE *(continued)*
  gastroenteritis
  gastroenterostomy
  gastroesophageal
  gel electrophoresis
  generator of excitation
  genome equivalent
G:E granulocyte to erythroid ratio
Ge
  Gerbich red cell antigen
  germanium
GEA gastroepiploic artery
GEC
  galactose elimination capacity
  glomerular epithelial cell
GED
  General Education Development (high school equivalency)
  graduated electronic decelerator
GEF
  gastroesophageal fundoplication
  glossoepiglottic fold
GEIN gradual elongation intramedullary nailing
GEJ gastroesophageal junction
GELS gravity extension locking system
GEN
  gender
  generation
  genetics (*See also* genet)
  genital (*See also* genit)
  gradual elongation nailing
gen. genus
gen-an general anesthesia
genet
  genetic
  genetics (*See also* GEN)
gen. et sp. nov. new genus and species [L. *genus et species nova*]
genit
  genital (*See also* GEN)
  genitalia
gen. nov. new genus [L. *genus novum*]
gen proc general procedure

GEP
  gastric emptying procedure
  gastroenteropancreatic
GEPG gastroesophageal pressure gradient
GEQ generic equivalent
GER
  gastroesophageal reflux
  granular endoplasmic reticulum
GERD gastroesophageal reflux disease
geriat
  geriatric
  geriatrics
geront gerontology
GES glucose-electrolyte solution
GE SPECT gradient-echo single-photon emission computed tomography
GEST gestation
GET
  gastric emptying time
  graded (treadmill) exercise test
GET1/2, GET½ gastric emptying half-time
GETA general endotracheal anesthesia
GEU
  geriatric evaluation unit
  gestation, extrauterine
GeV gigaelectron volt
GEX gas exchange
GF
  germ-free
  glass factor (tissue culture)
  glomerular filtration
  gluten-free
  grandfather
  growth factor
  growth failure
gf gram-force
GFA global force applicator
GFCL Goldmann fundus contact lens
GFD gluten-free diet
GFFF gravitational field-flow fractionation

GFFS glycogen- and fat-free solid
GFH glucose-free Hanks (solution)
GFI
glucagon-free insulin
ground-fault interrupter
GFM good fetal movement
GFP
gel-filtered platelet
glomerular-filtered phosphate
green fluorescent protein
GFR
glomerular filtration rate
grunting, flaring, and retracting (breathing)
GFS
glaucoma filtering surgery
global focal sclerosis
GFT gradient field transform
GFTA Goldman-Fristoe Test of Articulation
G-F-W Goldman-Fristoe-Woodcock (Auditory Skills Test Battery)
GG
gamma globulin
genioglossus
guar gum
GGA ground-glass attenuation
GGCT ground-glass clotting time
GGE gradient gel electrophoresis
GGM glucose-galactose malabsorption
GGO ground-glass opacity
GGS
glands, goiter, or stiffness (of neck)
group G streptococcus
GGVB glucose-gelatin Veronal buffer
GH
genetic hemochromatosis
genetic hypertension
geniohyoid
gingival hyperplasia

glenohumeral
growth hormone
GH3 Gerovital
GHAQ General High Altitude Questionnaire
GHBSS gelatin Hanks buffered salt solution
GHD growth hormone deficiency
GHI growth hormone insufficiency
GHIH, GH-IH growth hormone-inhibiting hormone
GHJ glenohumeral joint
GHK Goldman-Hodgkin-Katz (equation)
GHL glenohumeral ligament
GHRF, GH-RF growth hormone-releasing factor
GHRH, GH-RH growth hormone-releasing hormone
GHST growth hormone stimulation test
GHT geniculohypothalamic tract
GHz gigahertz
GI
gastrointestinal
gelatin infusion (medium)
General Inquiry
Gingival Index
glomerular index
glucose intolerance
granuloma inguinale
growth inhibiting
Gi gilbert (unit of magnetomotive force)
GIA
gastrointestinal anastomosis
gastrointestinal anisakiasis
GIB
gastric ileal bypass
gastrointestinal bleeding
GIBF gastrointestinal bacterial flora
GIC
gastric interdigestive contraction
general immunocompetence

141

GICA gastrointestinal cancer-associated antigen

GID
gastrointestinal distress
gender identity disorder

GIF
gonadotropin-inhibitory factor (somatostatin)
growth hormone-inhibiting factor

GIFT
gamete intrafallopian transfer
granulocyte immunofluorescence test

GIH
gastric-inhibitory hormone
gastrointestinal hemorrhage
gastrointestinal hormone
growth hormone-inhibiting hormone

GIK glucose-insulin-potassium (solution)

GING
gingiva
gingival
gingivectomy

g-ion gram-ion

GIP
gastric inhibitory peptide
gastrointestinal polyposis
giant (cell) interstitial pneumonia (pneumonitis)
glucose insulinotropic peptide

GIRMS gas isotope ratio mass spectrometry

GITS gut-derived infectious toxic shock

GITT
gastrointestinal transit time
glucose insulin tolerance test

GITUP glansplasty and in situ tubularization of urethral plate

GIWU gastrointestinal workup

GJ
gap junction
gastric juice
gastrojejunostomy

GJT gastrojejunostomy tube

GKNa glucose-potassium-sodium

GL
gastric lavage
germline
gland
glaucoma
glomerular layer
glucagon (*See also* GN)
glycolipid
granular layer
greatest length (fetus)
gustatory lacrimation

Gl glabella

g/L grams per liter

GLA
gamma linolenic acid
gene-linkage analysis
gingivolinguoaxial
glucose-lowering agents

glau glaucoma

GLB gay, lesbian, bisexual

GLC gas-liquid chromatography

GLC/MS gas-liquid chomatography/mass spectrometry

GLD globoid leukodystrophy

GLH
germinal layer hemorrhage
giant lymph node hyperplasia

GLIIRA green light induced infrared absorption

GLIM generalized linear interactive model

GLIO
glioblastoma
glioma

GLL glabellolambda line (craniometric point)

GLN glomerulonephritis

Gln glutamine (*See also* Q)

glob.
globular
globulin

GLOC gravity induced loss of consciousness

GLOF global level of functioning

GLORIA gold-labeled optical rapid immunoassay

GLP
good laboratory practice

grid laser photocoagulation
group-living program
GLPC gas-liquid phase
chromatography
GLPP, GL-PP glucose,
postprandial
GLR
graphic level recorder
gravity lumbar reduction
GLS
gait lock splint
generalized lymphadenopathy
syndrome
GLSH glucose, lactalbumin,
serum, and hemoglobin
GLTN glomerulotubulonephritis
GLTT glucose-lactate tolerance
test
Glu glutamate (*See also* E)
gluc glucose
GLUS granulomatous lesions of
unknown significance
Glx glutaminyl and/or glutamyl
(indicates uncertainty between
Glu and Gln)
GLY glycyl
Gly glycine (*See also* G)
glyc
glyceride
glycerin
glycerite
glycerol
GM
gastric mucosa
Geiger-Müller (counter)
genetically modified
geometric mean
gingival margin
grand mal
grandmother
grand multiparity
gray matter
growth medium
g/m gallon per minute
g-m gram-meter
GMA gross motor activity
gm/cc gram per cubic
centimeter

GM-CFU granulocyte-
macrophage colony-forming
unit
GM-CSF granulocyte-macrophage
colony-stimulating factor
GMD geometric mean diameter
GMFCS Gross Motor Function
Classification System (cerebral
palsy level I–V)
GML glabellomeatal line
g/mL gram per milliliter
GMN gradient moment nulling
GMO genetically modified
organism
g-mol gram-molecule
GMR
gallop, murmur, or rub
gradient moment reduction
(rephasing)
GMS
galvanic muscle stimulation
Grocott-Gomori methenamine
silver stain
GMSPS Glasgow Meningococcal
Septicemia Prognostic Score
GMT
geometric mean (antibody)
titer
gingival margin trimmer
Greenwich Mean Time
GMW gram molecular weight
GN
ganglioneuroma
gaze nystagmus
glomerulonephritis
glucagon (*See also* GL)
gnotobiote
gram-negative
G:N
glucose to nitrogen (ratio in
urine)
glucose to nitrogen (ratio in
water)
Gn
gnathion
gonadotropin
GNB
ganglioneuroblastoma

GNB *(continued)*
  gram-negative bacillus
  gram-negative bacteremia
GNC gram-negative cocci
GND gram-negative diplococcus
gnd ground
GNID gram-negative intracellular
  diplococcus
GNR gram-negative rod
GNRF guanine nucleotide-
  releasing factor
GnRF gonadotropin-releasing
  factor
GnRH, Gn-RH gonadotropin-
  releasing hormone
GNRP guanine nucleotide
  regulatory protein
GNS gram-negative sepsis
G/NS glucose in normal saline
GO Graves ophthalmopathy
G&O gas and oxygen
Go
  Golgi
  gonion (craniometrics)
GOBI growth monitoring, oral
  rehydration, breast feeding,
  and immunization
GOE gas, oxygen, and ether
  (anesthesia)
GOL glabelloopisthion line
GON
  gonococcal ophthalmia
  neonatorum
  greater occipital neuritis
GONA glaucomatous optic
  nerve atrophy
gonio gonioscopy
GOO gastric outlet obstruction
GO-POG gonion to pogonion
  (craniometrics)
GOQ glucose oxidation quotient
GORD gastro-oesophageal reflux
  disease (United Kingdom)
GOS Glasgow Outcome Scale
  (Score)
GOT glutamic-oxaloacetic
  transaminase (aspartate
  aminotransferase)
GOT-S glutamic-oxaloacetic
  transaminase, soluble

GP
  gastroplasty
  general paralysis
  general paresis
  geometric progression
  globus pallidus
  gutta-percha
G/P gravida/para
gp
  gene product
  glycoprotein
GPA gravida, para, abortus
GPAC gram-positive anaerobic
  coccus
GPB
  glossopharyngeal breathing
  gram-positive bacillus
  gram-positive bacteremia
GPC
  gel permeation
  chromatography
  giant papillary conjunctivitis
  G-protein coupled
  gram-positive cocci
  granular progenitor cell
GPCL gas permeable contact
  lens
GPGL gamma probe guided
  lymphoscintigraphy
GPI
  general paresis of insane
  Gingival-Periodontal Index
  globus pallidus interna
GPi gram-positive identification
GPJ glossopalatal junction
Gply gingivoplasty
GPMAL gravida, para, multiple
  births, abortions, live births
GPR
  good partial response
  gram-positive rod
GPRL gamma probe
  radiolocalization
GPS gray platelet syndrome
GP-ST group A streptococcus
  direct test
GPT glutamic-pyruvic
  transaminase
GR
  gamma ray (roentgen)

gastric resection
glucose response
granulocyte
growth rate
gr
grade
graft
grain
great
GRA
gated radionuclide angiography
glucocorticoid-remediable
aldosteronism
grad.
gradient
gradually
graduate
GRAE generally regarded as
effective
gran
granulated
granule
GRAS Generally Recognized As
Safe
GRASE Generally Recognized
as Safe and Effective
GRASS gradient-recalled
acquisition in a steady state
GRBAS grade, rough, breathy,
asthenic, strained (voice
quality)
GRD gender role definition
grd ground
GRE
graded resistive exercise
gradient-recalled echo
(technique)
GRFoma growth hormone-
releasing factor tumor
GRG glycine-rich glycoprotein
GRH glucocorticoid-remediable
hyperaldosteronism
GRN
granule
green
gros coarse [L. *grossus*]
grp group
GRPS glucose-Ringer-phosphate
solution

GRS
Graphic Rating Scale
gross
GRS&MIC gross and
microscopic
GRT
gastric residence time
giant retinal tear
glandular replacement therapy
GRV gastric residual volume
GRW giant ragweed (test)
GRWR graft-to-recipient weight
ratio
gr wt gross weight
GS
gallstone
gastrocnemius (and) soleus
(muscles)
generalized seizure
gestational sac
Gleason score
glomerular sclerosis
gluteal sets
graft survival
Gram stain
grip strength
g/s gallon per second
GSA
general somatic afferent
(nerve)
group-specific antigen
GSAP greatest single allergen
present
GSB graduated spinal block
GSC
gas-solid chromatography
gravity settling culture (plate)
GSCU geriatric skilled care unit
GSD
genetically significant dose
(of mutagenic radiation)
glycogen storage disease
GSE
general somatic efferent
(nerve)
genital self-examination
gluten-sensitive enteropathy
grips strong and equal

GSH
Green-Seligson-Henry (orthopedic nail)
growth-stimulating hormone
GSI
genuine stress incontinence
Global Severity Index
GSI-BSI Global Severity Index of Brief Symptom Inventory
GSIS glucose-stimulated insulin secretion
GSL goniosynechialysis
GSM gray-scale median
GSMD gestational sac and maternal date
GSP
galvanic skin potential
generalized social phobia
glycosylated serum protein
GSPECT gated single-photon emission computed tomography
GSPN greater superficial petrosal neurectomy
GSR
galvanic skin resistance
galvanic skin response
gastrosalivary reflex
generalized Shwartzman reaction
GSRA galvanic skin response audiometry
GSRS Gastrointestinal Symptom Rating Scale
GSS
gestational sac size
gloves and socks syndrome
GSSI Global Sexual Satisfaction Index
GST
gold salt therapy
graphic stress thermography
group striction
GSW gunshot wound
GSWA gunshot wound to abdomen
GSWH gunshot wound to head
GT
gait (training)
Gamow-Teller (strength)

gastrostomy
generation time
genetic therapy
gingiva treatment
Glanzmann thrombasthenia
glucagon test
glucose tolerance
granulation tissue
greater trochanter
great toe
g/t granulation time
gt. gutta (drop)
GTC, GTCS generalized tonic-clonic seizure
GTD gestational trophoblastic disease
GTE general therapeutic exercise
GTF
gastrostomy tube feeding
glucose tolerance factor
GTH gonadotropic hormone
GTN
gestational trophoblastic neoplasm
glomerulotubulonephritis
glyceryl trinitrate (nitroglycerin)
GTO Golgi tendon organ
GTR
galvanic tetanus ratio
generalized time reflex
granulocyte turnover rate
guided tissue regeneration
GTS
Gilles de la Tourette syndrome
glucose transport system
guided trephine system
GTT
gelatin-tellurite-taurocholate (agar)
gestational transient thyrotoxicosis
gestational trophoblastic tumor
glucose tolerance test
gtt. drops [L. *guttae*]
G-tube gastrostomy tube
GTV gross tumor volume

GU
- gastric ulcer
- genitourinary
- glucose uptake
- gonococcal urethritis
- gravitational ulcer

GUD genital ulcer disease

GUI genitourinary infection

guid guidance

GULHEMP general (physique), upper (extremity), lower (extremity), hearing, eyesight, mentality, personality

GUS
- genitourinary sphincter
- genitourinary system

GV
- gastric volume
- gentian violet
- germinal vesicle
- growth velocity

GVA general visceral afferent (nerve)

GVB gelatin-Veronal buffer

GVD graft vessel disease

GVE general visceral efferent (nerve)

GVF
- Goldman visual fields
- good visual fields

GVHD, GvHD graft-versus-host disease (grade 1–4)

GVL graft-versus-leukemia (effect)

GVS gastric vertical stapling

GVTY gingivectomy

GW
- gastric wrap
- germ warfare
- gigawatt

G/W glucose in water

GWBI General Well-Being Index

GWD Guinea worm disease

GWS Gulf War syndrome

GWX guide wire exchange

GX tumor grade cannot be assessed (TNM classification)

GXP graded exercise program

GXT graded exercise test

Gy, Gy rad gray (unit of absorbed dose of ionizing radiation)

GYN gynecology

H

deflection in His bundle in electrogram (spike)
Haemophilus
Hauch (motile bacteria with flagellum)
henry (electric inductance)
heroin
histidine (*See also* His)
hydrogen
hypermetropia
hyperopia
hyperphoria
per hypodermic
region of sarcomere containing only myosin filaments [Ger. *heller* lighter]
vectorcardiography electrode (neck)

H_1 histamine receptor type 1
H specific enthalpy
H^+ hydrogen ion

h

coefficient of heat transfer
hecto-
human
negatively staining region of chromosome

hν photon
h Planck constant
H1 protium (light hydrogen)
H2 deuterium (heavy hydrogen)
H_2 histamine receptor type 2
H2O water
H2O2 hydrogen peroxide
H3 tritium

HA

hallux abductus
height age
hemadsorption (test)
hemagglutination
hemolytic anemia
hepatic artery
heterophil antibody
hospital acquired

hyperalimentation
hypermetropic astigmatism
hyperopia, absolute
H:A head-to-abdomen ratio (fetal)
Ha

absolute hypermetropia
hahnium

HAA hepatitis associated antigen
HAAb hepatitis A antibody
HAAg hepatitis A antigen
HAART highly active antiretroviral therapy
HAc acetic acid
HACE

hepatic artery chemoembolization
high-altitude cerebral edema

HACEK *Haemophilus aphrophilus, Actinobacillus actinomycetemcomitans, Cardiobacterium hominis, Eikenella corrodens,* and *Kingella kingae*
HAd hemadsorption
HADD hydroxyapatite deposition disease
HAE

hepatic artery embolization
hereditary angioneurotic edema

hAFP human alpha-fetoprotein
HAGG hyperimmune antivariola gamma globulin
HAH high-altitude headache
HAIC hepatic arterial infusional chemotherapy
HAL

hand-assisted laparoscopy
hemorrhoidal artery ligation
hepatic artery ligation
hyperalimentation
hypoplastic acute leukemia

Hal halogen
HALK hyperopic automated lamellar keratoplasty
halluc hallucination

149

HALN hand-assisted laparoscopic (radical) nephrectomy

HALNU hand-assisted laparoscopic nephroureterectomy

HALO hours after light onset

HALS hand-assisted laparoscopic surgery

HAM

hearing aid microphone

helical axis of motion

human (T-cell lymphotropic virus type I-)associated myelopathy

hams. hamstrings

HAN heroin-associated nephropathy

HANE hereditary angioneurotic edema

HANES health and nutrition examination survey

hANP human atrial natriuretic peptide

HAP

hepatic arterial phase

hospital-acquired pneumonia

HAPD home automated peritoneal dialysis

HAPE high-altitude pulmonary edema

HAPO high-altitude pulmonary oedema (British)

HAPS hepatic arterial perfusion scintigraphy

HAPTO haptoglobin

HAQ

Headache Assessment Questionnaire

(Stanford) Health Assessment Questionnaire

HAQ DI Health Assessment Questionnaire Disability Index

HAR

high-altitude retinopathy

hyperacute rejection

HARH high-altitude retinal hemorrhage

harm. harmonic

HARP harmonic phase

HARPPS heat, absence of use, redness, pain, pus, swelling (symptoms of infection)

HART hyperfractionated accelerated radiation therapy

HARTS heat-activated recoverable temporary stent

HAS

high-amplitude sucking (technique)

hospitalized attempted suicide

hyperalimentation solution

hypertensive arteriosclerosis

HASCHD

hypertensive arteriosclerotic heart disease

hypertensive atherosclerotic heart disease

HASCI head and spinal cord injury

HASCVD

hypertensive arteriosclerotic cardiovascular disease

hypertensive atherosclerotic cardiovascular disease

HASTE half-Fourier acquisition single-shot turbo spin-echo

HAT

Halstead Aphasia Test

heparin-associated thrombocytopenia

hepatic artery thrombosis

heterophil antibody titer

human African trypanosomiasis (sleeping sickness)

HATT heparin-associated thrombocytopenia and thrombosis

HATTS hemagglutination treponemal test for syphilis

HAV

hallux abductovalgus

hepatitis A virus

HAZWOPER Hazardous Waste Operations and Emergency Response

HB

heart-beating (donor)

heart block

heel to buttock
His bundle
housebound
hyoid body
HB1° first-degree heart block
HB2° second-degree heart block
HB3° third-degree heart block
Hb hemoglobin (*See also* HGB, hgb)
HbA, Hb A hemoglobin A (adult, α-chain)
HbA° hemoglobin determination
HbA$_1$ major component of adult hemoglobin
HbA$_{1c}$ glycosylated hemoglobin
HbA$_2$ minor fraction of adult hemoglobin
HBAb hepatitis B antibody
HBAg, HbAg hepatitis B antigen
HbAS heterozygosity for hemoglobin A and hemoglobin S (sickle-cell trait)
HbB hemoglobin b (chain)
HbBC hemoglobin-binding capacity
HBC hereditary breast cancer
HbC, Hb C hemoglobin C
HB$_c$Ab, HB$_{cAb}$, HBcAb hepatitis B core antibody
HB$_c$Ag, HB$_{cAg}$, HBcAg hepatitis B core antigen
Hb$_{Chesapeake}$ hemoglobin Chesapeake
HbCO carboxyhemoglobin
HbCS hemoglobin Constant Spring
HBCT helical biphasic contrast-enhanced CT
HBD
  has been drinking
  heart-beating donor
  hypophosphatemic bone disease
HbD hemoglobin D (hemoglobin delta chain)
HBE
  His bundle electrogram

hypopharyngoscopy, bronchoscopy, and esophagoscopy
HB$_e$, HBe hepatitis B e antigen
HbE hemoglobin E (ε chain)
HB$_e$Ab, HB$_{eAb}$ hepatitis B early antibody
HB$_e$Ag, HBeAg hepatitis B early antigen
HbF, Hb F fetal hemoglobin (hemoglobin F)
HbG1 hemoglobin γ chain A
HbG2 hemoglobin γ chain G
HBGA had it before, got it again
HBGM home blood glucose monitoring
HbH hemoglobin H
Hb-Hp hemoglobin-haptoglobin (complex)
HBI
  hemibody irradiation
  hepatobiliary imaging
  Hutchins Behavior Inventory
HBIG, H-BIG, HBIg
  hepatitis B virus immunoglobulin
Hb$_{Kansas}$ hemoglobin Kansas
Hb$_{Lepore}$ hemoglobin Lepore
HBLP hyperbetalipoproteinemia
HBM
  human bone marrow
  hypertonic buffered medium
HbM hemoglobin M
HbMet methemoglobin
HBO hyperbaric oxygen (therapy)
HbO$_2$ oxyhemoglobin
HBOC hereditary breast and ovarian cancer
HBP high blood pressure
HbP primitive (fetal) hemoglobin
HBPM home blood pressure monitoring
HbR methemoglobin reductase
HBS
  Health Behavior Scale

H

151

HBS *(continued)*
  hyperkinetic behavior
    syndrome
HbS
  hemoglobin S
  sickle cell hemoglobin
HB$_s$Ab, HB$_{sAb}$, HBsAb
  hepatitis B surface antibody
HB$_s$Ag, HB$_{sAg}$, HBsAg
  hepatitis B surface antigen
HBSC hemopoietic blood stem
  cell
HbSC, HbsC sickle cell
  hemoglobin C
HBSS Hanks balanced salt
  solution
HbSS homozygosity for
  hemoglobin S
HBSSG Hanks balanced salt
  solution plus glucose
HbS-Thal hemoglobin S-
  thalassemia (sickle
  thalassemia)
HBT
  home-based telemetry
  human (blood) bilayer Tween
    (agar)
  hydrogen breath test
HBV
  hepatitis B virus
  honeybee venom
HBW high birth weight
H:BW
  heart to body weight ratio
  height-to-body weight ratio
HbZ hemoglobin Z (zeta,
  Zurich, ξ chain)
HC
  head circumference
  heart catheterization
  heavy chain
  heel cord
  hemochromatosis
  hemorrhage, cerebral
  hepatocellular cancer
  hippocampus
  histamine challenge
  histochemistry
  hospital course
  hot compress

  Huntington chorea
  hyaline cast
  hydranencephaly
  hydrocarbon
  hydrocephalus
  hyoid cornu
  hypercholesterolemia
  hypertrophic cardiomyopathy
H&C hot and cold
Hc hydrocolloid
HCA
  heel cord advancement
  hepatocellular adenoma
  heterocyclic antidepressant
  hypercalcemia
  hypothalamic chronic
    anovulation
  hypothermic circulatory arrest
HCC
  hepatitis contagiosa canis
    (virus)
  hepatocellular carcinoma
  history of chief complaint
HCC-CC clear cell
  hepatocellular carcinoma
HCD
  heavy-chain disease (protein)
  herniated cervical disc
  high caloric density
  higher cerebral dysfunction
  homologous canine distemper
    (antiserum)
  hydrocolloid dressing
H(c)ELISA hemagglutinin
  enzyme-linked immunosorbent
  assay
HCF Horsley-Clarke stereotactic
  frame
HCFA Health Care Financing
  Administration
HCFSH human chorionic
  follicle-stimulating hormone
hCG human chorionic
  gonadotropin
β-hCG beta-human chorionic
  gonadotropin
HCH hygroscopic condenser
  humidifier
hch hemochromatosis
HCHO formaldehyde

HCII heparin cofactor II
HCL
  hairy cell leukemia
  hard contact lens
HCl
  hydrochloric (acid)
  hydrochloride
HCLF high carbohydrate, low fiber (diet)
HCM
  health care maintenance
  heterogeneous cation-exchange membrane
  hypercalcemia of malignancy
  hypertrophic cardiomyopathy
HCMA hyperchloremic metabolic acidosis
HCMV human cytomegalovirus
HCN
  high calorie and nitrogen
  hydrocyanic acid
  hydrogen cyanide
HCO₃ bicarbonate (*See also* bicarb, CO₂)
HCP
  healthcare provider
  hearing conservation programs
  home chemotherapy program
HCPCS HCFA (Health Care Financing Administration) Common Procedure Coding System
HCPS hantavirus cardiopulmonary syndrome
HCR hysterical conversion reaction
hCRH human corticotropin-releasing hormone
h'crit hematocrit (*See also* HCT, crit)
HCRM home cardiorespiratory monitor
HCS
  heel-cord stretches
  hourglass contraction of stomach
  human cord serum
hCS human chorionic somatomammotropin

(somatotropin) (human placental lactogen)
HCT
  head computerized (axial) tomography
  heart-circulation training
  hematocrit (*See also* crit, h'crit)
  histamine challenge test
  homocytotrophic
  hydrocortisone
hCT
  human calcitonin
  human chorionic thyrotropin
HCTA helical computed tomographic angiography
HCTU home cervical traction unit
HCTZ hydrochlorothiazide
HCU homocystinuria
HCV hepatitis C virus
HCV EIA hepatitis C virus enzyme immunoassay
HCVR hypercapnic ventilatory response
HCV RNA hepatitis C virus RNA
Hcy homocysteine
HD
  hard corn [L. *heloma durum*]
  hearing distance
  heart disease
  Heller-Dor (procedure)
  hemidiaphragm
  hemodialysis
  hemolytic disease
  hepatic duct
  herniated disc
  hip disarticulation
  Hodgkin disease
  house dust
  hydatid disease
  mustard gas code name in WWI (mechlorethamine) (*See also* HN2)
HD# hospital day number
HDA
  heteroduplex analysis
  high-dose arm

153

HDAg hepatitis D antigen
HDC
    hand drive control
    high-dose chemotherapy
    human diploid cell
    hyperdiploid cell
    hypodermoclysis
HDC-SCR, HDC/SCR high-dose
    chemotherapy and stem cell
    rescue
HDCT high-dose chemotherapy
HDCV human diploid cell
    (culture rabies) vaccine
HDD
    half-dose depth
    high-dose depth
HDE Humanitarian Device
    Exemption (FDA)
HDF
    hemodiafiltration
    high dry field
HDG hydrogel (dressing)
HD-HIV Hodgkin disease and
    HIV infection
HDI
    hemorrhagic disease of infants
    high-definition imaging
HDIT high-dose
    immunosuppressive therapy
HDL high-density lipoprotein
HDL-C high-density lipoprotein-
    cholesterol
HDLW hearing distance, left,
    watch (distance from watch,
    heard by left ear)
HDM
    high-dose morphine
    house dust mite
HDN
    hemolytic (hemorrhagic)
      disease of newborn
    high-density nebulizer
hDNA deoxyribonucleic acid,
    histone
HDR
    high dose rate
    husband to delivery room
HDRB high dose rate
    brachytherapy

HDRV human diploid (cell
    strain) rabies vaccine
HDRW hearing distance, right,
    watch (distance from watch,
    heard by right ear)
HDS
    health delivery system
    hematuria-dysuria syndrome
    herniated disc syndrome
    HIV Dementia Scale
HDT
    hand dynamometer test
    hearing distraction test
    high-dose therapy
HDU head-drop unit (curare
    standard)
HDV hepatitis D (delta) virus
HDW hearing distance (with)
    watch
HDYF how do you feel
HE
    half-scan with extrapolation
    hard exudate
    Hektoen enteric (agar)
    hemoglobin electrophoresis
    hepatic encephalopathy
    human ehrlichiosis
    hyperextension
    hypogonadotropic
      eunuchoidism
    hypoxemic episode
H&E
    hematoxylin and eosin (stain)
    hemorrhage and exudate
    heredity and environment
He helium
HEADSS home (life), education
    (level), activities, drug (use),
    sexual (activity), suicide
    (ideation/attempts) (adolescent
    medical history)
hEAT human erythrocyte
    agglutination test
HEB hematoencephalic barrier
    (blood-brain barrier)
HEC
    health evaluation center
    human endothelial cell

HED
> hypohidrotic ectodermal dysplasia
> skin erythema dose [Ger. *Haut-Erythem-Dosis*]
> unit skin dose (of x-rays) [Ger. *Haut-Einheits-Dosis*]

HEDIS Health (Plan) Employer Data and Information Set

HEENT head, ears, eyes, nose, throat

HEG hemorrhagic erosive gastritis

hEGF, h-EGF human epidermal growth factor

HEIR
> health effects of ionizing radiation
> high-energy ionizing radiation

HEIS high-energy ion scattering

HeLa continuously cultured carcinoma cell line used for tissue cultures (named for patient, Henrietta Lacks)

heliox helium-oxygen mixture

HELLP hemolysis, elevated liver enzymes, low platelets

HEM, hem
> hematologist
> hematology
> hematuria
> hemolysis
> hemolytic
> hemorrhage
> hemorrhoid

hematem hematemesis

hemi
> hemiparalysis
> hemiparesis
> hemiplegia
> hemisphere

hemo hemophilia

hemocyt hemocytometer

hemorr hemorrhage

HEMOSID hemosiderin

HEMPAS hereditary erythroblastic multinuclearity with positive acidified serum

HEMS helicopter emergency medical services

HEN
> hemorrhages, exudates, and/or nicking
> home enteral nutrition

He-Ne, HeNe helium-neon

HEP
> hemoglobin electrophoresis
> heparin
> hepatic
> hepatoma
> high egg passage (virus)
> home exercise program

HEp human epithelial (cell)

hEP human endorphin

hep hepatitis

HEPA high-efficiency particulate air (filter)

hep A hepatitis A

hep B hepatitis B

hep C hepatitis C

Hep/Clav hepatoclavicular

hep E hepatitis E

hep lock heparin lock

HER2 human epidermal growth receptor 2

hered
> hereditary
> heredity

HERG human ether-a-go-go-related gene

hern
> hernia
> herniate

HER2/neu breast cancer gene

HERP human exposure (dose)/rodent potency

HES
> (acute) hypereosinophilic syndrome
> hematoxylin-eosin stain
> hypereosinophilic syndrome

HEs hypertensive emergencies

hES human embryonic stem (cell)

het
> heterophil (antibody)
> heterozygous

155

HETF home enteral tube feeding

HETP height equivalent to a theoretical plate (gas chromatography)

HE-TUMT high-energy transurethral microwave thermotherapy

HEV
health and environment
hemorrhagic endovasculitis
hepatitis E virus

HEx hard exudate

HF
Hageman factor
half
haplotype frequency
hard feces
hay fever
head of fetus
heart failure
hemofiltration
hemorrhagic fever
high-fat (diet)
high flow
high frequency
hollow filter (dialyzer)
hot flashes
human fibroblast
hyperflexion

Hf hafnium

HFA high-functioning autism

HFAK hollow-fiber artificial kidney

HFB high-frequency band

HFC
high-frequency current
histamine-forming capacity
hydrofluorocarbon

HFCB horizontal flow clean bench

HFCC high-frequency chest compression

HFD
high-fiber diet
high forceps delivery
high-frequency discharges
high-frequency Doppler
Human Figure Drawing

HFEC human foreskin epithelial cell

HFEE high-frequency epicardial echocardiography

HFF high-filter frequency

HFFI high-frequency flow interruption

HFG hand-foot-genital (syndrome)

HFH hemifacial hyperplasia

HFHL high-frequency hearing loss

HFI
half-Fourier imaging
Hand Functional Index

HFJV high-frequency jet ventilation

H flu *Haemophilus influenzae*

HFM
hand-foot-and-mouth (disease)
hemifacial microsomia

HFO high-frequency oscillation

HFOC high-flow oxygen conserver

HFOV high-frequency oscillatory ventilation

HFPPV high-frequency positive-pressure ventilation

HFPV high-frequency percussive ventilation

HFS
hand-foot syndrome
hemifacial spasm

hfs hyperfine structure

hFSH human follicle-stimulating hormone

HFST hearing for speech test

HFT
hemofiltration therapy
high-frequency transduction
high-frequency transfer

HFU
hand-foot-uterus (syndrome)
high-intensity focused ultrasound

HFV
hepatitis F virus
high-frequency ventilation
high-fruit/vegetable (diet)

HFX RT hyperfractionated radiation therapy

HG
hand grip (exercise)
herpes genitalis
herpes gestationis
Heschl gyrus
human gonadotropin
human growth (factor)
hypoglycemia

Hg mercury [L. *hydrargyrum* silver water] (*See also* hydrarg.)

hg hectogram

HGB, hgb hemoglobin (*See also* Hb)

Hgb ELECT hemoglobin electrophoresis

HgCl2 mercury chloride

HGE human granulocytic ehrlichiosis

hGG human gamma globulin

hGH
human (pituitary) growth hormone
somatotropin

HGI Human Genome Initiative

HGM home glucose monitoring

HGN hypogastric nerve

HGO hip guidance orthosis

HGSIL high-grade squamous intraepithelial lesion

HGV hepatitis G virus

HH
halothane hepatitis
healthy hemophiliac
hiatal hernia
home health
homonymous hemianopia (hemianopsia)
hyperhidrosis
hypogonadotropic hypogonadism
hyporeninemic hypoaldosteronism

H-H head-to-head sperm agglutination

H/H, H&H hemoglobin and hematocrit

HHA
hereditary hemolytic anemia
hypothalamic-hypophysial-adrenal (system)

HHB hypohemoglobinemia

HHb reduced hemoglobin

HHCS high-altitude hypertrophic cardiomyopathy syndrome

HHD
handheld dynamometer
home hemodialysis
hypertensive heart disease

HHFM high-humidity face mask

HHH hyperammonemia, hyperornithinemia, homocitrullinuria (syndrome)

HHHO hypotonia, hyperphagia, hypogonadism, obesity

HHIE, HHIE-S Hearing Handicap Inventory for the Elderly

HHM high-humidity mask

H-Hm compound hypermetropic astigmatism

HHN hand-held nebulizer

HHNC, HHNK hyperosmolar hyperglycemic nonketotic (coma)

HHPC hyperoxic-hypercapnic

HHS
Harris hip score
Hearing Handicap Scale
hereditary hemolytic syndrome
hyperglycemic hyperosmolar syndrome
hyperkinetic heart syndrome

HHT
head halter traction
hereditary hemorrhagic telangiectasia
heterotopic heart transplantation
hypertensive hypervolemic therapy

HHTC high-humidity tracheostomy collar

HHTM high-humidity tracheostomy mask

HHTS high-humidity
tracheostomy shield
HHTx head halter traction
HHV, HHV 1–8 human
herpesvirus (1–8)
HHV-8/KSHV human
herpesvirus 8/Kaposi sarcoma
herpesvirus
HHW hand-held weight
HI
harmonic imaging
head injury
hearing impaired
hemagglutination inhibition
(titer)
hepatobiliary imaging
homicidal ideation
hormone insensitive
hospital induced
human insulin
humoral immunity
hyperglycemic index
hypoglycemic index
hypomelanosis of Ito
hypothermic ischemia
Hi histamine
HIA
heat infusion agar
hemagglutination inhibition
assay
hyperventilation-induced
asthma
HIB
Haemophilus influenzae type
b
heart infusion broth
hemolytic immune body
hyperpnea-induced
bronchoconstriction
hypoxia, intussusception, brain
mass
HIC Human Investigation
Committee
hi-cal high calorie (diet)
H-ICD-A International
Classification of Diseases,
Adopted Code for Hospitals
HICHO high carbohydrate (diet)

HiCN
cyanmethemoglobin
hemoglobincyanide
HICROS high-frequency
contralateral routing of signals
HID
headache, insomnia, and
depression (syndrome)
herniated intervertebral disc
hyperkinetic impulse disorder
HIE hypoxic-ischemic
encephalopathy
HIFT high-frequency ventilation
trial
HIFU high-intensity focused
ultrasound
HIg hyperimmunoglobulin
hIg human immunoglobulin
HIHA high impulsiveness high
anxiety
HIL hypoxic-ischemic lesion
HILA high impulsiveness low
anxiety
HILP hyperthermic isolated
limb perfusion
HIM hepatitis-infectious
mononucleosis
HINT Harris Infant Neuromotor
Test
Hint. Hinton (flocculation test
for syphilis)
HIO
hepatic iron overload
hole-in-one (technique)
hypoiodism
HIPAA Health Insurance
Portability and Accountability
Act of 1996
HIPC hormone independent
prostate cancer
HiPro, HiProt high protein (diet)
HIS
high intermittent suction
hyperimmune serum
His histidine (*See also* H)
His- histidyl
-His histidino
hISG human immune serum
globulin

hist
> histidinemia
> history (*See also* Hx)

Histo-Dx histologic diagnosis

histol histology

HIT
> heparin-induced thrombocytopenia
> home infusion therapy

HITS high-intensity transient signal

HITT heparin-induced thrombocytopenia-thrombosis

HIV human immunodeficiency virus

HIV-Ab human immunodeficiency virus antibody

HIVAN human immunodeficiency virus nephropathy

HIVAT home intravenous antibiotic therapy

HIV-1C human immunodeficiency virus-1 subtype C

HIVD herniated intervertebral disc

HIV-D human immunodeficiency virus dementia

HIV-G human immunodeficiency virus gingivitis

HIVIg human immunodeficiency virus immunoglobulin

HiVit high vitamin

HIV-NHL human immunodeficiency virus non-Hodgkin lymphoma

HIV-P human immunodeficiency virus periodontitis

HIV-PARSE human immunodeficiency virus-patient-reported status and experience

HIV-SGD human immunodeficiency virus salivary gland disease

HJB
> high jugular bulb
> Howell-Jolly bodies

HJR hepatojugular reflux

H-K, H→K
> hand-to-knee (coordination)
> heel-to-knee (test) (*See also* HTK)

HK heat killed

HKAFO hip-knee-ankle-foot orthosis

HKAO hip-knee-ankle orthosis

HKMN Hickman (catheter)

HKO hip-knee orthosis (splint)

HKS heel-knee-shin (test)

HKT heterotopic kidney transplant

HL
> hairline
> hairy leukoplakia
> half-life (element, pharmaceutical)
> hallux limitus
> hearing level
> hearing loss
> hemilaryngectomy
> Hodgkin lymphoma
> human leukocyte
> human lymphocyte
> humerus length
> hypermetropia, latent

HL7 health level seven

H:L hydrophil to lipophil ratio

H&L heart and lungs

hL
> hectoliter
> hyperopia, latent

HLA
> heart, lungs, and abdomen
> histocompatibility leukocyte antigen
> horizontal long axial
> human leukocyte antigen (system)

HLA-A, HLA-B, HLA-C, HLA-D, HLA-DR
> varieties of human leukocyte antigen

HLB head, limbs, and body

159

HLD
  hepatolenticular degeneration
  herniated lumbar disc
HLF heat-labile factor
HLH
  helix-loop-helix
  hypoplastic left heart
    (syndrome)
hLH human luteinizing hormone
hLI human leukocyte
    (lymphocyte) interferon
HLK heart, liver, and kidneys
HLN hilar lymph node
HLP hyperlipoproteinemia
HLR
  heart to lung ratio
  heart-lung resuscitator
hLS human lung surfactant
HLT heart-lung transplantation
hlth health
HLV
  herpeslike virus
  hypoplastic left ventricle
HM
  hand motion (movement)
  harmonic mean
  head movement
  heart murmur
  heloma molle (soft corn)
  high magnification
    Holter monitor
  human milk
  human semisynthetic insulin
  humidity mask
  hydatidiform mole
  hypoxic-metabolic
Hm hyperopia, manifest
    (hypermetropia)
hm hectometer
hMAM RNA human
    mammaglobin RNA
HMBANA Human Milk Bank
    Association of North America
HMC heroin, morphine, and
    cocaine
HMD hyaline membrane disease
HME
  heat, massage, and exercise
    (*See also* HMX)

  heat/moisture exchanger
  human monocytic ehrlichiosis
HMETSC heavy metal screen
HMF human milk fortifier
HM/3ft hand motion at 3 feet
    (vision test)
hMG human menopausal
    gonadotropin
HMIS hallux
    metatarsophalangeal
    interphalangeal scale
HM & LP hand motion and
    light perception (vision test)
HMM heavy meromyosin (of
    muscle)
HMO
  health maintenance
    organization
  hypothetical mean organism
HMP hot moist pack
HMPAO-SPECT hexamethyl-
    propylene amine oxime
    single-photon emission
    computed tomography
HMR Hoechst Marion Roussel
    (stain)
H-mRNA H-chain messenger
    ribonucleic acid
1H-MRS proton magnetic
    resonance spectroscopy
HMRT hazardous materials
    response team
HMRU hazardous materials
    rsponse unit
HMS
  hypermobility syndrome
  hypodermic morphine sulfate
hMSC human mesenchymal
    stem cell
HMSN hereditary motor-sensory
    neuropathy (type IA, II,
    III–VII)
HMW high molecular weight
HMX heat, massage, and
    exercise (*See also* HME)
HN
  hematemesis neonatorum
  hemorrhage of newborn
  hereditary nephritis
  hilar node

160

home nursing
hypertensive nephrosclerosis
hypertrophic neuropathy
H&N head and neck
HN₂, HN2 nitrogen mustard
(mechlorethamine, mustard
gas) (*See also* HD)
HNA hypothalamoneurohypophy-
sial axis
HNC
head and neck cancer
hyperosmolar nonketotic coma
hyperoxic normocapnic
HNKDC hyperosmolar
nonketotic diabetic coma
HNKDS hyperosmolar nonketotic
diabetic state
H&N mot head and neck
motion
HNP herniated nucleus pulposus
HNPCC hereditary nonpolyposis
colorectal cancer
HNPP hereditary neuropathy
(with susceptibility to)
pressure palsy
hnRNA heterogeneous nuclear
ribonucleic acid
hnRNP heterogeneous nuclear
ribonucleoprotein
HNS
half-normal saline (0.45%
sodium chloride)
head, neck, and shaft (of
bone)
head and neck surgery
home nursing supervisor
HNSCC head and neck
squamous cell carcinoma
HNT Hantaan virus (hantavirus)
HNTD highest nontoxic dose
HNTLA Hiskey-Nebraska Test
of Learning Aptitude
HnTT heparin neutralized
thrombin time
HNU human *neu* unit
HNV has not voided
HNWG has not worn glasses
HO
hand orthosis

heterotopic ossification
high oxygen
hip orthosis
house officer
hypertrophic ossification
Ho
holmium
horse (slang for heroin)
horse (veterinary)
HOA
hip osteoarthritis
hypertrophic osteoarthritis
(osteoarthropathy)
Ho antigen low-frequency blood
group antigen
HoaTTG horse antitetanus
toxoid globulin
HOB head of bed
HOC
human ovarian cancer
hypertrophic obstructive
cardiomyopathy
HOCA high-osmolar contrast
agent
HOCM
high-osmolar contrast medium
hypertrophic obstructive
cardiomyopathy
HOD
hereditary opalescent dentin
hyperbaric oxygen drenching
HOF height of fundus
Hoff Hoffmann (reflex)
HOG halothane, oxygen, and
gas (nitrous oxide)
HOH
hand over hand
hard of hearing
HoIg horse immunoglobulin
HoLRP holmium laser resection
of the prostate
Homeo, Homeop homeopathy
HOMO highest occupied
molecular orbital
homolat homolateral
HONK hyperosmolar nonketotic
(coma)

161

HOOD, HOODS hereditary
onychoosteodysplasia
(osteoonychodysplasia)

HOP
high oxygen pressure
hypothyroxinemia of
prematurity

HOPE high oxygen percentage

HOPE-ROP high oxygen
percentage in retinopathy of
prematurity

hor, horiz horizontal

HORF high-output renal failure

HORS Hemiballism/Hemichorea
Outcome Rating Score

HOS
human osteosarcoma
hypoosmotic swelling

HoS horse serum

hosp hospital

HOST hypoosmotic shock
treatment

HOT
human old tuberculin
hypertension optimal treatment

HOW hypothermia oxygen
warmer

HOX homeobox (gene)

Ho:YAG holmium:yttrium-
aluminum-garnet

HP
handicapped person
Harding-Passey (melanoma)
hard palate
Harvard pump
hemiparesis
hemipelvectomy
hemiplegia
hemoperfusion
highly purified
high pressure
human pituitary
hydrogen peroxide
hyperphoria
hypersensitivity pneumonitis
hypoparathyroidism
hypopharynx

H→P heel-to-patella

H&P
history and physical
(examination)
Hodgen and Pearson
(suspension traction)

hp horsepower

HPA
Hereford Parental Attitude
(Survey)
human papillomavirus
hypothalamic-pituitary axis

HPAA hypothalamic-pituitary-
adrenal axis

HPAC high-performance affinity
chromatography

HPAT home parenteral
antibiotic therapy

HPC
heterotopic plate count
(bacteria)
history of present complaint
hydrophilic-coated (guidewire)

HPCE high-performance
capillary electrophoresis

HPD
hearing protection device
high-protein diet
home peritoneal dialysis

HPE
hemorrhage, papilledema,
exudate
holoprosencephaly

HPET *Helicobacter pylori*
eradication therapy

HPF
high-pass filter
high-power field
hypocaloric protein feeding

HPFH hereditary persistence of
fetal hemoglobin

hPFSH human pituitary follicle-
stimulating hormone

HPG hypothalamic-pituitary-
gonadal

hPG human pituitary
gonadotropin

HPH
halothane-percent-hour
hypoxia-induced pulmonary
hypertension

HPI history of present illness
HPIP history, physical, impression, and plan
HPL hyperplexia
hPL human placental lactogen
HPLC high-performance (pressure) liquid chromatography
HPLO *Helicobacter pylori*-like organism
HPM hemiplegic migraine
HPMC high-performance membrane chromatography
HPN home parenteral nutrition
HPNI hemodialysis prognostic nutrition index
HPO
  high-pressure oxygen
  hydrophilic ointment
  hypothalamic-pituitary-ovarian
HPOA hypertrophic pulmonary osteoarthropathy
HPP
  hereditary pyropoikilocytosis
  history (of) presenting problems
2HPP two-hour postprandial (blood sugar)
hPP human pancreatic polypeptide
HPPM hyperplastic persistent pupillary membrane
HPPO high partial pressure of oxygen
hPrL human prolactin
HPRT hot plate reaction time
HPS
  hantavirus pulmonary syndrome
  hematoxylin-phloxine-saffron (stain)
  hepatopulmonary syndrome
  high-protein supplement
  His-Purkinje system
  hypertrophic pyloric stenosis
  hypothalamic pubertal syndrome
HpSA *Helicobacter pylori* stool antigen

HPT
  heparin protamine titration
  histamine provocation test
  home pregnancy test
  hyperparathyroid(ism)
  hypothalamic-pituitary-thyroid
HPTD highly permeable transparent dressing
hPTH human parathyroid hormone
HPTM home prothrombin time monitoring
HPTX hemopneumothorax
hPUTH human placental uterotropic hormone
HPV
  hepatic portal vein
  human papillomavirus
  human parvovirus
HPX
  hypophysectomized
  partial hepatectomy
Hpx hemopexin (serum protein)
H. pylori *Helicobacter pylori*
HPZ high-pressure zone
HQL health-related quality of life
HR
  hallux rigidus
  Harrington rod
  hemorrhagic retinopathy
  heterosexual relations (scale)
  high resolution
  high risk
  hyperimmune reaction
  hypertensive retinopathy
H&R hysterectomy and radiation
H₂R histamine-2 receptor
hr 0 zero hour (when treatment starts)
hr hour
HRA
  heart rate audiometry
  histamine-releasing activity
HRAE high right atrium electrocardiogram
HRBC high-risk breast cancer

HRC
  help-rejecting complainer
  high-resolution chromatography
  human rights committee
HRCT high-resolution computed
  tomography
HRE
  high-resolution
    electrocardiography
  high-resolution electrophoresis
HREC hepatic reticuloendothelial
  cell
HREM high-resolution electron
  microscopy
HRES high-resolution
  endoluminal sonography
HRF
  Harris return flow
  high-resolution fingerprint
  hypertensive renal failure
HRH hypothalamic-releasing
  hormone
HRHS hypoplastic right heart
  syndrome
HRI
  Harrington rod instrumentation
  high-resolution infrared
    (imaging)
3H-RIA 3H (tritium)
  radioimmunoassay
HRIG human rabies immune
  globulin
HRL head rotation to left
HRLM high-resolution light
  microscopy
HRMPC hormone-refractory
  metastatic prostate cancer
HRMS high-resolution mass
  spectrometry
HRP
  high right parasternal (view)
  high-risk pregnancy
HRPC hormone-refractory
  prostate cancer
HRQL, HRQOL health-related
  quality of life
HRR
  Hardy-Rand-Ritter (color
    vision test kit)
  head rotation to right

  heart rate range
  high-risk recipient
HRS
  hepatorenal syndrome
  Hodgkin-Reed-Sternberg (cells)
  hormone receptor site
  humeroradial synostosis
HRS-D Hamilton Rating Scale
  for Depression
HRST
  heat, reddening, swelling, or
    tenderness
  heavy resistance strength
    training
HRSV human respiratory
  syncytial virus
HRT
  half relaxation time
  heart rate
  Heidelberg retina tomograph
  heparin response test
  hormone replacement therapy
  hyperfractionated radiation
    therapy
HRTEM high-resolution
  transmission electron
  microscopy
HRV
  heart rate variability
  human rotavirus
HS
  half-scan
  half strength
  hamstring sets
  hand surgery
  Hartmann solution
  healthy subject
  heart sounds
  heat stable
  heel spur
  heel stick
  heme synthetase
  hereditary spherocytosis
  herpes simplex
  hidradenitis suppurativa
  human serum
  hyperplastic synovium
  hypersensitivity
  hypertonic saline
  hypertrophic scar

H→S heel-to-shin (test) (*See also* HTS)

H:S helper to suppressor (cell) ratio

H&S
hearing and speech
hemorrhage and shock
hysterectomy and sterilization

Hs hypochondriasis

h.s. at bedtime [L. *hora somni hour of sleep*]

HSA
Hazardous Substances Act
hypersomnia-sleep apnea (syndrome)

HSAN hereditary sensory and autonomic neuropathy (types I-IV)

HSAS hydrocephalus (due to congenital) stenosis of aqueduct of Sylvius

HSBG heel-stick blood gas

HSC
hematopoietic stem cell
horizontal semicircular canal

HSCL-90 Hopkins Symptom Checklist-90

HSCT hematopoietic stem cell transplantation

HSD hypoactive sexual desire (disorder)

HSE
hemorrhagic shock and encephalopathy
herpes simplex encephalitis
hypertonic saline-epinephrine (solution)

Hse homoserine

HSG
herpes simplex genitalis
hysterosalpingogram
hysterosonography

hSGF human skeletal growth factor

hSGP human sialoglycoprotein

HSGYV heat, steam, gum, yawn, and Valsalva maneuver (treatment for otitis media)

H-SIL, HSIL high-grade squamous intraepithelial lesion

HSK herpes simplex keratitis

HSL herpes simplex labialis

HSLC high-speed liquid chromatography

HSM
hepatosplenomegaly
holosystolic murmur

HSMN hereditary sensory motor neuropathy (type I–III)

HSN
Hansen-Street nail
heart sounds normal
herpes simplex neonatorum

HSP
heat shock protein
hemostatic screening profile
Henoch-Schönlein purpura
hereditary spastic paraplegia

HSQ Health Status Questionnaire

HSR
heated serum reagent
homogeneous staining region (of chromosome)
hypersensitivity reaction
hypofractionated stereotactic radiotherapy

HSRA high-speed rotational atherectomy

HSRD hypertension secondary to renal disease

HSRS Health-Sickness Rating Scale

HSSE high soapsuds enema

HSSG hysterosalpingosonography

HST
health screening test
Hemoccult slide test
horseshoe tear

HSV herpes simplex virus

HSVE herpes simplex virus encephalitis

HT
hammertoe
Hashimoto thyroiditis
head trauma
heart

165

HT *(continued)*
  heart tones
  height *(See also* ht.)
  histotechnology
  hormone therapy
  hydrotherapy *(See also* hydro)
  hyperopia, total
    (hypermetropia) *(See also* Ht)
H&T hospitalization and treatment
H/T heel and toe (walking)
H(T) intermittent hypertropia
Ht
  hyperopia, total
    (hypermetropia, total) *(See also* HT)
  hypothalamus
ht. height *(See also* HT)
3-HT 3-hydroxytyramine (dopamine)
5-HT 5-hydroxytryptamine (serotonin)
HTA
  hypertension (French)
  hypophysiotropic area (of hypothalamus)
hTAT human tetanus antitoxin
HTB hot tub bath
HTC
  heated tracheostomy collar
  homozygous typing cells
  hypertensive crisis
HTCMS home telecare management system
HTCP Hendler Test for Chronic Pain
HTD human therapeutic dose
HTDW heterosexual development of women
HTG
  high-tension glaucoma
  hypertriglyceridemia
hTg human thyroglobulin
HTH helix-turn-helix
HTHD hypertensive heart disease
hTIG, hTIg homologous (human) tetanus immune globulin

HTK heel-to-knee (test) *(See also* H-K)
HTL
  hearing threshold level
  histotechnologist
  honey-thick liquid (diet consistency)
  human T-cell leukemia (lymphoma)
HTLV human T-cell lymphotropic (leukemia) virus
HTN hypertension
HTNV Hantaan virus (hantavirus)
HTO
  heterotropic ossification
  high tibial osteotomy
HTP
  hypothalamic, pituitary, thyroid
  hypothromboplastinemia
5-HTP, 5HTP 5-hydroxytryptophan
HTPN home total parenteral nutrition
HTR
  hard tissue replacement
  hypermetropia, right
hTR human thyroid hormone receptor
HTR-MFI hard tissue replacement-malleable facial implant
hTRT human telomerase reverse transcriptase
HTS
  hammertoe syndrome
  head trauma syndrome
  heel-to-shin (test) *(See also* H→S)
  hemangioma-thrombocytopenia syndrome
HtSDS height standard deviation score (pediatrics)
hTSH human thyroid-stimulating
HTST high temperature-short time (pasteurization)
HTT hand thrust test
HTVD hypertensive vascular disease

HTx
  heart transplantation
  hemothorax
HU
  head unit
  hemagglutinin unit
  hemolytic unit
  Hounsfield unit
  human urine
  hyperemia unit
  hypertensive urgency
hUAEC human umbilical artery endothelial cells
HUAM home uterine activity monitor(ing)
hUCB human umbilical cord blood
huEPO human erythropoietin
hu-FSH human urinary follicle-stimulating hormone
HuGE Human Genome
HuGe Index Human Gene Expression Index
HuGENet Human Genome Epidemiology Network
HUI Harris uterine injector
HUIFM human leukocyte interferon Meloy
HuIFN human interferon
HUIS high-dose urea in invert sugar
HUM heat (or hot packs), ultrasound, and massage
hum. humerus
HUMAN hyper utilities mechatronic assistant (microscopic neurosurgical manipulator
HUMARA human androgen receptor assay (locus)
HUMI Harris-Kronner uterine manipulator-injector
HUS
  head ultrasound
  hemolytic uremic syndrome
HuSA human serum albumin
husb husband

HUS/TTP hemolytic uremic syndrome/thrombotic thrombocytopenia purpura
HUT head-up tilt (table test)
HUV human umbilical vein
HUVEC human umbilical vein endothelial cells
HV
  hallux valgus
  heart volume
  hepatic vein
  herpesvirus
  high voltage
  hyperventilation
  hypervolemic
H&V hemigastrectomy and vagotomy
HVA hallux valgus angle
HVC high voltage can
HVDO hypovitaminosis D osteopathy
HVE
  high-voltage electrophoresis
  high-volume evacuator
HVEM high voltage electron microscope
HVES high-voltage electrical stimulation (physical therapy)
HVF Humphrey visual field
HVG
  hematoxylin and van Gieson (stain)
  host-versus-graft (disease, response)
HVGS high-voltage galvanic stimulation (physical therapy)
HVI hollow viscus injury
HVID horizontal visible iris diameter
HVI-DHP hepatic venous isolation by direct hemoperfusion
HVL half-value layer
HVLA high-velocity low-amplitude
HVLP high-volume low-pressure
HVM
  high-velocity missile

HVM *(continued)*
 hypothalamic ventromedial (nucleus)
HVO hallux valgus orthosis
HVOD hepatic venoocclusive disease
HVOT Hooper Visual Organization Test
HVPC high-voltage pulsed current
HVPE high-voltage paper electrophoresis
HVPG hepatic venous pressure gradient
HVPGS high-voltage pulsed galvanic stimulation
HVPS high-voltage pulsed stimulation
HVPT hyperventilation provocation test
HVR hypoxic ventilatory response
HVSA high-voltage slow activity
H vs A home versus (against) advice
HVSD hydrogen-detected ventricular septal defect
HVT
 half-value thickness
 high-voltage therapy
HVTEM high-voltage transmission electron microscopy
HWB hot water bottle
HWE hot water extract
HWG has worn glasses
HWOK heel walking normal (OK)
HWP
 hepatic wedge pressure
 hot wet pack
HWPG has worn prescription glasses
HWS hot water soluble
HX hydrogen exchange

Hx history (*See also* hist)
HXIS hard x-ray imaging spectrometer
Hy
 hydrostatics
 hypermetropia
 hyperopia
hydrarg. mercury (*See also* Hg)
hydro hydrotherapy (*See also* HT)
hyd and tur hydration and turgor
hyg hygiene
hyp
 hypalgesia
 hyperresonance
 hypertrophy
 hypophysis
hyper
 above
 higher than
hyperal, hyper-al hyperalimentation
hyper K hyperkalemia
hyper T&A hypertrophy of tonsils and adenoids
hypes hypesthesia
hypno hypnosis
hypo
 below
 hypodermic
 lower than
hypo A hypoactive
hypo K hypokalemia
hypopit hypopituitarism
HYs healthy years of life
hys, hyst
 hysterectomy
 hysteria
HZ herpes zoster
Hz hertz
HZD herpes zoster dermatitis
HZFO hamster zona-free ovum (male fertility test)
HZO herpes zoster ophthalmicus
HZV herpes zoster virus

I

incisor (deciduous, permanent)
inosine (*See also* Ino)
inspired (gas)
iodine
isoleucine (*See also* Ile)
isotropic (band, disc)
moment of inertia
vector cardiography electrode
(right midaxillary line)

I-10-S invert sugar (10%) in saline

IA

ideational apraxia
image amplification
impedance angle
infantile apnea
inferior angle
intraalveolar
intraamniotic
intraaortic
intraarterial
intraarticular
intraatrial

I&A irrigation and aspiration

IAA ileoanal anastomosis

IAB

incomplete (induced) abortion
intermittent androgen blockade
intraabdominal

IABC intraaortic balloon catheter

IABCP intraaortic balloon counterpulsation

IAC

indwelling arterial catheter
internal auditory canal
interposed abdominal
compression (CPR adjunct)
intraarterial chemotherapy

IACD

implantable automatic
cardioverter-defibrillator
intraatrial conduction defect

IAD

implantable atrial defibrillator

inactivating dose
intermittent androgen
deprivation
internal absorbed dose

IADH inappropriate (secretion of) antidiuretic hormone

IADL Instrumental Activities of Daily Living

IAds immunoadsorption

IADSA intraarterial digital subtraction angiogram

IAE intraatrial electrocardiogram

IAFI infantile amaurotic familial idiocy

IAH implantable artificial heart

IAHC intraarterial hepatic chemotherapy

IAI

intraabdominal infection
intraabdominal injury
intraamniotic infection

IAIA immune adherence immunosorbent assay

IAM internal auditory meatus

IAN inferior alveolar nerve

IAP

intermittent acute porphyria
intraabdominal pressure
intracarotid amobarbital
procedure
intrapartum antibiotic
prophylaxis

IAPG interatrial pressure gradient

IAR

inhibitory anal reflex
iodine-azide reaction

IART intraatrial reentrant tachycardia

IAS

interatrial septum
interatrial shunting
intermittent androgen
suppression
internal anal sphincter

169

IAS *(continued)*
    intraabdominal sepsis
    intraamniotic saline (infusion)
IASA interatrial septal aneurysm
IASD interatrial septal defect
IAT
    immunoaugmentative therapy
    indirect antiglobulin test
IATT intraarterial thrombolytic
    therapy
IAV
    interactive video
    intermittent assisted ventilation
IAVB incomplete atrioventricular
    block
I-B interbody (vertebral)
IB
    ileal bypass
    inclusion body
    infantile botulism
    inferior basal
    irradiated bone
    isolation bed
I band isotropic band (striated
    muscle fiber) *(See also* I disc)
IBB intestinal brush border
IBC
    inflammatory breast cancer
    iron-binding capacity
IBD
    infectious bowel disease
    inflammatory bowel disease
    ischemic bowel disease
IBDQ Inflammatory Bowel
    Disease Questionnaire
IBF
    immature brown fat (cell)
    Insall-Burstein-Freeman (total
        knee instrumentation)
IBG
    iliac bone graft
    insoluble bone gelatin
IBI
    intermittent bladder irrigation
    internal border zone infarct
    ischemic brain infarction
ibid. in the same place [L.
    ibidem]
IBILI indirect bilirubin
IBL immunoblastic lymphoma

IBM
    ideal body mass
    inclusion body myositis
    isotonic-isometric brief
        maximum
IBOW intact bag of waters
IBP iron-binding protein
IBPS Insall-Burstein posterior
    stabilizer
IBR
    immediate breast
        reconstruction
    Infant Behavior Record
IBS
    irritable bowel syndrome
    isobaric solution
IBT
    immune-based therapy
    immunobead test
    ink blot test (Rorschach test)
    interblinking time
    intracavitary brachytherapy
IBW ideal body weight
IC
    ileocecal
    iliac crest
    iliococcygeal
    immune complex
    immunocompromised
    impedance cardiogram
    incipient cataract (grade 11
        to 41)
    indirect Coombs (test)
    inhibitory concentration
    inner canthal (distance)
    inspiratory capacity
    intercarpal
    intermittent claudication
    internal capsule
    internal carotid
    internal cerebral
    internal conjugate (diameter)
    interstitial cystitis
    Isaacson classification
    isovolumic contraction
ICA
    ileocolic anastomosis
    immunocytochemical assay
    internal carotid artery
    intracranial aneurysm

ICAM intercellular adhesion molecule
ICB intracranial bleeding
ICBG iliac crest bone graft
ICC
immunocompetent cell
immunocytochemistry
Indian childhood cirrhosis
interchromosomal crossing-over
intermittent clean catheterization
interstitial cells of Cajal
islet cell carcinoma
ICCE intracapsular cataract extraction
ICCEc̄PI intracapsular cataract extraction with peripheral iridectomy
ICD
implantable cardioverter-defibrillator
indigo carmine dye
intercanthal distance
intracervical device
ischemic coronary disease
ICD-10 International Classification of Diseases (and Related Health Problems), 10th Edition
ICDCD International Classification of Diseases and Causes of Death
ICD-CM International Classification of Diseases–Clinical Modification
ICD-O International Classification of Diseases for Oncology
ICE
ice, compression, and elevation
intracardiac echocardiography
iridocorneal endothelial (syndrome)
ICEEG intracranial electroencephalography
I-cell inclusion cell
ICES ice, compression, elevation, support

ICEUS intracaval endovascular ultrasound
ICF
interciliary fluid
intracellular fluid
IC fx intracapsular fracture
ICG
indocyanine green (dye)
isotope cisternography
ICGA indocyanine green angiography
ICH
immunocompromised host
intracerebral hematoma
intracerebral hemorrhage
intracerebral hypertension
intracranial hemorrhage
intracranial hypertension
ICHD ischemic coronary heart disease
ICI
intracardiac injection
intracranial injury
IC-IC intracranial to intracranial (anastomosis)
ICIDH International Classification of Impairments, Disabilities, and Handicaps
ICISS International Classification of Diseases (9th Ed.) Injury Severity Score
ICIT intracavernosal injection therapy
ICJ ileocecal junction
ICL
implantable contact lens
intracorneal lens
intracorporeal laser lithotripsy
ICLE intracapsular lens extraction
ICM
infracostal margin
intercostal margin
intercostal muscle
interference-contrast microscopy
intracytoplasmic membrane
ipsilateral competing message

ICMA immunochemiluminescence assay
ICN inferior calcaneonavicular ligament
ICO
impedance cardiac output
intracellular organism
ICP
inductively coupled plasma
intercostal position (for chest lead)
intermittent catheterization protocol
intracranial pressure
intrahepatic cholestasia of pregnancy
↑**ICP** increased intracranial pressure
ICPC intracranial pressure catheter
ICPMM incisors, canines, premolars, and molars (permanent dentition formula)
ICP-MS inductively-coupled plasma-mass spectrometer
ICP-OES inductively-coupled plasma-optical emission spectrometry
ICR
intercostal retractions
international calibrated ratio
intracardiac catheter recording
intracavitary radium
intrastromal corneal ring
ion cyclotron resonance
ICrH intracranial hemorrhage
ICRT intracoronary radiation therapy
ICRU International Commission on Radiation Units (and Measurements)
ICS
ileocecal sphincter
immotile cilia syndrome
intercostal space
intracranial stimulation
ICSD International Classification of Sleep Disorders: (Diagnostic and Coding Manual)

ICSHI intracytoplasmic sperm head injection
ICSI intracytoplasmic sperm injection
ICT
icterus
indirect Coombs titer
insulin coma therapy
insulin convulsive therapy
intracranial tumor
intradermal cancer test
islet cell transplant
ict ind icterus index
ICTX intermittent cervical traction
ICUS intracoronary ultrasound
ICV
internal cerebral vein
intracellular volume
intracerebroventricular
ICX immune complex
ID
identification
immunodeficiency
immunodiffusion (test)
inclusion disease
infant death
infectious disease (*See also* inf dis)
infective dose
inhibitory dose
inner diameter
inside diameter
internal derangement
internal diameter
interstitial disease
intraduodenal
I&D
incision and drainage
irrigation and debridement
Id
idiotypic
infradentale
interdentale
id. the same [L. *idem*]
IDA iron-deficiency anemia
IDAV immunodeficiency-associated virus
IDC
infiltrating ductal carcinoma

interdigitating dendritic cell
intervertebral disc calcification
IDCF immunodiffusion
complement fixation
IDD iodine-deficiency disorder
IDDM insulin-dependent diabetes
mellitus
IDDS implantable drug delivery
system
IDDT immunodouble diffusion
test
IDE Investigational Device
Exemption
IDEA Individuals with
Disabilities Education Act
ID:ED internal diameter to
external diameter (cardiac
valve replacement ratio)
IDEM ischemic, drug,
electrolyte, metabolic (effect)
IDG interdental groove
IDI
induction to delivery interval
intractable diarrhea of infancy
I disc isotropic disc (striated
muscle fiber) (*See also* I
band)
IDK internal derangement of
knee (joint)
IDL
Index to Dental Literature
intensity difference limen
intermediate-density lipoprotein
IDM infant of diabetic mother
IDMC interdigestive motility
complex
ID-MS isotope dilution-mass
spectrometry
IDNA iron-deficient, not anemic
IDPN intradialytic parenteral
nutrition
IDR
idiosyncratic drug reaction
intradermal reaction
IDS infectious disease service
IDSA intraoperative digital
subtraction angiography
IDT
immune diffusion test

interdisciplinary team
intradermal test
IDTP immunodiffusion tube
precipitin
IDU
intravenous drug use
Ivy dog unit
IDUS intraductal ultrasound
IDV intermittent demand
ventilation
IDVC indwelling venous
catheter
Idx cross-reactive idiotype
IE
immunizing unit [Ger.
immunitäts Einheit] (*See also*
IU)
inner (internal) ear
intake energy (unit of food)
international unit (European
abbreviation)
intraepithelial
I-E internal versus external
I&E internal and external
I:E inspiratory to expiratory
ratio
i.e. that is [L. *id est*]
IEA
immediate early antigen
immunoelectroadsorption
immunoelectrophoretic analysis
inferior epigastric artery
IEC
injection electrode catheter
intradiscal electrothermal
coagulation
ion-exchange chromatography
IED improvised explosive
device
IEE inner enamel epithelium
IEF isoelectric focusing
(electrophoresis)
IEHL intracorporeal
electrohydraulic lithotripsy
IEI isoelectric interval
IEL intimal elastic lamina
IEM
immune electron microscopy

IEM *(continued)*
  inborn error of metabolism
  internal elastic membrane
IEMG integrated electromyogram
IEOP immunoelectroosmophoresis
IET infantile estropia
IF
  immersion foot
  indirect fluorescence
  inferior facet
  inspiratory force
  internal fixation
  intrinsic factor
  involved field
IFA
  immunofluorescent antibody
    (assay)
  incomplete Freund adjuvant
IFAT indirect fluorescent
  antibody test
IFC interferential current
IFCL intermittent flow
  centrifugation leukapheresis
IFE
  immunofixation electrophoresis
  in-flight emergency
IFG inferior frontal gyrus
IFI
  indirect immunofluorescence
  intrafollicular insemination
IFIX immunofixation
IFM
  internal fetal monitoring
  intrafusal muscle
IFN
  immunoreactive fibronectin
  interferon
IFP intrapatellar fat pad
IFR inspiratory flow rate
IFRA indirect fluorescent rabies
  antibody (test)
IFROS ipsilateral frontal routing
  of signals
IFSA individualized functional
  status assessment
IFSE internal fetal scalp
  electrode
IFT
  immunofluorescence test

International Frequency Tables
inverse Fourier transform
I-G insulin-glucagon
IG
  image guide
  intragastric
Ig immunoglobulin
IgA immunoglobulin A
IgA-IFA IgA immunofluorescent
  antibody
IGBB image-guided breast
  biopsy
IgD immunoglobulin D
IGE impaired gas exchange
IgE immunoglobulin E
IGF insulinlike growth factor
IgF immunoglobulin F
IG-FESS image-guided
  functional endoscopic sinus
  surgery
IgG immunoglobulin G
IGHL inferior glenohumeral
  ligament
IgIM immunoglobulin,
  intramuscular
IgIV immunoglobulin,
  intravenous
IgM immunoglobulin M
IgM-IFA IgM
  immunofluorescent antibody
IGPA infragenicular popliteal
  artery
IgQ immunoglobulin quantitation
IGR
  immediate generalized reaction
  intrauterine growth retardation
IGS image-guided surgery
IGSS immunogold-silver staining
IH
  immediate hypersensitivity
  indirect hemagglutination
  industrial hygiene
  infantile hydrocephalus
  infectious hepatitis
  inguinal hernia
  inner half
  intermittent heparinization
  intimal hyperplasia
  intracerebral hematoma
  intracranial hypertension

intramural hematoma
intraretinal hemorrhage

IHA
indirect hemagglutination antibody (test)
infusion hepatic arteriography
intrahepatic atresia

IHB incomplete heart block

IHb hemoglobin content index

IHBT incompatible hemolytic blood transfusion

IHC
immobilization hypercalcemia
immunohistochemistry
inner hair cell (of cochlea)
intrahepatic cholestasis

IHD
intermittent hemodialysis
intraheptic duct(ule)
ischemic heart disease

IHG ichthyosis hystrix gravior

IHP
interhospitalization period
inverted hand position

IHPS infantile hypertrophic pyloric stenosis

IHR inguinal hernia repair

IHS
Idiopathic Headache Score
inactivated horse serum

IHSA iodinated human serum albumin

IHT
insulin hypoglycemia test
intravenous histamine test
ipsilateral head turning

IHW inner heel wedge

II
image intensifier
irradiated iodine

I or I illness or injuries

IIA internal iliac artery

IIC integrated ion current

IIEF International Index of Erectile Function

IIF
immune interferon
indirect immunofluorescence

IIGR ipsilateral instinctive grasp reaction

IIH iodine-induced hyperthyroidism

IIS local involvement of the spleen (Ann Arbor staging for Hodgkin disease)

IIM intracortical interaction mapping

IINB ilioinguinal-iliohypogastric nerve block

IIP indirect immunoperoxidase

IIS
intensive immunosuppression
intermittent infusion set

IIT integrated isometric tension

IJ
ileojejunal
internal jugular (vein)
intrajejunal

IJC internal jugular catheter

IJD inflammatory joint disease

IJP
inhibitory junction potential
internal jugular pressure

IJR idiojunctional rhythm

IJT idiojunctional tachycardia

IK
immobilized knee
infusoria killing (unit) (*See also* IKU)

IKE ion kinetic energy

IKI iodine potassium iodide (Lugol solution)

IKU infusoria killing unit

IL
ileum (bowel)
iliolumbar
ilium (bone)
immature lung
incisolingual
interleukin
intralipid
intralumbar

Il illinium (promethium)

ILA inferior lateral angle

ILa incisolabial

ILAP interstitial laser ablation of the prostate

ILB incidental Lewy body

ILC
  incipient lethal concentration
  interstitial laser coagulation

ILCP interstitial laser
  coagulation of the prostate

ILD
  immature lung disease
  intermediate density
    lipoproteins
  interstitial lung disease
  ischemic limb disease

ILDL intermediate low-density
  lipoprotein

Ile isoleucine (*See also* I)

ILHP ipsilateral
  hemidiaphragmatic paresis

ILI influenzalike illness

ILL
  inequality in leg length
  intracorporeal laser lithotripsy

ILLE inverted (position with)
  lower limbs extended

ILM
  insulinlike material
  internal limiting membrane

ILMA intubating laryngeal mask
  airway

ILMC immature living male
  child

ILo iodine lotion

ILP
  inadequate luteal phase
  interstitial laser
    photocoagulation
  interstitial lymphocytic
    pneumonia
  intralesional laser
    photocoagulation
  isolated limb perfusion

ILR irreversible loss rate

ILS
  increase in life span
  infrared liver scanner
  intralobular sequestration
  intraluminal stapler

ILSS integrated life support
  system

ILUS intraluminal ultrasound

IM
  immunosuppression method
  intramedullary
  intramuscular (injection)

IMA
  immunometric assay
  inferior mesenteric artery
  intermetatarsal angle
  internal mammary artery

IMAC image management
  archiving and communications

IMAGE integrated molecular
  analysis of gene expression

IMARD immunomodulating
  antirheumatic drug

IMAX internal maxillary artery

IMB intermenstrual bleeding

IMC
  index of marrow conversion
  intermittent catheterization
  intramedullary catheter

IMD
  immune-mediated diabetes
  immunologically mediated
    disease
  inherited metabolic disorder

ImD$_{50}$ immunizing dose
  sufficient to protect 50% of
  subjects

IMDC intramedullary metatarsal
  decompression

IME independent medical
  examination

IMET isometric endurance time

IMF
  inframammary fold
  intermaxillary fixation

IMG
  inferior mesenteric ganglion
  internal mammary graft

IMGG intramuscular gamma
  globulin

IMH
  indirect microhemagglutination
    (test)
  intramural hemorrhage

IMI
  indirect membrane
    immunofluorescence

inferior myocardial infarction
intermeal interval
IMIG intramuscular
immunoglobulin
IML
intermetacarpal ligament
internal mammary
lymphoscintigraphy
IMLA, IMLAD intramural left
anterior descending (artery)
IMLC incomplete mitral leaflet
closure
IMM
immunization
internal medial malleolus
immed immediately
immobil immobilize
immunol immunology
IMN
internal mammary (lymph)
node
intramedullary nailing
IMP
iatrogenic multiple pregnancy
incomplete male
pseudohermaphroditism
intramuscular (compartment)
pressure
IMPA incisal mandibular plane
angle
IMPEX immediate postexercise
IMPT intensity-modulated proton
therapy
Impx impacted
IMR
individual medical record
infant mortality rate
IMRA immunoradiometric assay
IMRAD, IMRD introduction,
materials and methods,
results, and discussion (formal
structure of scientific article)
IMRT intensity-modulated
radiation therapy
IMS
immunosuppressants
incurred in military service
IMSC intramedullary
supracondylar

IMSS in-flight medical support
system
IMT
inspiratory muscle training
intimal-medial thickness
ImU international milliunit
IMV
inferior mesenteric vein
intermittent mechanical
ventilation
IMVC, IMViC, imvic
indole, methyl red, Voges-
Proskauer, and citrate (test)
IN
icterus neonatorum
impetigo neonatorum
infundibular nucleus
intermediate nucleus
interneuron
interstitial nephritis
intranasal
In
indium
inion
inulin
in. inch
in² square inch
in³ cubic inch (*See also* cu in)
INA inferior nasal artery
INAD investigational new
animal drug
INB
intercostal nerve blockade
ischemic necrosis of bone
inbr inbreeding
INC
illuminated near card
incisal
incision
incomplete
inconclusive
incontinent
inside-the-needle catheter
interstitial nucleus of Cajal
Inc Ab incomplete abortion
incl including
incompl incomplete
incont incontinent

IND
> indirect treatment
> induced
> internodal distance
> Investigational New Drug

ind
> index
> indigo

INDA Investigational New Drug
> Application

indic indication

indig indigestion

INDIV individual

Ind Med Index Medicus

INEX inexperienced

INF
> infant
> infantile
> infarction
> infected (infection) (*See also* infx)
> inferior
> infundibulum (of neurohypophysis)
> infused, infusion

inf dis infectious disease (*See also* ID)

inflamm
> inflammation
> inflammatory

INFM, inf mono infectious mononucleosis

info information

infra- below

infx infected (infection) (*See also* INF)

ING
> inguinal
> isotope nephrogram

INH isonicotinic acid hydrazide (isoniazid)

inhal inhaler, inhalation

inhib inhibiting, inhibition

INI
> intranasal insulin
> intranuclear inclusion (agent)

inj injured, injury

inject. injection

INN International Nonproprietary Name

innerv innervate

INO
> inhaled nitrous oxide
> internuclear ophthalmoplegia

Ino inosine (*See also* I)

iNO inhaled nitric oxide

INOC inoculate

INOP internodal ophthalmoplegia

inop inoperable

inorg inorganic

iNOS inducible nitric oxide synthetase

Inox inosine, oxidized

INPAV intermittent negative pressure-assisted ventilation

INQ inferior nasal quadrant

INR international normalized ratio

INREM internal roentgen equivalent, man (radiation dose)

INS
> inspection
> insulin
> insurance

INS Ab insulin antibody

insem insemination

insol insoluble

insp inspect

inspir inspiration

INSS International Neuroblastoma Staging System

INST instrument (delivery)

insuf
> insufficiency, insufficient
> insufflation

INT
> intermediate
> intermittent
> intermittent needle therapy
> internal

INTEG integument

internat international

INTERP interpretation

intertroch intertrochanteric

intest intestinal, intestine

int/ext internal/external (rotation)

int hist interval history

int mon internal monitor

int obst intestinal obstruction

intol intolerance
INTOX intoxication
INTR intermittent
int rot internal rotation
int trx intermittent traction
intub intubation
INV inferior nasal vein
inv invalid
inver
    inversion
    inverted
invest. investigation
inv/ev inversion/eversion
inv ins inverted insertion
invol involuntary
INVOS in vivo optical
    spectroscopy
IO
    inferior oblique (eye muscle)
    inferior olive
    initial opening (pressure)
    inside-out (vesicle)
    internal os (cervix)
    intraocular (pressure)
    intra-Ommaya (reservoir)
    intraoperative
    intraosseous
I&O intake and output
Io ionium (slope of thorium)
IOA inner optic anlage
IOCG intraoperative
    cholangiogram
IOCM isosmolar contrast
    medium
IOD
    injured on duty
    integrated optical density
    interorbital distance
IOE
    intraoperative echocardiography
    intraoperative endoscopy
    intraoperative enteroscopy
IOEBT intraoperative electron
    beam therapy
IOECS intraoperative electrical
    cortical stimulation
IOF intraocular fluid
IOFB intraocular foreign body
IOI intraosseous infusion

IOL
IOLI intraocular lens
    implantation
IOLP intraocular lens power
IOM
    infraorbital margin
    interosseous membrane
    intraocular muscle
    intraoperative neurophysiologic
    monitoring
IOML infrabitomeatal line
ION ischemic optic neuropathy
IONTO iontophoresis
IOOA inferior oblique
    overaction
IOP intraocular pressure
IOR
    ideas of reference
    index of response
    inferior oblique recession
IORT intraoperative (electron
    beam) radiotherapy
IOS intraoperative sonography
IOT
    intraocular tension
    intraocular transfer
    ipsilateral optic tectum
IOTEE intraoperative
    transesophageal
    echocardiography
IOU international opacity unit
IOUS
    intraocular ultrasound
    intraoperative ultrasound
IP
    ileoproctostomy
    iliopsoas (muscle)
    immune precipitate
    immunoperoxidase
    incisoproximal
    incisopulpal
    incontinentia pigmenti
    induced potential
    induction period
    infundibular process
    infundibulopelvic (ligament)
    International Pharmacopoeia
    interstitial pneumonia
    (pneumonitis)

IP *(continued)*
ionization potential
isoelectric point
in plaster
I/P iris and pupil
IPA
International Phonetic
Alphabet
intrapulmonary artery
IPAA ileal pouch anal
anastomosis
IPAP inspiratory positive airway
pressure
IPB infrapopliteal bypass
IPC
intermittent pneumatic
compression
interpeduncular cistern
intraductal papillary carcinoma
ion-pair chromatography
IPCS intrauterine progesterone
contraceptive system
IPCT intraperitoneal
chemotherapy
IPD
incomplete pancreas divisum
inflammatory pelvic disease
intermittent peritoneal dialysis
interpupillary distance
IPE
interstitial pulmonary
emphysema
iris pigment epithelium
IPEUS intraportal endovascular
ultrasonography
IPF interstitial pulmonary
fibrosis
IPFD intrapartum fetal distress
IPG
impedance phlebograph
impedance plethysmography
implantable pulse generator
inspiratory phase gas
IPI
infertility perceptions
inventory
International Prognostic Index
interphonemic interval
interpulse interval
intraperitoneal insemination

IPITx isolated pancreatic islet
transplantation
IPJ interphalangeal joint
IPKD infantile polycystic kidney
disease
IPL
interpupillary line
intrapleural
IPLS intense pulsed light
source
IPM
impulse per minute
interventional pain
management
intrauterine pressure monitor
IPN interpeduncular nucleus
IPO improved pregnancy
outcome
IPOF immediate postoperative
fitting
IPOM intraperitoneal onlay
mesh (hernia repair)
IPOP immediate postoperative
prosthesis
IPP
inferior point of pubic (bone)
inflatable penile prosthesis
intrahepatic portal pressure
intrapleural pressure
IPPA inspection, palpation,
percussion, and auscultation
IPPB intermittent positive-
pressure breathing
IP-PDT intraperitoneal
photodynamic therapy
IPPO intermittent positive-
pressure (inflation with)
oxygen
IPPR intermittent positive-
pressure respiration
IPPV intermittent positive-
pressure ventilation
IPR
immediate phase reaction
insulin production rate
IPS
impulse per second
initial prognostic score
intermittent photic stimulation
(electroencephalography)

Interpersonal Perception Scale
intraparietal sulcus
intraperitoneal shock
intraurethral prostaglandin
  suppository
ischiopubic synchondrosis
ips inch per second
IPSB intrapartum stillbirth
IPSF immediate postsurgical
  fitting (of prosthesis)
IPSS International Prostate
  Symptom Score
IPT
  immunoprecipitation
  industrial physical therapist
  inflammatory pseudotumor
  intraductal papillary tumor
IPTX intermittent pelvic traction
IPV
  intrapulmonary percussive
    ventilation
  intrapulmonary vein
IPVD index of pulmonary
  vascular disease
IPW interphalangeal width
IQ intelligence quotient
IQR interquartile range
IR
  ileal resection
  immediate release (tablets)
  immunoreactive (*See also* ir)
  incisal ridge
  index of response
  individual reaction
  inferior rectus (muscle)
  infrared (light)
  inspiratory reserve
  inspiratory resistance
  integer ratio
  intelligence ratio
  internal reduction
  internal rotation
  intrastent restenosis
  inversion recovery
  ionizing radiation
  isotonic reversal
  isovolumetric relaxation
I-R Ito-Reenstierna (reaction,
  test)

I/R ischemia and reperfusion
I&R insertion and removal
Ir iridium
ir
  immunoreactive (*See also* IR)
  intrarectal
  intrarenal
IRA
  ileorectal anastomosis
  immunoradioassay
  immunoregulatory α-globulin
IR-ACTH immunoreactive
  adrenocorticotropic hormone
IRAK integrated reference air-
  kerma
IRB institutional review board
IRBC irradiated red blood cells
IRC
  indirect radionuclide
    cystography
  inspiratory reserve capacity
IRD isorhythmic dissociation
IRDA intermittent rhythmic
  delta activity (EEG)
IRDM insulin-resistant diabetes
  mellitus
IRDS infant respiratory distress
  syndrome
IRE internal rotation in
  extension
IRED infrared emission
  detection
IRF
  interferon regulatory factor
  internal rotation in flexion
IRG immunoreactive glucagon
IRH intraretinal hemorrhage
IRhCG immunoreactive human
  chorionic gonadotropin
IRhCS immunoreactive human
  chorionic somatomammotropin
IRhGH immunoreactive human
  growth hormone
IRhPL immunoreactive human
  placental lactogen
IRI
  immunoreactive insulin
  insulin resistance index
IRIA indirect radioimmunoassay

irid iridescent

IRIg insulin-reactive immunoglobulin

IRIS intensified radiographic imaging system

IRKO insulin receptor knockout (gene)

IRLT intravascular red light therapy

IRM
innate releasing mechanism
intermediate restorative material
magnetic resonance imaging (French)

IRMA
immunoradiometric assay
intraretinal microvascular abnormality

IRMS isotope ratio mass spectrometry

IROS ipsilateral routing of signal

IROX iridium oxide

IRP
immunoreactive plasma
incus replacement prosthesis
International Reference Preparation
interstitial radiation pneumonitis

IR-PCR interrepeat polymerase chain reaction

IR-PEP inspiratory resistance and positive expiratory pressure

IRR
infrared radiation
infrared refractometry
intrarenal reflux
irregular rate and rhythm

irr
irradiation
irritation

irreg irregular

IRRIG irrigate

IRS
infrared spectrophotometry
insulin-resistance syndrome

IRSB intravenous regional sympathetic block

IRSE inversion recovery spin-echo sequence

IRT
interresponse time
interstitial radiation therapy
intracoronary radiation therapy
isometric relaxation time
item response theory (psychologic testing)

IRV
inferior radicular vein
inspiratory reserve volume
inverse-ratio ventilation

IS
ileal segment (intestine)
ilial segment (bone)
iliosacral
immune serum
immunosuppression
incentive spirometer
index of sexuality
infant size
infrahyoid strap
insertion sequence
insufficient signal
interictal spike (in electroencephalography)
international standard
interspace
interstitial space
intracardial shunt
Ionescu-Shiley (artificial cardiac valve)
ipecac syrup
ischemic score
in situ (in original place) [L. *in situ*]

is.
island
islet

ISA
ileosigmoid anastomosis
induced sputum analysis
intraoperative suture adjustment
iodinated serum albumin
irregular spiking activity (in electroencephalography)

ISA$_5$ internal surface area (of lung at volume of) five (liters)

ISAGA immunosorbent agglutination assay

ISAM infant of substance-abusing mother

ISB incentive spirometry breathing

ISBP interscalene brachial plexus

ISC
immunoglobulin-secreting cell
indwelling subclavian catheter
infant servo-control
infant skin control
insoluble collagen
intensive supportive care
intermittent self-catheterization
intermittent straight catheterization
International Statistical Classification
intershift coordination
interstitial cell
intersystem crossing
irreversible sickle cell
Isolette servo control

ISCCO intersternocostoclavicular ossification

ISCF interstitial cell fluid

ISCM intramedullary spinal cord metastasis

ISCN International System for (Human) Cytogenetic Nomenclature

ISCOM immunostimulating complex

ISCP infection surveillance and control program

ISD
immunosuppressive drug
inhibited sexual desire
initial sleep disturbance
intensity (of service), severity (of illness), discharge (screen)
isosorbide dinitrate

ISDB indirect self-destructive behavior

ISE
inhibited sexual excitement
integrated square error
ion-selective electrode

ISEDP intraspinal epidural pressure

ISEL in situ end labeling

ISF interstitial fluid

ISFET ion-specific field effect transducer

ISFV interstitial fluid volume

ISG immune serum globulin

ISH
icteric serum hepatitis
isocapnic hyperventilation
isolated septal hypertrophy
isolated systolic hypertension
in situ hybridization

ISHH in situ hybridization histochemistry

ISI
infarct size index
initial slope index
injection scan interval
injury severity index
International Sensitivity Index
International Slope Index
interstimulus interval

ISIH interspike interval histogram

ISK
immune stromal keratitis
isokinetic

ISKD intramedullary skeletal kinetic distractor

ISL
interscapular line
interspinous ligament

Is of Lang islets of Langerhans

ISM intersegmental muscle

IS-5-MN, Is-5-Mn isosorbide-5-mononitrate

ISMP Institute for Safe Medication Practices

ISNA iron-sufficient, not anemic

ISO
  isodose
  isotropic
ISO2, ISO$_2$ oxygen saturation
  indices
ISOE isoetharine
ISOF isoflurane (Florane)
ISOK isokinetic
Isol Isolette
isol isolation
isom
  isometric
  isometropic
8-iso-PGF$_{2alpha}$ 8-iso-prostaglandin
  F_{2alpha}
IsoRAS isorenin-angiotensin
  system
isox isoxsuprine
ISP
  distance between iliac spines
  immunoreactive substance P
  immunosuppressed protocol
  inferior spermatic plexus
  input signal processor
IS-PCR in situ polymerase
  chain reaction
ISPT interspecies (ovum)
  penetration test
isp-Tx intrasplenic transplantation
ISPX Ionescu-Shiley pericardial
  xenograft
ISR
  injection site reaction
  in-stent restenosis
  insulin secretion rate
  integrated secretory response
ISS
  Individual Self-Rating Scale
  inferior sagittal sinus
  Injury Severity Scale (Score)
  Integrated Summary of Safety
  ion-scattering spectroscopy
IS10S 10% invert sugar in
  0.9% sodium chloride (saline)
  injection
ISSI interspinous segmental
  spinal instrumentation
  (technique)
ISSLC International Staging
  System for Lung Cancer

IST
  immunosuppressive therapy
  injection sclerotherapy
  insulin sensitivity test
  insulin shock therapy
ISTD insulin standard
ISUB immunosubtraction
IS10W 10% invert sugar
  injection (in water)
ISY intrasynovial
IT
  iliotibial
  immunotherapy
  immunotoxin therapy
  incentive therapy
  inferior temporal
  inferior turbinate
  inhalation therapy
  inspiratory time
  insulin treatment
  intensive therapy
  intentional tremor
  internal thoracic
  intolerance and toxicity
  intracellular tachyzoite
  intradermal test
  ischial tuberosity
  isomeric transition (of
  radioactive isotopes)
I/T intensity/time (duration of
  contractions)
ITA
  individual treatment
  assessment
  inferior temporal artery
  internal thoracic artery
ITB iliotibial band
ITBFS iliotibial band friction
  syndrome
^{131}I-TBS iodine-131 total body
  scan
ITC
  infrared thermographic
  calorimetry
  in-the-canal (hearing aid)
  isothermal titration calorimetry
ITc International Table calorie
ITCL interosseous talocalcaneal
  ligament
ITD insulin-treated diabetic

ITE
    insufficient therapeutic effect
    in-the-ear (hearing aid)
ITET isotonic endurance test
ITFF intertrochanteric femoral
    fracture
ITFS
    iliotibial tract friction
      syndrome
    incomplete testicular
      feminization
ITGV intrathoracic gas volume
ITH immediate-type
    hypersensitivity
ITh, i-thec intrathecal (anesthesia
    injection)
ITI
    intertrial interval
    intratubal insemination
I-time inspiratory time
ITLC instant thin-layer
    chromatography
ITLC-SG instant thin-layer
    chromatography-silica gel
ITM improved Thayer-Martin
    (medium)
ITOP intentional termination of
    pregnancy
ITP immune thrombocytopenic
    purpura
ITPV intratracheal pulmonary
    ventilation
ITQ
    Infant Temperament
      Questionnaire
    inferior temporal quadrant
ITR
    intraocular tension recorder
    intratracheal
ITS isometric trunk stabilization
ITT
    identical twins (raised)
      together
    insulin tolerance test
    internal tibial torsion
    iron tolerance test
ITTP idiopathic
    thrombocytopenic purpura

ITV
    impedance threshold valve
    inferior temporal vein
ITX
    immunotoxin(s)
    intertriginous xanthoma
IU
    immunizing unit
    International Unit
    intrauterine
    in utero
IUC intrauterine catheter
IUD
    intrauterine (contraceptive)
      device
    intrauterine death
IUDE in utero drug exposure
IUFB intrauterine foreign body
IUFD
    intrauterine fetal demise
    intrauterine fetal distress
IUFGR intrauterine fetal growth
    retardation
IUFT intrauterine fetal
    transfusion
IUG
    infusion urogram
    intrauterine gas
    intrauterine gestation
    intrauterine growth
IUGR
    intrauterine (fetal) growth rate
    intrauterine (fetal) growth
      restriction
IUI
    intrauterine infection
    intrauterine insemination
      (catheter)
IU/L International Unit per liter
IUM
    internal urethral meatus
    intrauterine (fetally)
      malnourished
    intrauterine membrane
IU/min International Unit per
    minute
IUP intrauterine pregnancy
IUPC intrauterine pressure
    catheter

IUPD intrauterine pregnancy, delivered

IUPM infectious units per million

IUPTB intrauterine pregnancy, term birth

IUP,TBCS intrauterine pregnancy, term birth, cesarean section

IUP,TBLC intrauterine pregnancy, term birth, living child

IUP,TBLI intrauterine pregnancy, term birth, living infant

IUT intrauterine transfusion

IUTD immunizations up-to-date

IV
  intravenous
  in vitro
  in vivo

IVA
  integrated visual and auditory
  intraoperative vascular angiography

IVAC intravenous accurate control (device)

IVAD implantable vascular access device

IVAP
  in vitro antibody production (assay)
  in vivo adhesive platelet

IVB intravitreal blood

IVBC intravascular blood coagulation

IVC
  indwelling venous catheter
  inferior vena cava
  inspiratory vital capacity
  intravascular coagulation
  intravenous chemotherapy
  intraventricular conduction
  isovolumic contraction

IVCC intravascular consumption coagulopathy

IVCD intraventricular conduction defect (delay)

IVCh intravenous cholangiogram

IVCP inferior vena cava pressure

IVCT
  inferior vena cava thrombosis
  intravenously (enhanced) computed tomography
  isovolumic contraction time

IVCU isotope voiding cystourethrography

IVCV inferior venacavogram

IVD
  intervertebral disc
  intravenous drip

IVDA intravenous drug abuse

IVDSA intravenous digital subtraction angiography

IVDU intravenous drug use(r)

IVF
  in vitro fertilization
  in vivo fertilization

IVFA intravenous fluorescein angiography

IVF-ET in vitro fertilization-embryo transfer

IVFT intravenous fetal transfusion

IVG isotopic ventriculogram

IVGG intravenous gamma globulin

IVGTT intravenous glucose tolerance test

IVH
  intravenous hyperalimentation
  intraventricular hemorrhage (grade 1–4)

IVI intravaginal insemination

IVIg intravenous immunoglobulin

IVJC intervertebral joint complex

IVL
  indwelling venous line
  intravenous lock

IVLBW infant of very low birth weight

IVM
  immediate visual memory
  intracranial venous malformation
  intravascular mass

IVN intravenous nutrition

IVNF intravitreal neovascular frond
IVO intraoral vertical osteotomy
IVOTTS Irvine viable organ-tissue transport system
IVOX intravascular oxygenator
IVP
intravenous pyelogram
intraventricular pressure
intravesical pressure
IVp intravenous push (dose)
IVPB intravenous piggyback (drug administration)
IVPF isovolume pressure flow (curve)
IVR
idioventricular rhythm
interactive voice-response (system)
intravenous rider
IVRA intravenous regional anesthesia
IVRAP intravenous retrograde access port
IVRG intravenous retrograde (procedure)
IV-RNV intravenous radionuclide venography
IVRO intraoral vertical ramus osteotomy
IVRP isovolumetric relaxation period

IVRT isovolumic relaxation time
IVS
interventricular septum
intervillous space
irritable voiding syndrome
IVSO intraoral vertical segmental osteotomy
IVT
index of vertical transmission
intravenous transfusion
intraventricular
isovolumic time
IVU intravenous urogram
IVUC intravenous ultrasound catheter
IVUS
intracoronary vascular ultrasound
intravascular ultrasound
IW
inner wall
inspiratory wheeze
I-5-W invert sugar 5% in water
IWL insensible water loss
IWP ischial weightbearing prosthesis
IWT
ice water test
impacted wisdom teeth
IX iodine-binding capacity
IZ infarction zone

J
joule
juvenile
polypeptide chain in
    polymeric immunoglobulins
reference point following
    QRS complex, at beginning
    of ST segment

JA
joint aspiration
juvenile arthritis
juxtaarticular

JAFAR Juvenile Arthritis
Functional Assessment Report

JAI juvenile amaurotic idiocy

JAK/STAT Janus kinase/signal
transducer and activator of
transcription

JAM joint alignment and
motion

JAN Japanese Accepted Name

JAS joint activated system

jaund jaundice

JBE Japanese B encephalitis

JBS Johanson Blizzard
syndrome

JC
Jakob-Creutzfeldt (disease)
joint contracture

J/C joule per coulomb

JCAHO Joint Commission on
Accreditation of Healthcare
Organizations

JCE job capacity evaluation

JCGC Japanese Classification
for Gastric Carcinoma

J/cm joule per centimeter

J/cm² joule per centimeter
squared

JD
jejunal diverticulitis
jugulodigastric (node)
juvenile delinquent

JDM juvenile diabetes mellitus

JDMS/PM juvenile
dermatomyositis/polymyositis

JE Japanese encephalitis

JEB junctional escape beat

JEE Japanese equine
encephalitis

JEJ jejunum

JER
Japanese erection ring
junctional escape rhythm

JET
jejunal extension tube
junctional ectopic tachycardia

JE-VAX Japanese encephalitis
virus vaccine

JF
joint fluid
jugular foramen
junctional fold

JG
June grass (test)
juxtaglomerular

JGA juxtaglomerular apparatus

JGI
jejunogastric intussusception
juxtaglomerular granulation
index

JHR Jarisch-Herxheimer reaction

JI
jejunoileal (bypass)
jejunoileitis
jejunoileostomy

JIH joint interval histogram

JJ
jaw jerk
jejunojejunostomy

J1–J3 Jaeger test type number
1–3

J/kg joule per kilogram

JL
jet length
Judkins left (catheter)

JM
jugomaxillary
juxtamembrane

JMC Jansen metaphyseal
chondrodysplasia

JMD juvenile macular degeneration
JMH John Milton Hagen (human blood group, antibody, antigen)
JMML juvenile myelomonocytic leukemia
JMR Jones-Mote reactivity
JMS Juberg-Marsidi syndrome
JNB jaundice of newborn
JND just noticeable difference
jnt joint (*See also* Jx)
JNVD jugular neck vein distention
JOAG juvenile open-angle glaucoma
JODM juvenile-onset diabetes mellitus
JOMAC judgment, orientation, memory, abstraction, and calculation
JOR jaw-opening reflex
JP
    Jackson-Pratt (drain)
    Jobst pump
    joint protection
    juvenile periodontitis
    juvenile polyposis
JPB junctional premature beat
JPBS Jackson-Pratt to bulb suction
JPC junctional premature contraction
JPD juxtapapillary diverticulum
JPS joint position sense
JR
    jaw reflex
    Jolly reaction
    Judkins right (catheter)
    junctional rhythm

JRA juvenile rheumatoid arthritis (type I, II)
jrnl journal
JROM joint range of motion
JS
    jejunal segment
    junctional slowing
J/s joule per second
JSF Japanese spotted fever
JSU Junkman-Schoeller unit (of thyrotropin)
JT
    jejunostomy tube
    junctional tachycardia
J/T joule per tesla
JTA job task analysis
jt asp joint aspiration
JTF jejunostomy tube feeding
JTJ jaw-to-jaw (position)
J-tube jejunostomy tube
Ju jugale (craniometric point)
jug. jugular
jug. comp. jugular compression (test)
junct junction (*See also* Jx)
juv juvenile
juxt. near [L. *juxta*]
JV jugular vein
JVC jugular venous catheter
JVD jugular venous distention
JVP
    jugular venous pressure
    jugular venous pulse
JWS Jackson-Weiss syndrome
Jx
    joint (*See also* jnt)
    junction (*See also* junct)

K

burst of diphasic slow waves in response to stimuli during sleep (in electroencephalography)

capsular antigen [Ger. *Kapsel* capsule]

carrying capacity (genetics)

constant

cornea curvature

Kell blood group, system, factor

kelvin (SI fundamental unit of temperature)

keratometric power

kerma

ketamine (Super K)

Klebsiella

kosher

lysine (*See also* Lys)

phylloquinone

potassium [L. *kalium*] (*See also* kal)

ratio of curvature of flattest meridian of apical cornea (in fitting of contact lens)

vitamin K.

k

kilo-

thousand

K24H potassium in 24-hour (urine)

KA ketoacidosis

K:A ketogenic to antiketogenic ratio

K$_a$

acid ionization (dissociation) constant

equilibrium association constant

kA kiloampere

KAB knowledge, attitude, behavior

KABINS knowledge, attitude, behavior, and improvement in nutritional status

KACT kaolin-activated clotting time

KAFO knee-ankle-foot orthosis

KAIT Kaufman Adolescent and Adult Intelligence Test

kal potassium [L. *kalium*] (*See also* K)

KAO knee-ankle orthosis

KAP knowledge, aptitudes, (and) practices (fertility)

KASH knowledge, abilities, skills, (and) habits

KASS Kaneda anterior spinal/scoliosis system

KAST Kindergarten Auditory Screening Test

KAT kinesthetic ability trainer

kat katal (enzyme unit of measurement)

kat/L katal per liter

KAU King-Armstrong unit

K-B Kleihauer-Betke (test)

KB

human oral epidermoid carcinoma cells

ketone body

knee-bearing

knee brace

knuckle-bender (splint)

K$_b$, *K$_b$*

base ionization constant

dissociation constant of a base

kB kilobyte

kb kilobase

K-BIT Kaufman Brief Intelligence Test

kbp kilobase pair (nucleic acid molecules)

kBq kilobecquerel

KBr potassium bromide

KC

keratoconjunctivitis

keratoconus

knees to chest

Kupffer cell

191

kC kilocoulomb

kc kilocycle

kcal kilocalorie

KCCT kaolin-cephalin clotting time

KCD kinestatic charge detector

K cell killer cell

KCG kinetocardiogram

kCi kilocurie

KCl potassium chloride

K complex slow waves related to sleep arousal (in electroencephalography)

kc/sec, kc/s kilocycle per second

KD
ketogenic diet
kidney donor
killed
knee disarticulation
knitted Dacron
knowledge deficit

K$_d$
dissociation constant of an acid
distribution coefficient
partition coefficient

KDA known drug allergies

kDa kilodalton

KDS Kaufman Development Scale

KDSS Kurtzke Disability Status Scale

kdyn kilodyne

KE
first order elimination rate constant in hour-1 (*See also* kel)
Kendall compound E (cortisone)
kinetic energy

kel elimination rate constant (*See also* KE)

kemo Tx chemical therapy (chemotherapy)

K$_{eq}$ equilibrium constant

KER keratin

kera keratitis

kerma kinetic energy released in the medium

KET ketones

keV kiloelectron volt

KF
Kenner fecal (medium)
kidney function
Klippel-Feil (syndrome)

kf flocculation rate in antigen-antibody reaction

KFA kinetic fibrinogen assay

K factor gamma-ray dose (roentgens per hour at 1 cm from 1-mCi point source of radiation)

KFAO knee-foot-ankle orthosis

KFD Kikuchi-Fujimoto disease

KFR Kayser-Fleischer ring

KG-1 Koeffler Golde-1 (cell line)

kG kilogauss

kg kilogram (*See also* kilo)

kg-cal kilogram-calorie

kg/cm^2 kilogram per square centimeter

kgf kilogram-force

kg/L kilogram per liter

kg/m^2 kilogram per meter squared

kg-m kilogram-meter

kg-m/s^2 kilogram-meter per second squared

Kgn kininogen

KGS ketogenic steroid

kg/s kilogram per second

kGy kilogray

KH Krebs-Henseleit (cycle)

KHB Krebs-Henseleit bicarbonate (buffer)

KHb potassium hemoglobinase

KHC
kinetic hemolysis curve
knot holding capacity

KHD kinky-hair disease

KHE kaposiform hemangioendothelioma

KHF Korean hemorrhagic fever

KHM keratoderma hereditaria mutilans

KHN Knoop hardness number (of solids)

KHS
kinky hair syndrome
Krebs-Henseleit solution
kHz kilohertz
KI
karyopyknotic index
knee immobilizer
Krönig isthmus
potassium iodide
K_I
dissociation of enzyme-inhibitor complex
inhibition constant
Kliger iron agar (medium)
KIDS Kent Infant Development Scale
kilo kilogram (*See also* kg)
KJ knee jerk
kJ kilojoule
KJR knee jerk reflex
KK
kallikrein-kinin
knee kick
knock-knee
kkat kilokatal
KL
kidney lobe
kit ligand
Klebs-Löffler (bacillus)
kL kiloliter
kl musical overtone (ringing, in acoustics) [Ger. *Klang*]
K level lowest level (of x-rays)
KLH keyhole-limpet hemocyanin
KLS kidneys, liver, spleen
KLST Kindergarten Language Screening Test
KM keratomileusis
Km Michaelis constant
km kilometer
km² square kilometer
kMc kilomegacycle
kMc/s, kMcps kilomegacycle per second
KMEF keratin, myosin, epidermin, and fibrin (class of proteins)
KMG kangaroo mother care
KMnO4 potassium permanganate

KMO Kaiser-Meyer-Olkin (measure of statistical sampling adequacy)
KMS kwashiorkor-marasmus syndrome
Kn
knee
Knudsen number (low-pressure gas flow)
kN kilonewton
KNF model Koshland-Némethy-Filmer model
knork knife and fork (physical medicine)
KO
keep on (continue)
keep open
killed organism
knee orthosis
knock out (mouse, gene)
KO'd knocked out
KOH potassium hydroxide (stain)
KOR keep open rate
KP
Kaufmann-Peterson (base)
keratitic precipitate
keratitis punctata
keratoprecipitate
kidney punch (trauma)
kinetic perimetry
knowledge of performance
Köbner phenomenon
kPa kilopascal
kPas/L kilopascal-second per liter
KPB kalium (potassium) phosphate buffer
KPE Kelman phacoemulsification
KPR key pulse rate
KPS Karnofsky performance score (status)
KPT
kidney punch test (physical exam)
Kuder Performance Test
KPTT kaolin partial thromboplastin time

K

KPV
  killed parenteral vaccine
  killed polio vaccine
KR
  knowledge of result
  Kopper Reppart (medium)
Kr krypton
kR kiloroentgen
KRB, KRBB Krebs-Ringer
  bicarbonate (buffer)
KRBG Krebs-Ringer bicarbonate
  (buffer) with glucose
KRBS Krebs-Ringer bicarbonate
  solution
KRD kinetic rehab device
K readings keratometric
  readings
K-rod Küntscher rod
KRP Kolmer (test with) Reiter
  protein (antigen)
KRPS Krebs-Ringer phosphate
  solution
KS
  Kaposi sarcoma
  ketosteroid
  kidney stone
  Kveim-Siltzbach (test)
17-KS 17-ketosteroid
ks kilosecond
KSA knowledge, skills, and
  abilities
KSBOP Kaderavek-Sulzby
  Bookreading Observational
  Protocol
KSE knee sling exercises
KSHV Kaposi sarcoma
  herpesvirus
KS/OI Kaposi sarcoma and
  opportunistic infections
KSP kidney-specific protein
K$_{sp}$ potassium solubility product
KSW knife stab wound
KT
  kinesiotherapy
  known to
  Kuder test
KTC knee-to-chest

KTP potassium titanyl
  phosphate (laser)
KTU known to us
KTx kidney transplantation
KU
  Karmen unit
  Kimbrel unit
Ku kurchatovium
KUB
  kidneys, ureters, bladder (x-
  ray)
  kidney ultrasound biopsy
KUS kidneys, ureters, and
  spleen (x-ray)
KV killed vaccine
kV kilovolt
kVA kilovolt-ampere
KVBA kanamycin-vancomycin
  blood agar
kVcp kilovolt constant potential
KVE Kaposi varicelliform
  eruption
KVLBA kanamycin-vancomycin
  laked blood agar
KVO keep vein open (IV
  lines)
KVO C D5W keep vein open
  with 5% dextrose in water
kVp
  kilovoltage peak
  kilovoltage potential
KW
  Keith-Wagener (classification
  of eye ground findings)
  (*See also* KWB)
  kidney weight
  Kruskal-Wallis (test)
K$_w$ dissociation constant of
  water
kW kilowatt
KWB Keith-Wagener-Barker
  (classification of eye ground
  findings) (*See also* KW)
kWh, kW-hr kilowatt-hour
K wire Kirschner wire
kyph kyphosis

L

angular momentum
Avogadro constant/number (*See also* NA)
boundary [L. *limes*] (*See also* LIM)
coefficient of induction
diffusion length
fifty (Roman numeral)
inductance
lambert (unit of luminance)
latent (heat)
Latin
left
lethal (Erlich's symbol for fatal)
leucine (*See also* Leu)
levorotatory
lewisite
ligament, ligamentum (*See also* lig)
light (chain of protein molecules) (*See also* LT)
light sense
lilac (indicator color)
limes (*See also* LIM)
lingual (*See also* ling)
linking (number)
liquor
liter
longitudinal (section)
lumbar
luminance
lung (*See also* LU)
lysosome
radiance
self-inductance
syphilis (lues)

L/3 lower third (of long bone)
L₊ limes tod (toxin-antitoxin mixture that contains one fatal dose in excess)
L₀ limes zero (neutralized toxin-antitoxin mixture) [L. *limes nul*]
l- levorotatory

L-I, L-II, L-III
stages of lues (syphilis)
LA
lactic acid
language age
laparoscopic appendectomy
latex agglutination
left atrium
leukemia antigen
levator ani (muscle)
lichen amyloidosis
linguoaxial
local anesthesia
long acting
lymphocyte antibody
La lanthanum
LA50 total body surface area of burn that will kill 50% of patients (lethal area)
L&A, L+A, l&a
light and accommodation
living and active (family history)
LAA leukemia-associated antigen
LA:A left atrial to aortic ratio
LAAH laparoscopic-assisted abdominal hysterectomy
LAAL lower anterior axillary line
LAARD long-acting antirheumatic drug
lab laboratory
LABA laser-assisted balloon angioplasty
LABD linear IgA bullous dermatosis
LABS laboratory admission baseline studies
LAC
laceration
lactose
left antecubital
left atrial contraction
linguoaxiocervical
locally advanced cancer
long arm cast

LAC *(continued)*
  low amplitude contraction
  lung adenocarcinoma cell
  lupus anticoagulant
LaC labiocervical
lac & cont laceration and
  contusion
lacr lacrimal
LAD
  language acquisition device
  left anterior descending
    (coronay artery)
LADA
  laboratory animal dander
    allergy
  left acromiodorsoanterior
    (position of fetus)
LADD lacrimoauriculodentodigital
  (syndrome)
LADH
  lactic acid dehydrogenase
  liver alcohol dehydrogenase
LADME liberation, absorption,
  distribution, metabolism, and
  excretion (drug system)
LADP left acromiodorsoposterior
  (position of fetus)
LAE
  left atrial enlargement
  long above-elbow (cast)
LAEI left atrial emptying index
LAER late auditory evoked
  response
LAF
  laminar air flow
  left atrial enlargement
  leukocyte (lymphocyte)
    activating factor
LAFR laminar air flow room
LAG
  labiogingival
  linguoaxiogingival
  lymphangiography
LAH
  laparoscopic-assisted
    hepatectomy
  left anterior hemiblock
  left atrial hypertrophy

LA-HFOV liquid-assisted high-
  frequency oscillatory
  ventilation
LAI
  labioincisal
  laboratory-acquired infection
  latex (particle) agglutination
    inhibition
  left atrial involvement
  left atrial isomerism
  leukocyte adherence inhibition
    (assay)
LAK lymphokine-activated killer
  (cell)
LAL
  left axillary line
  low air loss
LaL labiolingual
L-Ala L-alanine
LALT
  larynx-associated lymphoid
    tissue
  low air loss therapy
    (mattress)
LAM
  lactation amenorrhea method
    (birth control)
  laminectomy
  laser-assisted myringotomy
  limb accurate measurement
  lymphangioleiomyomatosis
  lymphangiomyomatosis
LAM-1 leukocyte adhesion
  molecule-1
LAMA laser-assisted
  microanastomosis
LA–MAX maximal left atrial
  (dimension)
LAMB lentigines, atrial
  myxomas, cutaneous papular
  myxomas, blue nevi
  (syndrome)
lam & fus laminectomy and
  fusion
LAMMA laser microprobe mass
  analyzer
LAMP lysosomal membrane
  glycoprotein
LAN
  local area network

long-acting neuroleptic
lymphadenopathy
lang language
L ANT left anterior
LAO
    left anterior oblique
    left anterior occipital
LAP
    laparoscopy
    laparotomy
    laser-assisted palatoplasty
    leukocyte alkaline phosphatase
      (stain)
    low atmospheric pressure
    lower abdominal pain
LAP-1 Los Angeles preservation
    solution 1
LAP APPY laparoscopic
    appendectomy
LAP CHOLE laparoscopic
    cholecystectomy
lap Nissen laparoscopic Nissen
    fundoplication
LAQ long arc quad
LAR
    laryngeal adductor reflex
    laryngology
    late asthmatic response
    left arm, reclining (blood
      pressure, pulse measurement)
    long-acting release
    low anterior resection
LARC leukocyte automatic
    recognition computer
LARD lacrimoauriculoradiodental
    (syndrome)
LARS laparoscopic antireflux
    surgery
LARSI lumbar anterior-root
    stimulator implant
LAS
    lateral amyotrophic sclerosis
    laxative abuse syndrome
    left anterior superior
    left arm, sitting (blood
      pressure, pulse measurement)
    long arm splint
    low-amplitude signal
    lower abdominal surgery

lymphadenopathy syndrome
lymphangioscintigraphy
LASA
    left anterior spinal artery
    Lisfranc articular set angle
LASE laser-assisted spinal
    endoscopy
LASEC left atrial spontaneous
    echo contrast
laser light activation by
    stimulated emission of
    radiation
LASGB laser adjustable silicone
    gastric banding
LASIK laser-assisted in situ
    keratomileusis
LASS Linguistic Analysis of
    Speech Samples
LASV Lassa virus
LAT
    latent
    lateral
    latex agglutination test
    limbal autograft transplantation
LATC lateral talocalcaneal
    (angle)
LATCH lower anchors and
    tethers for children
lat & loc lateralizing and
    localizing
L·atm liter-atmosphere
lat men lateral meniscectomy
LATS long-acting thyroid-
    stimulating (hormone)
lats latissimus dorsi (muscle)
LAUP laser-assisted
    uvulopalatoplasty
LAV lymphadenopathy-associated
    virus
LAVH laparoscopic-assisted
    vaginal hysterectomy
LAW LDH, AST, WBC (blood
    tests)
lax.
    laxative
    laxity
LB
    lamellar body
    large bowel

LB *(continued)*
    lateral basal
    lateral bending
    lipid body
    live birth
    liver biopsy
    living bank
    loose body
    low back
    low breakage
    lung biopsy
    lymphoid body
L-B Liebermann-Burchard (test for cholesterol)
L&B left and below
lb. pound [L. *libra*]
LBA
    laser balloon angioplasty
    left basal artery
lb. avdp. avoirdupois pound [L. *libra avoirdupois*]
LBB
    long back board
    low back bend
LBC
    lamellar body count
    lidocaine blood concentration
    locoregional breast cancer
    lymphadenosis benigna cutis
LBCF Laboratory Branch Complement Fixation (test)
LBCL large B-cell lymphoma
L/B/Cr electrolytes, blood urea nitrogen, and serum creatinine
LBD
    lamellar body density
    left border dullness (of heart to percussion)
    Lewy body dementia
    low back disability
LBF
    Lactobacillus bulgaricus factor (pantetheine)
    limb blood flow
    liver blood flow
lbf pound-force
lbf-ft pound-force foot
lb-ft pound-foot
LBG Landry-Guillain-Barré (syndrome)

LBH length, breadth, height
LBM
    lean body mass
    little brown mushroom
    lung basement membrane
LBP
    lipopolysaccharide binding protein
    low back pain
    low blood pressure
LBQC large base quad cane
LBRF louse-borne relapsing fever
LBS
    lactobacillus selector (agar)
    low back syndrome
LBT
    loaded breathing test
    low back tenderness
    lupus band test
LBW
    lean body weight
    low birth weight
LC
    inductance-capacitance
    Laënnec cirrhosis
    lamina cortex
    Langerhans cell
    left (ear), cold (stimulus)
    lethal concentration
    light chain
    lingual cusp
    linguocervical
    locus ceruleus
    long-chain (triglycerides)
    longus capitis (muscle)
    lung cancer
    lymphangitic carcinomatosis
    lymph capillary
    lymphocyte count
    lymphocytic colitis
    lymphoma culture
3LC triple-lumen catheter
LCA
    lateral cricoarytenoid
    Leber congenital amaurosis
    leukocyte common antigen
    light contact assist
    lithocholic acid

lymphocyte chemoattractant
activity
lymphocytotoxic antibody
LCAT lecithin-cholesterol
acyltransferase
LCB lymphomatosis cutis
benigna
LCBF local cerebral blood flow
LCC
large cell change
liver cell carcinoma
long calcaneocuboid
LCCA
left common carotid artery
leukocytoclastic angiitis
LCCS lower cervical cesarean
section
LCD
lipochondral degeneration
liquid crystal display
liquor carbonis detergens
(coal tar solution)
localized collagen dystrophy
low-calcium diet
LC-DCP, LCDCP low-contact
dynamic compression plate
LCDD light-chain deposition
disease
LCDE laparoscopic common
duct exploration
LCE
laparoscopic cholecystectomy
left carotid endarterectomy
lower completely edentulous
LC-EMR lift-and-cut endoscopic
mucosal resection
LCF
left common femoral (artery)
low-frequency current field
lymphocyte chemoattractant
factor
lymphocyte culture fluid
LCFA long-chain fatty acid
LCFA-CoA long chain fatty
acyl-coenzyme A
LCFM laser cell and flare
meter
LCFU leukocyte colony-forming
unit

LCG
Langerhans cell
granulomatosis
liquid chemical germicide
LCH Langerhans cell
histiocytosis
L chain light chain
(polypeptides with low
molecular weight)
LCIS lobular carcinoma in situ
LCL
large cell lymphoma
lateral collateral ligament
Levinthal-Coles-Lillie
(cytoplasmic inclusion body)
localized cutaneous
leishmaniasis
lymphocytic lymphosarcoma
lymphoid cell line
LCLC large cell lung
carcinoma
LCM
laser-capture microdissection
leukocyte-conditioned medium
lowest common multiple
lymphocytic choriomeningitis
LCMG long-chain
monoglyceride
L/cm H₂O liter per centimeter
of water
LCMI left ventricular mass
index
LCN
lateral cervical nucleus
left caudate nucleus
LCNB large-core needle biopsy
LCNST late central nervous
system toxicity
LCOS low cardiac output
syndrome
LCPD Legg-Calvé-Perthes
disease
LCPS
leukocytapheresis
long-chain polysaturated (fatty
acid)
long, closed, posterior
(cervix)

199

LCPUFA long-chain polyunsaturated fatty acid

LCR
laryngeal cough reflex test
ligamentous and capsular repair
ligase chain reaction

LCS
laser correlational spectroscopy
lateral crural steal
Leydig cell stimulation
lichen chronicus simplex
low constant (continuous) suction
low-contact stress

LCSS Lung Cancer Symptom Score

LCT
Leydig cell tumor
liquid crystal thermography
liver cell tumor
long-chain triglyceride
lung capillary time
lymphocytotoxin

LCTA lungs clear to auscultation

LCU laparoscopic contact ultrasonography

LCV
leukocytoclastic vasculitis
low cervical vertical (incision)

LCVA left hemisphere cerebrovascular accident

LCVP laser coagulation vaporization procedure

LD
labyrinthine defect
learning disability
Legionnaire disease
Leishman-Donovan (body)
lethal dose
lichenoid dysplasia
light-dark
light differentiation
light duty
linear dichroism
linguodistal
lipodystrophy
liver disease
living donor

loading dose
Lombard-Dowell (agar)
Lyme disease
lymphocyte depletion

L&D
labor and delivery
light and distance (in ophthalmology)

L:D light to dark amplitude ratio

LD$_{50}$ median lethal dose (lethal for 50% of test subjects)

LD$_{50/30}$ dose that is lethal dose for 50% of test subjects within 30 days

LD$_{100}$ lethal dose in all exposed subjects

LDA
laser Doppler anemometry
lateral disc attachment
left dorsoanterior (fetal position)
limiting dilution analysis
linear discriminant analysis
low density area

LDAR latex direct agglutination reaction

LDB
lamb dysentery bacillus
Legionnaire disease bacillus
ligand-binding domain

LDC
leukocyte differential count
lymphoid dendritic cell

L-DC Langerhans-dendritic cell

LDCI low-dose continuous infusion

LDD
laser disc decompression
lead locking device
light-dark discrimination
low drain (class) D

LDDS local dentist

LD-EYA Lombard-Dowell egg yolk agar

LDF
laser Doppler flowmetry
limit dilution factor
lumbodorsal fascia

LDG lingual developmental groove

LDH
lactate dehydrogenase
lactic (acid) dehydrogenase
low-dose heparin

LDIH left direct inguinal hernia

LDIR low-dose of ionizing radiation

LDI-TOF-MS laser desorption/ionization time-of-flight-mass spectrometer

LDL
loudness discomfort level
low-density lipoprotein

LDLA low-density lipoprotein apheresis

LDL-C low-density lipoprotein-cholesterol

LDLT living donor liver transplantation

LDM lactate dehydrogenase, muscle

LDMA lymphocyte detected membrane antigen

LDN laparoscopic donor nephrectomy

LD-NEYA Lombard-Dowell neomycin egg yolk agar

LDNF lung-derived neurotrophic factor

L-DOPA, l-dopa levodopa

LDP
late diastolic potential
left dorsoposterior (fetal position)

LDR
labor, delivery, and recovery
length to diameter ratio
long-duration response
low-dose rate

LDRP labor, delivery, recovery, postpartum

LDS
late dumping syndrome
ligate-divide-staple

LDSST low-dose short synacthen test

LDT left dorsotransverse (fetal position)

LDV
large dense-cored vesicle
laser Doppler velocimetry
lateral distant view

LE
left ear (*See also* A.S.)
left eye (*See also* O.L., O.S.)
lens extraction
leukocyte esterase
leukoerythrogenic
live embryo
lupus erythematosus (cell)

Le
Lewis antibody
Lewis number (diffusivity:diffusion coefficient of a fluid)

LEA
lower extremity amputation
lumbar epidural anesthesia

LEAD lower extremity arterial disease

LEADER Lightweight Epidemiological Advanced Detection and Emergency Response (System)

LEAP
latex ELISA for antigen protein
lens epithelial cell
leukoencephalitis
Lewis expandable adjustable prosthesis
low-energy charged (particle)

LEC Life Experiences Checklist

LECP low-energy charged particle

LED
light-emitting diode
lowest effective dose
lupus erythematosus disseminatus

LEDC low energy direct current

LEEDS low-energy electron diffraction spectroscopy

LEEP loop electrocautery excision procedure

LEF
lower extremity fracture
lupus erythematosus factor

LEFS Lower Extremity Functional Scale

leg com
legal commitment
legally committed

LEIS low-energy ion scattering

LEJ ligation of esophagogastric junction

LEL
low-energy laser
lowest effect level (of toxicity)

LEM
lateral eye movement
Leibovitz-Emory medium
light electron microscope

LEMO lowest empty molecular orbital

LEMS Lambert-Eaton myasthenic syndrome

LENI lower extremity noninvasive (procedure)

lenit.
gently [L. *leniter*]
lenitive

LEOD lens extraction, oculus dexter (right eye)

LEOPARD lentigines, electrocardiographic (conduction abnormalities), ocular (hypertelorism), pulmonary (stenosis), abnormal (genitalia), retardation (of growth), and deafness (syndrome)

LEOS lens extraction, oculus sinister (left eye)

LEP
leptospirosis
lethal effective phase (leptospirosis)
limited English proficiency
lipoprotein electrophoresis

low egg passage (strain of virus)
lower esophageal pressure

L$_{EPN}$ effective perceived noise level

LEPT leptocyte

LEPTOS leptospirosis agglutinins

Leq loudness equivalent

LERG local electroretinogram

LES
Lawrence Experimental Station (agar)
lesser esophageal sphincter
Life Experience Survey
Locke egg serum (medium)
lower esophageal sphincter
low excitatory state
lumbar epidural steroids
lupus erythematosus, systemic

LESEP lower extremity somatosensory evoked potential

LESS lateral electrical spine stimulation

LET
language enrichment therapy
left esotropia
leukocyte esterase test
lidocaine, epinephrine, tetracaine (topical ansthesia)
linear energy transfer
low energy transfer

LETZ loop excision of the transformation zone

LEU leukocyte equivalent unit

Leu leucine (*See also* L)

leuk, leuko leukocyte

LEV
levator (muscle)
lower extremity venous

LF
labile factor
laparoscopic fundoplication
laryngofissure
Lassa fever
latex fixation
lethal factor
ligamentum flavum
lingual fossa

living female
low-fat (diet)
low frequency

Lf

limes flocculation (unit, dose
of toxin per mL)
limit of flocculation

LFA

left frontoanterior (fetal
position)
leukotactic factor activity
low friction arthroplasty
lymphocyte function-associated
antigen

LFAC low frequency alternating
current

LFB

lingual-facial-buccal
liver, iron, and B complex
low frequency band

LFC

lateral femoral cutaneous
living female child
low fat and cholesterol (diet)

LFCS low flap cesarean section

LFCT lung-to-finger circulation
time

LFD

lactose-free diet
large for dates
late fetal death
lateral facial dysplasia
least fatal dose
low-fat diet
low-fiber diet
low forceps delivery
lunate fossa depression

LFER linear free-energy
relationship

LFF low-filter frequency

LFH left femoral hernia

LFIT low-friction ion treatment
(prosthesis)

LFL left frontolateral

LFLA lactoferrin latex bead
agglutination

LFM

laser flare meter
lateral force microscopy

LFN lactoferrin

LFOV large field of view

LFP left frontoposterior position
(fetal)

LFPPV low-frequency positive
pressure ventilation

LFS

lateral facet syndrome
leukemia-free survival
limbic forebrain structure

LFT

lateral femoral torsion
latex flocculation test
left frontotransverse (fetal
position)
liver function test
localized fibrous tumor
low flap transverse
low-frequency tetanic
(stimulation)
low-frequency transduction
low-frequency transfer

LFU

lipid fluidity unit
lost to follow-up

LFV

large field of view
low-frequency ventilation

L fx linear fracture

L-G Lich-Gregoire
(ureteroneocystostomy)

LG

lactoglobulin
lamellar granule
large
laryngectomy
lateral ground
lingual groove
linguogingival
lipoglycopeptide
liver graft
low glucose
lymph gland
lymphocytic gastritis
lymphography

LGA

large for gestational age
left gastric artery
low-grade astrocytoma

LGB
  Landry-Guillain-Barré
    (syndrome)
  lateral geniculate body
LGD low-grade dysplasia
LGd dorsal lateral geniculate
    (nucleus)
LGE linear gingival erythema
LGG low-grade glioma
LGH
  lactogenic hormone
  little growth hormone
LGI
  large glucagon
    immunoreactivity
  lower gastrointestinal
LGIB lower gastrointestinal
    bleeding
LGL
  large granular leukocyte
  lobular glomerulonephritis
  low grade lymphoma
  Lown-Ganong-Levine
    (syndrome)
LGMD limb-girdle muscular
  dystrophy
LGN
  lateral geniculate nucleus
  lobular glomerulonephritis
LG-NHL low-grade non-Hodgkin
  lymphoma
LGP labioglossopharyngeal
LGS
  Langer-Giedion syndrome
  limb-girdle syndrome
  low Gomco suction
LGSIL low-grade squamous
  intraepithelial lesion
LGV
  large granular vesicle
  lymphogranuloma venereum
LgX lymphogranulomatosis X
LH
  lateral hypothalamus
  learning handicap
  loop of Henle
  lower half
  lues hereditaria (hereditary
    syphilis)
  luteinizing hormone
  lutropin
L/H lymphocytic/histiocytic (cell)
LHA
  lateral hypothalamic area
  left hepatic artery
LHB long head of biceps
LHb lateral habenular
LHBT lactose hydrogen breath
  testing
LHBV left heart blood volume
LHC
  Langerhans cell histiocytosis
  left heart catheterization
  left hypochondrium
LHCG luteinizing hormone-
  (human) chorionic
  gonadotropin (hormone)
LHD
  lateral head displacement
  left-hand dominant
  left hemisphere (brain)
    damage
LHF
  left heart failure
  ligament of head of femur
LHFA lung Hageman factor
  activator
LH-FSH luteinizing
  hormone/follicle-stimulating
  hormone
LH/FSH-RF luteinizing
  hormone/follicle-stimulating
  hormone-releasing factor
LHH left homonymous
  hemianopia
LHL
  left hemisphere lesion
  left hepatic lobe
LHN lateral hypothalamic
  nucleus
LHON Leber hereditary optic
  neuropathy
LHP
LHPZ lower (esophageal) high-
  pressure zone
LH-RF luteinizing hormone-
  releasing factor
LH-RH luteinizing hormone-
  releasing hormone

LHS
  long-handled sponge
  lymphatic and hematopoietic
    system
LHT left hypertropia
LI
  lactose intolerance
  lacunar infarction
  lamellar ichthyosis
  laser iridotomy
  learning impaired
  linguoincisal
  liver involvement
  loop ileostomy
Li
  labrale inferius
  lithium
LIA
  laser interference acuity
  local infiltrative anesthesia
  lock-in amplifier
  lysine-iron agar
LIB left in bottle
LIBC latent iron-binding
  capacity
LIC
  left iliac crest
  limiting isorrheic concentration
LICA
  laser image custom
    arthroplasty
  left internal carotid artery
LICU laparoscopic intracorporeal
  ultrasound
LID
  late immunoglobulin
    deficiency
  lymphocytic infiltrative disease
LIDC low-intensity direct
  current
LIDO lidocaine
LIE
  labioincisal edge
  linguoincisal edge
LIF
  laser-induced fluorescence
  leukemia-inhibiting factor
  leukocyte infiltration factor
  leukocyte inhibitory factor

  leukocytosis-inducing factor
  liver (migration) inhibitory
    factor
  local intraarterial fibrinolysis
LIFE
  laser-induced fluorescence
    emission
  lung imaging fluorescent
    endoscopy
LIFEC lumbar intersomatic
  fusion expandable cage
L-IFN human lymphoblastoid
  interferon
LIFS laser-induced fluorescence
  spectroscopy
LIFT laser-assisted internal
  fabrication technique
LIG
  leukemia inhibitory factor
  lymphocyte immune globulin
lig
  ligament, ligamentum (*See
    also* L)
  ligate
ligg ligaments, ligamenta (plural)
LIH
  laparoscopic inguinal
    herniorrhaphy
  left inguinal hernia
LIHA low impulsiveness, high
  anxiety
LIJ left internal jugular
LILA low impulsiveness, low
  anxiety
LILI low-intensity laser
  irradiation
LIM
  boundary [L. *limes*] (*See also*
    L)
  limited toxicology screening
LIMA left internal mammary
  artery (graft)
LIN laryngeal intraepithelial
  neoplasia
lin
  linear
  liniment
LINAC linear accelerator
  (system)

LINCL late infantile neural ceroid lipofuscinosis

ling
lingual (*See also* L)
lingular

LIO
laser-indirect ophthalmoscope
left inferior oblique (muscle)

LIOU laparoscopic intraoperative ultrasound

LIP
lipoid interstitial pneumonitis
lymphocytic interstitial pneumonia (pneumonitis)

LIPA
line probe assay
lysosomal acid lipase A

LIPB lysosomal acid lipase B

LIPV left inferior pulmonary vein

LIQ lower inner quadrant

liq liquid [L. *liquor*]

liq oz liquid ounce

LIS
lateral intercellular space
left intercostal space
lobular in situ (carcinoma)
locked-in syndrome
low intermittent suction
low ionic strength
lung injury score

LISL laser-induced intracorporeal shock wave lithotripsy

LISS low ionic strength solution (medium test)

LIT
literature
liver injury test

LITA left internal thoracic artery

LITH lithotomy

litho lithotripsy

LITT laser-induced thermography

LITx liver and intestinal transplantation

LIV
law of initial value
liver
louping ill virus

liv live

LIVC left inferior vena cava

LJ left jugular

LJL lateral joint line

LJM
limited joint mobility
Löwenstein-Jensen medium

LJP localized juvenile periodontitis

LK
left kidney
lichenoid keratosis

LKPD Lillehei-Kaster pivoting disc

LKS liver, kidneys, and spleen

LKSB liver, kidneys, spleen, and bladder

LKTx liver and kidney transplantation

LKV laked kanamycin vancomycin (agar)

LL
laser lithotripsy
lateral lemniscus
lepromatous leprosy
Lewandowski-Lutz (syndrome)
lid lag
lines (plural)
long leg
loudness level
lumbar laminectomy
lumbar length

L1–L5 first through fifth lumbar vertebrae or lumbar nerve

L&L lids and lashes

LLA
lids, lashes, and adnexa
limulus lysate assay

L lat left lateral

LLB
left lower border
long leg brace
lower lobe bronchus

LLC
labrum-ligament complex
laparoscopic laser cholecystectomy
Lewis lung carcinoma
liquid-liquid chromatography

long leg cast
lymphocytic leukemia, chronic
LLD
left lateral decubitus
(position)
limb length discrepancy
liquid-liquid distribution
long-lasting depolarization
LLDF *Lactobacillus lactis*
Dorner factor (vitamin B_{12})
LLE
left lower extremity (*See also*
LLX)
Little League elbow
LLETZ large loop excision of
transformation zone
LLF
Laki-Lorand factor (factor
XIII)
left lateral femoral (site of
injection)
left lateral flexion
LLFG long leg fiberglass (cast)
LLG left lateral gaze
LLI leg length inequality
LLLE lower lid, left eye (*See
also* LLOS)
LLLI La Leche League
International
LLLL lids, lashes, lacrimals,
lymphatics
LLLT low-level laser therapy
LLNA local lymph-node assay
LLO
Legionella-like organism
lower limb orthosis
LLOD
lower lid, oculus dexter
(right eye) (*See also* LLRE)
lower limit of detection
LLOS lower lid, oculus sinister
(left eye) (*See also* LLLE)
LLP
late luteal phase
long-lasting potentiation
long leg plaster (cast)
lower limb prosthesis
LLPS
low-load prolonged stress

low-load prolonged stretch
low-pressure plasma spray
LLQ left lower quadrant
LLR
large local reaction
left lumbar region
LLRE lower lid, right eye (*See
also* LLOD)
LLS
lateral loop suspensor
lazy leukocyte syndrome
long leg splint
LLT left lateral thigh
LLVP left lateral ventricular
preexcitation
LLW low-level waste
LLX left lower extremity (*See
also* LLE)
LM
labiomental
lactose malabsorption
laryngeal muscle
lateral malleolus
legal medicine
lemniscus medialis
leptomeningeal
light microscope
lingual margin
linguomesial
liquid membrane
living male
lower motor (neuron) (*See
also* LMN)
lung metastases
lymphatic malformation
lm lumen
LMA
lactose malabsorption
laryngeal mask airway
left mentoanterior (fetal
position) (*See also* MLA)
limbic midbrain area
liver (cell) membrane
autoantibody
LMB
left main stem bronchus
leiomyoblastoma
LMBD lingular mandibular bony
defect

LMC
   large motile cell
   lateral motor column
   left main coronary (artery)
   left middle cerebral (artery)
   living male child
   lymphocyte-mediated cytolysis
LMCAD left main coronary
   artery disease
LMCAT left middle cerebral
   artery thrombosis
LMD
   left main disease (cardiology)
   local medical doctor
LMDF lupus miliaris
   disseminatus faciei
LME left mediolateral
   episiotomy
LMF
   left middle finger
   leukocyte mitogenic factor
lm/ft² lumen per square foot
lm-hr unlumen hour
LMI
   lateral medullary infarction
   leukocyte migration inhibition
   (assay)
LMIF leukocyte migration
   inhibition factor
L/min liter per minute
LMJA longitudinal midtarsal
   joint axis
LML
   left middle lobe
   lower midline
LMM
   Lactobacillus maintenance
   medium
   lentigo maligna melanoma
lm/m² lumen per square meter
LMN lower motor neuron (*See
   also* LM)
LMP
   last menstrual period
   left mentoposterior (fetal
   position) (*See also* MLP)
LMP-1 latent membrane protein-
   1

LMR
   left medial rectus (eye
   muscle)
   linguomandibular reflex
LMRM left modified radical
   mastectomy
LMS
   lateral medullary syndrome
   leiomyosarcoma (*See also* LS)
lm·s lumen-second
LMT
   left main trunk
   left mentotransverse (fetal
   position)
   leukocyte migration technique
   light moving touch
   luteomammotrophic (hormone)
LMTA Language Modalities
   Test for Aphasia
LMV larva migrans visceralis
LMW low molecular weight
lm/W lumen per watt
LMWD low molecular weight
   dextran
LMWH low molecular weight
   heparin
LN
   labionasal
   laminin
   latent nystagmus
   lipoid nephrosis
   lobular neoplasia
   lupus nephritis
   lymph node
LN₂ liquid nitrogen
LNA linolenic acid
LNa low sodium
LNAB large-needle aspiration
   biopsy
LNaCl low salt
LNB
   Lyme neuroborreliosis
   lymph node biopsy
LNC
   large noncleaved
   lymph node cell
LND lymph node dissection
LNF laparoscopic Nissen
   fundoplication
LNG liquified natural gas

LNH large number hypothesis
LNKS low natural killer (cell) syndrome
LNL
    lower normal limit
    lymph node lymphocyte
LNMP last normal menstrual period
LNR lymph node region
LNS
    lateral nuclear stratum
    localized nodular synovitis
    lymph node sampling
LO
    lateral oblique (x-ray view)
    linguo-occlusal
    low
    lumbar orthosis
LOA
    leave of absence
    Leber optic atrophy
    left occipitoanterior (fetal position) (*See also* OLA)
    looseness of associations
    lysis of adhesions
LOAEL lowest observed adverse effect level
LOB loss of balance
LOC loss of consciousness
LOCA low-osmolar contrast agent
LoCa low calcium (diet)
lo cal low-calorie (diet)
loc. cit. in the place cited [L. *loco citato*]
LOCD local cementoosseous dysphasia
LoCHO low carbohydrate
LoChol low cholesterol
LOCM low-osmolar contrast medium
LOCS Lens Opacification Classification System
LOD
    limit of detection
    line of duty
    logarithm of odds (method of genetics linkage analysis)
LOE left otitis externa

LOF
    leaking of fluid
    low outlet forceps (delivery)
log. logarithm
LOH
    loop of Henle
    loss of heterogeneity
    loss of heterozygosity
LOI
    level of incompetence
    level of injury
    limit of impurities
    loss of imprinting
LoK low kalium (potassium)
LOL left occipitolateral (fetal position)
LOM
    left otitis media
    limitation of movement
    loss of motion
LoNa$^+$ low sodium
LOO length of operation
LOP
    laparoscopic orchiopexy
    left occipitoposterior (fetal position) (*See also* OLP)
    left occiput posterior (fetal position) (*See also* OLP)
    level of pain
LoPro low protein
LOQ
    limit(s) of quantitation
    lower outer quadrant
LOR
    loss of resistance
    loss of righting (reflex)
LORS-1 Level of Rehabilitation Scale 1
LOS
    length of stay
    loss of sight
    low (cardiac) output syndrome
    lower oesophageal sphincter (pressure) (British)
LOT
    lateral olfactory tract
    left occipitotransverse (fetal position) (*See also* OLT)

LOV · LPO

LOV
large opaque vesicle
loss of vision
LOVA loss of visual acuity
LOWBI low-birth-weight infant
lox. liquid oxygen
LOZ lozenge
LP
lamina propria
laryngopharyngeal
latex particle
levator palati
lichen planus
ligamentum patellae
light perception
linguopulpal
lipid panel
lipoprotein
low potency
low power (microscopy)
lumbar puncture
lumboperitoneal
lung parenchyma
lung perfusion
(nucleus) lateralis posterior
L:P
acetate to pyruvate ratio
liver to plasma (concentration ratio)
lymphocyte to polymorph ratio
lymph to plasma ratio
LPc̄P light perception with projection
LPA
latex particle agglutination
left pulmonary artery
lymphocyte proliferation assay
LPB low-profile bioprosthesis
LPC
laser photocoagulation
leukocyte-poor cell
limiting precursor cell
LPD
leiomyomatosis peritonealis disseminata
low potassium dextran
low-protein diet
luteal phase defect
lymphoproliferative disease

LPDA left posterior descending artery
LPDF lipoprotein-deficient fraction
LPE lower partially edentulous
LPEP left preejection period
LPF
leukopenia factor
lipopolysaccharide factor
liver plasma flow
localized plaque formation
low-power field
LPFN low–pass-filtered noise
LPFS low–pass-filtered signal
LPG liquified petroleum gas
LPH
left posterior hemiblock
lipotropic pituitary hormone (lipotropin)
LPHD lymphocyte-predominant Hodgkin disease
LPHS loin pain-hematuria syndrome
LPI
laser iridotomy
laser peripheral iridectomy
left posterior-inferior
leukotriene pathway inhibitor
long process of incus
LPL
lamina propria lymphocyte
laparoscopic pelvic lymphadenectomy
left posterolateral
lichen planus-like lesion
long plantar ligament
LPLC low-pressure liquid chromatography
LPLND laparoscopic pelvic lymph node dissection
LPM
latent primary malignancy
lateral pterygoid muscle
left posterior measurement
liver plasma membrane
localized pretibial myxedema
lymphoproliferative malignancy
LPO
lateral preoptic (area)
left posterior oblique

210

left posterior occipital
light perception only
lobus parolfactorius
LPOA lateral preoptic area
L POST left posterior
LPP
  lateral pterygoid plate
  leak point pressure
  lichen planopilaris
LP&P light perception and
  projection
LPPH late postpartum
  hemorrhage
LPPS low-pressure plasma-
  sprayed
LPR
  lactate-pyruvate ratio
  late-phase reaction
LPS
  last Pap smear
  levator palpebrae superioris
    (muscle)
  linear profile scan
  lipase
  lipopolysaccharide
LPSP light perception without
  projection
LPT
  lateral position test
  lipotropin
LPV lymphopathia venereum
LQ
  linear-quadratic (equation)
  longevity quotient
  lordosis quotient
  lower quadrant
LQTS long QT syndrome
LR
  laboratory reference
  labor room
  lactated Ringer (solution)
  laser resection
  lateral rectus (eye muscle)
  lateral rotation
  leishmaniasis recidivans
  light reflex
  limit of reaction
  lingual ridge
  lingual root

livedo reticularis
local recurrence
L:R left to right ratio
L-R left to right
L&R left and right
Lr
  lawrencium
  limes reacting (dose of
    diphtheria toxin)
LRD
  limb reduction defects
  living related donor
  living renal donor
LRDTx living related donor
  transplant
LRE
  lamina rara externa
  least restrictive environment
  leukemic reticuloendotheliosis
  localization-related epilepsy
LREH low renin essential
  hypertension
LRF
  left rectus femoris
  left ring finger
  local-regional failure
LRFS local recurrence-free
  survival
LRHTx living related hepatic
  transplantation
LRI
  lamina rara interna
  lower respiratory (tract)
    infection (*See also* LRTI)
LRL long radiolunate
LRM
  left radical mastectomy
  local regional metastases
LRMP last regular menstrual
  period
LRN
  laparoscopic radical
    nephrectomy
  lateral reticular nucleus
LRNA low renin, normal
  aldosterone
LRND left radical neck
  dissection
LRO long range objective

211

Lrot left rotation
LROU lateral rectus, both eyes
LRP
>laparoscopic radical
>prostatectomy
>lichen ruber planus
>locking reconstruction plate
>long-range planning
>lung-resistance protein

LRQ lower right quadrant
LRR
>labyrinthine righting reflex
>light reflection rheography

LRRFS locoregional recurrence-free survival
LRRT locoregional radiotherapy
LRS
>lactated Ringer solution
>lateral recess stenosis
>lumboradicular syndrome
>lymphoreticular system

LR-SH left-right shunt
LRT
>living-related (donor) transplantation
>local radiation therapy
>lower respiratory tract
>low-risk tumor

LRTD living relative transplant donor
LRTI lower respiratory tract infection (*See also* LRI)
LRTx
>living related transplant
>living renal transplant

LS
>lateral septal
>lateral suspensor (ligament)
>legally separated
>leiomyosarcoma (*See also* LMS)
>light sensitive
>light sleep
>Likert scale
>liminal sensation
>linear scleroderma
>liver scan
>lower segment
>Lowe syndrome

>lumbosacral
>lung sounds

L5-S1 lumbar fifth vertebra to sacral first vertebra
L&S
>ligation and stripping (varicose veins)
>liver and spleen

L:S
>lactase to sucrase ratio
>lecithin to sphingomyelin ratio
>liver to spleen ratio

LSA
>left sacroanterior (fetal position) (*See also* SLA)
>left subclavian artery
>leukocyte-specific activity

LS&A lichen sclerosus et atrophicus
LSB
>long spike burst
>lower sternal border
>lumbar spinal block
>lumbar sympathetic block

LSC
>last sexual contact
>late systolic click
>left-sided colon (cancer)
>lichen simplex chronicus
>liquid scintillation counting
>liquid-solid chromatography
>lower segment cesarean (section)

LSCA, LScA
>left scapuloanterior (fetal position)
>left subclavian artery

LSCM laser-scanning confocal microscopy
LSCP, LScP left scapuloposterior (fetal position)
LSCV left subclavian vein
LSD
>low-salt diet
>lysergic acid diethylamide

LSE
>lifestyle education
>living skin equivalent
>local side effect

L/sec liter per second
LSed level of sedation
LSEP left somatosensory evoked
  potential
LSF
  line-spread function
  low saturated fat
  lymphocyte-stimulating factor
LSG
  labial salivary gland
  lymphoscintigraphy
LSH
  laparoscopic supracervical
    hysterectomy
  lutein-stimulating hormone
  lymphocyte-stimulating
    hormone
LSI
  large-scale integration
  light scattering index
  Limb Salvage Index
  lumbar spine index
LSIL, L-SIL low-grade squamous
  intraepithelial lesion
LSK liver, spleen, and kidneys
LSL
  left sacrolateral (fetal
    position)
  left short leg (brace)
LSLF low sodium, low fat
  (diet)
LSM
  laser scanning microscope
  late systolic murmur
  lifestyle modification
LSMT life-sustaining medical
  treatment
LSO
  lateral superior olive (of
    brain)
  left salpingo-oophorectomy
  left superior oblique
  lumbosacral orthosis
LSP
  left sacroposterior (fetal
    position) (*See also* SLP)
  liver-specific protein
LSp life span

LS-PACS low-speed picture
  archive and communication
  system
L-spine lumbar spine
LSR laser skin resurfacing
LSS
  lexical-syntactic syndrome
  limb sparing surgery
  liver-spleen scan
  lumbar spinal stenosis
  scapholunate ligament
LSSS Liverpool Seizure Severity
  Scale
LST
  laser tomography scanner
  lateral spinothalamic tract
  left sacrotransverse (fetal
    position) (*See also* SLT)
  lysis, storage, and
    transportation
Ls & Ts lines and tubes
LSU lactose-saccharose-urea
  (agar)
LSV lateral sacral vein
LSVC left superior vena cava
LSW left-sided weakness
LSWA large amplitude, slow
  wave activity (in EEG)
LT
  (heat-)labile toxin
  laminar tomography
  length-tension curve
  less than
  lethal time
  Levin tube
  levothyroxine
  low transverse
  lues test
  lumbar traction
  lung transplantation
  lunotriquetral
  lymphotoxin
LT3, LT$_3$ liothyronine
LT4, LT$_4$
  levothyroxine
  l-thyroxine
LTA
  laryngeal tracheal anesthesia
  laryngotracheal applicator

LTA *(continued)*
  lateral thoracic arteries
  local tracheal anesthesia
LTAF local tissue advancement flap
LTB
  laparoscopic tubal banding
  laryngotracheobronchitis
  life-threatening behavior
LTC
  lateral talocalcaneal ligament
  long thick closed (cervix)
  low transverse cesarean
  lysed tumor cell
LTCF long-term care facility
LTCS low transverse cervical (cesarean) section
LTD
  largest tumor dimension
  Laron-type dwarfism
  leg transfer device
  limited
  long-term disability
LTE laryngotracheoesophageal
LTF
  lipotropic factor
  lost to followup
  lymphocyte-transforming factor
LTFU long-term follow-up
LTG low-tension glaucoma
LTH
  local tumor hyperthermia
  low-temperature holding (pasteurization)
  luteotropic hormone
LTK laser thermal keratoplasty
LTL laparoscopic tubal ligation
LTM long-term memory
LTP
  laryngotracheoplasty
  laser trabeculoplasty
LTR
  laryngotracheal reconstruction
  local twitch response
  long terminal repeat (sequence)
  lower trunk rotation
  lymphocyte transfer reaction
LTRA leukotriene receptor antagonist

LTS
  laparoscopic tubal sterilization
  laryngotracheal stenosis
  long tract sign (neurology)
LTT
  lactose tolerance test
  lateral tibial torsion
  leucine tolerance test
  limited treadmill test
LTx lung transplant
LU
  left upper (limb)
  left ureteral
  loudness unit
  lung (*See also* L)
L&U lower and upper (extremities)
Lu lutetium
LUE left upper extremity
LUFS luteinized unruptured follicle syndrome
LUL
  left upper (eye)lid
  left upper limb
  left upper lobe (lung)
  left upper lung
LUO left ureteral orifice
LUOB left upper outer buttock
LUOQ left upper outer quadrant
LUP
  left ureteropelvic (junction)
  low urethral pressure
LUPP laser uvulopalatoplasty
LUQ left upper quadrant
LURD living unrelated donor
LUS
  laparoscopic ultrasound
  lower uterine segment
LUSB
  left upper scapular border
  left upper sternal border
LUST lower uterine segment transverse (cesarean section)
LUT lower urinary tract
LUTT lower urinary tract tumor
LV
  Lactobacillus viridescens
  lactoovovegetarian

laryngeal vestibule
left ventricle
left ventricular
 (echocardiography images)
liquid ventilation
low vertical
low volume
lumbar vertebra
lung volume

LVA
left vertebral artery
low vision aid

LVAD left ventricular assist
device

LV Angio left ventricular
angiogram

LVBP left ventricle bypass
pump

LVC
laser vision correction
low-viscosity cement

LVCS low vertical cesarean
section

LVD
left ventricular dimension
left ventricular dysfunction

LVDP left ventricular diastolic
pressure

LVE
left ventricular ejection
left ventricular enlargement

LVED left ventricular end
diastole

LVEF left ventricular ejection
fraction

LVF
left ventricular failure
left ventricular function
left visual field
low-voltage foci

LVFA low-voltage fast activity

LVG
left ventriculogram
left ventrogluteal

LVH left ventricular
hypertrophy

LVI
large-vessel infarction

left ventricular insufficiency
 (ischemia)
lymph vessel invasion

LVIV left ventricular inflow
volume

LVL
large volume leukapheresis
left vastus lateralis (muscle)

LVLG left ventrolateral gluteal
(injection site)

LVM
lateral ventromedial (nucleus)
left ventricular mass
lymphaticovenous malformation

LVMI left ventricular mass
index

LVMM left ventricular muscle
mass

LVN
lateral ventricular nerve
lateral vestibular nucleus

LVOT left ventricular outflow
tract

LVOV left ventricular outflow
volume

LVP
large-volume paracentesis
large-volume parenteral
 (infusion)
left ventricular pressure
levator veli palatini (muscle)

LVR
left ventricular reduction
limb vascular resistance
lung volume reduction

LVS
lateral venous sinus
live vaccine strain

LVSD left ventricular systolic
dysfunction

LVSI lymphovascular space
invasion

LVSO left ventricular systolic
output

LVSP left ventricular systolic
pressure

LVST lateral vestibulospinal
tract

LVSW left ventricular septal
  wall
LVT left ventricular tension
LVV
  left ventricular volume
  LeVeen valve
LVW
  lateral vaginal wall
  lateral ventricular width
  left ventricular wall
LVWMA left ventricular wall
  motion abnormality
LW
  lateral wall
  left (ear), warm (stimulus)
  Leri-Weill (syndrome)
  lung weight
  lung width
L/W, L&W
  Lee and White (clotting time)
  living and well
LWAQ Living with Asthma
  Questionnaire
LWD living with disease
LWK large white kidney

LWOP leave without pay
LWOT left without treatment
LWS Lowry-Wood syndrome
LX
  latex
  local irradiation
  lower extremity
lx
  larynx
  lux
LX, L0, L1 lymphatic invasion
  (TNM classification)
LXT left exotropia
LYEL lost years of expected
  life
LYM lymph
lymph lymphocyte
lyo lyophilized
LYP lactose, yeast, and peptone
  (agar)
Lys
  lysine (*See also* K)
  lysosome
lytes electrolytes

M

blood factor in the MNS blood group system
chin [L. *mentum*]
death [L. *mors*]
dullness (of sound) [L. *mutitas*]
macerate [L. *macerare*]
masked (audiology)
mega-
meta-
methionine (*See also* Met)
million
molar (concentration mol/L solution)
molar (permanent tooth)
morgan (unit of gene separation)
muscular (response to electrical stimulation of motor nerve)

MΩ megohm

m

meter
milli-
minim

M1 left mastoid
M2 right mastoid
M₁ mitral first sound (slight dullness)
M₂

mitral second sound (marked dullness)
promyelocyte

m² square meter
M/3 middle third (of long bones) (*See also* mid/3)
M₃

mitral third sound (absolute dullness)
myelocyte at third stage of maturation

m³ cubic meter
M/10 tenth molar solution
M/100 hundredth molar solution

M₄ myelocyte at fourth stage of maturation
M₅ metamyelocyte
M₆ band form in sixth stage of myelocyte maturation
M₇ polymorphonuclear neutrophil

MA

masseter
matrix
megaampere
menstrual age
mental age
mentum anterior (fetal position)
metatarsus adductus
microcytotoxicity assay
microscopic agglutination
Miller-Abbott (tube)

M/A

male, altered (animal) (*See also* MALT)
mood and/or affect

mA

meter-angle
milliampere
milliangstrom

MAA

mandibular advancement appliance
monoarticular arthritis

MAb monoclonal antibody
MABP mean arterial blood pressure
MAC

MacConkey (agar)
maximal acid concentration
membrane attack complex
minimal anesthetic concentration
minimal antibiotic concentration
minimum alveolar concentration
Minimum Auditory Capabilities Test
monitored anesthesia control

MAC *(continued)*
   multiaccess catheter
   Mycobacterium avium-
     intracellulare complex
1-MAC 1-minimum alveolar
   concentration
Mac
   Macintosh (laryngoscope
     blade)
   macula
MAC AWAKE minimal
   alveolar (anesthetic)
   concentration (patient
   recovering from general
   anesthesia able to respond to
   instructions)
MACE major adverse cardiac
   event
MACIS metastasis, age,
   completeness of resection,
   local invasion, and tumor
   size
macro
   macrocyte
   macroscopic
macro-EMG macroelectromy-
   ography
MACTAR McMaster-Toronto
   Arthritis Patient Reference
   (Disability Questionnaire)
MAD
   major affective disorder
   mandibular advancement
     device
   maximal allowable dose
   maximum accumulated dose
   maximum acid output
   mind-altering drug
   minimal average dose
   moderate atopic dermatitis
MADGE microliter array
   diagonal gel electrophoresis
MADL mobility activities of
   daily living
MADRS Medicare automated
   data retrieval system
MAE
   medical air evacuation
   moves all extremities

Multilingual Aphasia
   Examination
MAF
   macrophage-activating factor
   macrophage-agglutinating factor
   master apical file
   minimum acceptable field
   minimum audible field
MAFA movement-associated
   fetal (heart rate) accelerations
MAFO molded ankle-foot
   orthosis
MAFP maternal alpha
   fetoprotein
MAG
   medication administration
     guideline (record)
   myelin-associated glycoprotein
mag
   large [L. *magnus*]
   magnesium
   magnification
   magnify
mag cit magnesium citrate
MAGF male accessory gland
   fluid
MAGPI
   meatal advancement
     glansphalloplasty
   meatal advancement and
     glanuloplasty
mag sulf magnesium sulfate
mA-h milliampere-hour
MAHA microangiopathic
   hemolytic anemia
MAI
   microscopic aggregation index
   movement arousal index
   movement assessment of
     infants
   Mycobacterium avium-
     intracellulare
MAIN medication induced,
   autoimmune, infectious,
   neoplastic (diseases associated
   with antiphospholipid
   antibodies)
MAL
   malaria vaccine

malfunction

midaxillary line

mal

ill [L. *malum*]

maleate

MALA malarial parasites

MALAR malaria

MALDIMS matrix-assisted laser desorption and ionization mass spectrometry

MALDI-TOFMS matrix-assisted laser desorption ionization-time-of-flight mass spectrometry

malig malignant

MALL massive all layer liposuction

MALT

male, altered (animal) (*See also* M/A)

mucosa-associated lymphoid tissue

MALToma mucosa-associated lymphoid tissue lymphoma

M-Am compound myopic astigmatism

MAMC mean arm muscle circumference

MAmg medial amygdaloid (nucleus)

mA-min milliampere-minute

mammo mammogram

MAN magnocellular nucleus (of anterior neostratum)

Man mannose

man.

handful [L. *manipulus*] (*See also* manip.)

manipulate

MANCOVA multivariate analysis of covariance

mand

mandible

mandibular

MANE Morrow Assessment of Nausea and Emesis

manip.

handful [L. *manipulus*] (*See also* man.)

manipulation

MANOVA multivariate analysis of variance

MAO

maximal acid output

medical ankle orthosis

monoamine oxidase

MAODP Medic Alert Organ Donor Program

MAOI monoamine oxidase inhibitor

MAP

magnesium, ammonium, and phosphate (feline struvite stones)

mean airway pressure

mean aortic pressure

mean arterial pressure

microlithiasis alveolarum pulmonum

microtubule-associated protein

minimum audible pressure

mitogen-activating protein

monophasic action potential

morning after pill (oral contraceptives)

Multiaxial Assessment of Pain

Muma Assessment Program (student assessment)

muscle-action potential

Musical Aptitude Profile

MAR

marasmus

mean atrial rate

medication administration record

minimal angle resolution

MARE manual active-resistive exercise

MARS motion artifact rejection system

marX marker X

MAS

meconium aspiration syndrome

mesoatrial shunt

M

MAS *(continued)*
    mobile arm support
    motion analysis system
mA-s milliampere second
MASA mutant allele specific amplification
MASDA multiple allele specific diagnostic assay
MASE microsurgical extraction of sperm from epididymis
MASER microwave amplification by stimulated emission of radiation
MASH mobile Army surgical hospital
MAST
    military antishock trousers
    motion artifact suppression technique
    multiple antigen stimulation test
    multithread allergosorbent test
MAT
    maternal
    maternity
    mature
    microagglutination test
    Miller-Abbott tube
    motivation analysis test
MATPP Medical Audiologic Tinnitus Patient Protocol
MAV minute alveolar volume
MAVA multiple abstract variance analysis
max
    maxilla
    maximal
    maximum
MAX A maximum assist (assistance)
MAxL midaxillary line
MB
    Mallory body
    mammillary body
    mandible
    margin, buccal
    Marsh-Bendall (factor)
    medulloblastoma
    megabyte
    mesiobuccal

    methylene blue
    microbubble
    muscle balance
    muscle-brain
Mb
    mandible body
    myoglobin
mb millibar
MBC
    male breast cancer
    maximum bladder capacity
    maximum breathing capacity
    mesiobuccal cusp
    metastatic breast cancer
    microcrystalline bovine collagen
    minimum bactericidal concentration
MB-CK M and B subunits of creatine kinase
MBCL monocytoid B-cell lymphoma
MBCR mesiobuccal cusp ridge
MBCU metallic bead-chain cystourethrograph
MBD
    maximum bactericidal dilution
    metabolic bone disease
    methylene blue dye
    minimal brain dysfunction (syndrome)
MBDG mesiobuccal developmental groove
MBE may be elevated
MBEST modulus blipped echo-planar single-pulse technique
MBF
    meat base formula
    medullary blood flow
    muscle blood flow
    myocardial blood flow
MBFC medial brachial fascial compartment
MBFLB monaural bifrequency loudness balance
MBH medial basal hypothalamus
MBL
    medium brown loose (stool)

menstrual blood loss
minimal bactericidal level
MBM
mineral basal medium
mother's breast milk
MBNW multiple-breath nitrogen washout
MBO mesiobuccoocclusal
MbO₂ oxymyoglobin
MBP
mean blood pressure
medullary bone pain
melitensis, bovine, porcine (antigen from *Brucella melitensis*, *B. bovis* and *B. suis*)
mesiobuccopulpal
Münchhausen by proxy
myelin basic protein (assay)
MBPS multigated (cardiac) blood pool scanning
MBq megabecquerel
MBR
major breakpoint region
mesiobuccal root
methylene blue, reduced
MBRT methylene blue reduction time
MBRVO macular branch retinal vein occlusion
MBS
Martin-Bell syndrome
modified barium swallow
MBSD maple bark stripper disease
MBT
maternal blood type
mixed bacterial toxin
multiple blunt trauma
MBV mitral balloon valvotomy
MC
macroglobulinemia
male child
mass casualty
maximal concentration
medium-chain (triglyceride)
megacoulomb
megacycle
Merkel cell

mesiocervical
mesocaval (shunt)
metacarpal
metatarsocuneiform
microcirculation
midcarpal
mineralocorticoid
minilaparotomy cholecystectomy
mitotic cycle
mitral commissurotomy
molluscum contagiosum
mycelial phase (of fungi)
myocarditis
Mc mandible coronoid
mC millicoulomb
MCA
mesial contact area
middle cerebral artery
middle colic artery
motorcycle accident
multichannel analyzer
multiple congenital abnormalities
MCAT
middle cerebral artery thrombosis
myocardial contrast appearance time
MCB
midcycle bleeding
middle chamber bubbling
McB McBurney (point)
mCBF mean cerebral blood flow
MCC
metacarpocarpal (joint)
midstream clean catch (urine)
mucocutaneous candidiasis
McC
McCarthy (panendoscope)
McCoy (antibody)
McCi microcurie
MCD
mean central dose
medullary collecting duct
MCDT multiple choice discrimination test

MCE myocardial contrast echocardiography

MCF
median cleft face
medium corpuscular fragility
microcomplement fixation
most comfortable frequency
multicentric foci
myocardial contractile force

MCFA medium-chain fatty acid

MCG
magnetocardiogram
mesencephalic central gray

mcg microgram

MCH
melanin-concentrating hormone
muscle contraction headache

MCHC
maternal and child health care
mean cell hemoglobin concentration
mean corpuscular hemoglobin concentration
mean corpuscular hemoglobin count

MCI
mean cardiac index
mild cognitive impairment

MCi megacurie

mCi millicurie

MCID minimum clinically important difference(s)

MCKD multicystic kidney disease

MCL
mantle cell lymphoma
maximal comfort level
maximal containment laboratory
medial collateral ligament
midclavicular line
midcostal line
most comfortable loudness

mcL microliter (1/1,000 of a mL)

MCLL most comfortable loudness level

MCL1–MCL4 modified chest lead 1–4 (modification of V1–V4)

MCL-N midclavicular line to nipple

mcmol micromole

MCP
mean carotid pressure
metacarpophalangeal (joint)
mitotic-control protein
mucopolysaccharidoses

MCPT Monte Carlo photon transport

MCR
mesial cusp ridge
message competition ratio
metabolic clearance rate
midcarpal-radial
minor cluster region
mother-child relationship
mutation cluster region

MCS
malignant carcinoid syndrome
mesocaval shunt
microculture and sensitivity
middle coronary sinus
moderate constant suction
multiple chemical sensitivity

Mc/s megacycles per second

M-CSF macrophage colony-stimulating factor

MCSW male commercial sex worker

MCT
manual cervical traction
mean circulation time
mean colonic transit
medium-chain triglyceride
medullary collecting tubule
microwave coagulation therapy
motor coordination test
mucociliary transport

MCTC metrizamide computed tomography cisternography

MCTD mixed connective-tissue disease

MCTT mucociliary clearance time

MCU
micturating cystourethrography

midcarpal-ulnar
motor cortex unit
mcU microunit
MCUG micturating
cystourethrogram
MCV
mean cell volume
mean corpuscular volume
motor conduction velocity
mcV microvolt
MCx main circumflex (artery)
MD
macula densa
macular degeneration
maintenance dialysis
major depression
mammary dysplasia
mandibular
Mantoux diameter
Marek disease (poultry)
maternal deprivation
Meckel diverticulum
medialis dorsalis (nucleus)
mediastinal disease
mediodorsal
mesiodistal
moderately differentiated
monocular deprivation
movement disorder
muscular dystrophy
myeloproliferative disease
myocardial disease
myotonic dystrophy
Md mendelevium
MDA
manual dilatation of anus
micrometastases detection
assay
motor discriminative acuity
multivariant discriminant
analysis
right mentoanterior (fetal
position) [L.
mentodextroanterior] (*See
also* RMA)
MDAC multidose activated
charcoal
MDAD mineral dust airways
disease

MDBP mean resting diastolic
blood pressure
MDC
Major Diagnostic Category
medial dorsal cutaneous
(nerve)
minimum detectable
concentration
MDCN medial dorsal cutaneous
nerve
MDD
major depressive disorder
mean daily dose
mesial developmental
depression
MDE major depressive episode
MDF mean dominant frequency
MDH medullary dorsal horn
MDI metered-dose inhaler
MDIT mean disintegration time
MDL master drug list
MDM
medical decision making
middiastolic murmur
MDMA 3,4-methylenedioxy-
methamphetamine
mDNA mitochondrial
deoxyribonucleic acid
MDO
mentally disordered offender
mesiodistocclusal
MDP
mandibular dysostosis and
peromelia
muscular dystrophy,
progressive
right mentoposterior (fetal
position) [L. *mento-dextra
posterior*] (*See also* RMP)
MDPD maximal dose
permissible dose
MDPI maximal daily
permissible intake
MDQ minimal detectable
quantity
MDR
Medical Device Reporting
(regulation)

M

223

MDR *(continued)*
    minimum daily requirement
    multiple drug-resistant
MDRH multidisciplinary
    rehabilitation hospital
MDR-TB multidrug-resistant
    tuberculosis
MDS
    maternal deprivation syndrome
    microsurgical drill system
    minimum data set
    myelodysplastic syndrome
MDSBP mean daily supine
    blood pressure
MDSO mentally disordered sex
    offender
MDT
    maggot debridement therapy
    mast (cell) degeneration test
    mean dissolution time
    motion detection threshold
    multidisciplinary team
    multidrug therapy
    right mentotransverse (fetal
      position) [L.
      mentodextrotransverse] (*See
      also* RMT)
MDU microvascular Doppler
    ultrasonography
MDV
    multiple dose vial
    myocardial Doppler velocity
MDY month, date, year
Mdyn megadyne
ME
    macular edema
    maximal effort
    median eminence
    medical evidence
    meningoencephalitis
    metabolic and electrolyte
      (disorder)
    metabolic energy
    microembolization
    middle ear
    muscle energy
    myalgic encephalomyelitis
M:E myeloid to erythroid ratio
Me
    megakaryocytic

    menton
    methyl
ME$_{50}$ 50% maximal effect
MEA
    microwave endometrial
      ablation
    multiple endocrine
      adenomatosis
MEB muscle-eye-brain (disease)
MEC
    meconium
    median effective concentration
    middle ear canal
    minimum effective
      concentration
MED
    medial
    median
    medical
    medication
    medicine
    medium
    minimal effective dose
    minimal erythema dose
    multiple epiphyseal dysplasia
MEDEVAC medical evacuation
MEDEX, Medic military medical
    corpsmen [Fr. *medicin
    extension*]
MEDICS
    meat, eggs, dairy, invisible
      fat, condiments, snacks
    Medical Examination and
      Diagnostic Coding System
med men
    medial meniscectomy
    medial meniscus
MED NEC medically necessary
MEDS
    medications
    microsurgical extraction of
      ductal sperm
MedSurg medicine and surgery
Med Tech medical technology
MEE
    measured energy expenditure
    middle ear effusion
    multilocus enzyme
      electrophoresis
M-EEG magnetoencephalogram

MEF
maximum expiratory flow
middle ear fluid
midexpiratory flow

MEF$_{50}$ maximum expiratory flow at 50% vital capacity

MEFR maximum expiratory flow rate

MEFV maximum expiratory flow volume

MEG magnetoencephalogram

MEI
medical economic index
metastatic efficiency index
middle ear implantable

MEIA microparticle capture enzyme immunoassay

MEKS Mediterranean Kaposi sarcoma

MEL
melatonin
metabolic equivalent level

MEM
(Eagle) minimum essential medium
memory

MEN
meningococcal (*Neisseria meningitidis*) (serogroups unspecified) vaccine
multiple endocrine neoplasia

men. meninx, pl. meninges

MENS microamperage electrical nerve stimulation

menst
menstrual
menstruate

MEP
maximum expiratory pressure
mean effective pressure
motor end plate
motor evoked potential
multimodality evoked potential

MEPAS mobility assist for paralyzed, amputee, and spastic (patients)

MEPS means-end problem solving

mEq milliequivalent

mEq/L milliequivalent per liter

MER
mean ejection rate
medical evidence of record
motor-evoked response
multimodality-evoked response

MERAC musculoskeletal evaluation, rehabilitation and conditioning

MERG macular electroretinogram

MERRF myoclonus epilepsy with ragged red fibers

MES
maintenance electrolyte solution
maximal electroshock seizure
mesial
myoelectric signal

Mes mesencephalon

MESA microsurgical epididymal sperm aspiration

MeSH Medical Subject Heading

MESI Mangled Extremity Syndrome Index

MESP maximal exercise systolic pressure

MESS Mangled Extremity Severity Score

MET
medical emergency treatment
metamyelocyte
metastasis
midexpiratory time
minimum elicitation threshold
multistage exercise test

Met methionine (*See also* M)

met metallic (chest sounds)

meth methamphetamine (*See also* crystal meth)

METS
metabolic equivalents (multiples of resting oxygen consumption)
metastases
Metzenbaum (scissors)

MEV maximal exercise ventilation

MeV megaelectron volt

MEWDS multiple evanescent white dot syndrome

MF
magnification factor
medium frequency
megafarad
melamine-formaldehyde (resin)
mesial facial
microfilament
multifactorial
multiplication factor
mutation frequency
mycosis fungoides
myelofibrosis
myocardial fibrosis
myofibrillar

M:F
male to female ratio
moment to force ratio

Mf
maxillofrontal
microfilaria

mF millifarad

MFA
malaise, fatigue, and anorexia
multifocal functional autonomy
multiple factor analysis
Musculoskeletal Function Assessment

MFAT multifocal atrial tachycardia

MFB
medial forebrain bundle
metallic foreign body
multiple-frequency bioimpedance

MFC
medial femoral condyle
minimal fungicidal concentration

m-FC membrane fecal coli (broth)

MFD
mandibulofacial dysostosis
midforceps delivery
milk-free diet
minimal fatal dose
monorhythmic frontal delta (EEG)

multiple fractions per day (radiotherapy)

MFF metal fume fever

MFG
magnetic field gradient
manofluorography
middle frontal gyrus

MFI
malleable facial implant
mean fluorescent intensity

M-FISH multispectral fluorescent in situ hybridization

MFM
millipore filter method
multifidus muscle

MFMN multifocal motor neuropathy

MFPR multifetal pregnancy reduction

MFPVC multifocal premature ventricular contractions

MFR
mean flow rate
midforceps rotation
myofascial release

MFRL maximal force at rest length

MFS
mitral first sound
monofixation syndrome

MFT
multifocal atrial tachycardia
muscle function test

MFU medical followup

MFVD midforceps vaginal delivery

MFVPT Motor-Free Visual Perception Test

MFW multiple fragment wounds

MG
mesiogingival
Michaelis-Gutmann (body)
muscle group
myasthenia gravis

Mg magnesium
mG milligauss
mg milligram
mg% milligram percent

MGA
>malposition of great arteries
>medical gas analyzer

MGB medial geniculate body

Mgb myoglobulin

MGC
>minimal glomerular change
>multinucleated giant cell

MgCO₃ magnesium carbonate

MGD
>meibomian gland dysfunction
>mixed gonadal dysgenesis

mg/dL milligram per deciliter

mg-el milligram-element

MGES multiple gated
equilibrium scintigraphy

MGG May-Grünwald-Giemsa
(staining)

MGH microglandular hyperplasia

mg/h milligram per hour

MGHL middle glenohumeral
ligament

MGI magnetically guided
intubation

MGJ mucogingival junction

mg/kg milligram per kilogram

mg/kg d milligram per
kilogram per day

mg/kg hr milligram per
kilogram per hour

mg/L milligram per liter

MGM maternal grandmother

MGN medial geniculate nucleus

MgO magnesium oxide

MGP
>Marcus Gunn pupil
>methyl green pyronin (dye)

MGR
>multiple gas rebreathing
>murmur, gallop, rub

MGS metric gravitational system

MGSD mean gestational sac
diameter

MgSO₄ magnesium sulfate
(Epsom salt)

mgtt minidrop (60 minidrops =
1 mL)

MGUS monoclonal gammopathy
of undetermined significance

MGW multiple gunshot wound

MGXT multistage graded
exercise test

mGy milligray

MH
>macular hemorrhage
>macular hole
>malignant hyperpyrexia
>malignant hypertension
>malignant hyperthermia
>medial hypothalamus
>menstrual history
>mental health
>mutant hybrid
>myohyoid

M/H microcytic hypochromic
(anemia)

Mh mandible head

mH millihenry

MHA
>May-Hegglin anomaly
>microhemagglutination assay
>middle hepatic artery
>mixed hemadsorption
>Mueller-Hinton agar

MHA-TPA microhemagglutina-
tion-*Treponema pallidum* assay

MHb
>medial habenular
>methemoglobin
>myohemoglobin

MHC
>major histocompatibility
complex
>myosin heavy chain

m/hct microhematocrit

MHD
>maintenance hemodialysis
>maximal human dose
>mean hemolytic dose
>minimal hemolytic dilution

MHI
>Mental Health Index
(information)
>mild head injury

MHN
>Mohs hardness number
>morbus hemolyticus
neonatorum

M

mho siemens unit (ohm spelled backward)

MHP
maternal health program
monosymptomatic hypochondriacal psychosis

MHR
malignant hyperthermia resistance
maximal heart rate

MHSA microaggregated human serum albumin

MHT
meningohypophyseal trunk
multiphasic health testing

MHV
magnetic heart vector
middle hepatic vein
minimal height velocity

MHx medical history

MHz megahertz

MI
mesioincisal
myocardial infarction

MIA
medically indigent adult
missing in action

MIBI-SPECT methoxyisobutyl isonitrile single-photon emission computed tomography

MIC
maternal and infant care
methacholine inhalation challenge
microscopic
minimal isorrheic concentration
minimum inhibitory concentration

MICABG minimally invasive coronary bypass grafting

microbiol microbiology

microgram (*See also* mcg)

MID
maximum inhibiting dilution
mesioincisodistal
minimal infective dose
minimal inhibitory dilution
minimal irradiation dose

Modular Internal Distraction (orthopedics)
multiinfarct dementia

mid
middle
midposition

mid/3 middle third (of long bone) (*See also* M/3)

MIDAS
medical image display and analysis system
Medical Information Data Analysis System

MIDCAB minimally invasive direct coronary artery bypass

MID EPIS midline episiotomy

MIDI Microbial Identification System

midsag midsagittal

MIE maximum inspiratory effort

MIF
macrophage-inhibiting factor
melanocyte-inhibiting factor
merthiolate, iodine, formalin (solution)
microimmunofluorescence (test)
migration-inhibiting factor
mixed immunofluorescence
müllerian-inhibiting factor

MIg
malaria immunoglobulin
measles immunoglobulin

MIGET multiple inert gas elimination technique

MIH
minimal intermittent (dosage of) heparin
myointimal hyperplasia

Mik Mikulicz (disease, clamp)

MIL
mesial, incisal, lingual (surface)
military
mother-in-law

MIM Mendelian Inheritance in Man

MIN
medial interlaminar nucleus
mineral

minimum
minor
minute
MIN A minimal assistance (assist)
mini-FES mini functional endoscopic sinus
minilap, mini-lap minilaparotomy
mini-MUD mini matched unrelated donor (stem cell transplant)
MIO monocular indirect ophthalmoscopy
MIP
    maximum-intensity projection (radiology)
    mean intravascular pressure
    minimally invasive procedure
MIPcor coronal maximum-intensity projection
MIPS myocardial isotopic perfusion scan
MIRBI Mini Inventory of Right Brain Injury
MIRD medical internal radiation dosimetry
MIS
    melanoma in situ
    microbial identification system
    minimally invasive surgery
    moderate intermittent suction
misc
    miscarriage
    miscellaneous
MISH multiple in situ hybridization
MISS
    minimally invasive spine surgery
    modified injury severity score (scale)
MIT
    male impotence test
    mean input time
    melodic intonation therapy
    Motor Impersistence Test
    multiple injection therapy (of insulin)
MIU million International Units

mIU milli-International unit (one-thousandth of an International Unit)
MIVR minimally invasive valve repair (replacement)
MJ megajoule
mJ millijoule
MJA mechanical joint apparatus
MJL medial joint line
MJS medial joint space
MK
    menaquinone (vitamin K_2)
    myokinase
M-K McCarey-Kaufman (medium)
Mk monkey
mkat millikatal
mkat/L millikatal per liter
mkg meter-kilogram
MKS, mks meter-kilogram-second
M-L Martin-Lewis (medium)
ML
    mediolateral
    mesiolingual
    middle lobe
    midline
    motor latency
    mucolipidosis
    muscular layer
    myeloid leukemia
M:L
    maltase to lactase ratio
    monocyte-lymphocyte ratio
mL milliliter
MLA left mentoanterior (fetal position) [L. *mento-laeva anterior*] (*See also* LMA)
MLa mesiolabial
MLAB Multilingual Aphasia Battery
MLAC minimum local analgesic concentration
MLAI, MLaI mesiolabioincisal
MLAP mean left atrial pressure
MLaP mesiolabiopulpal
MLB monaural loudness balance (test)
mLb millilambert

M

MLBW moderately low birth weight

MLC
Marginal Line Calculus (Index)
mesiolingual cusp
minimum lethal concentration

MLCR mesiolingual cusp ridge

MLCT metal-to-ligand charge transfer

MLD
manual lymph drainage
masking level difference
metachromatic leukodystrophy
microsurgical lumbar discectomy
minimal lethal dose

MLD$_{50}$ median lethal dose

MLDG mesiolingual developmental groove

mL/dL milliliter per deciliter

MLE maximal likelihood estimation

MLEE multilocus enzyme electrophoresis

MLEpis
mediolateral episiotomy
midline episiotomy

MLF
medial longitudinal fasciculus
mesiolingual fossa

MLG mesiolingual groove

MLI mesiolinguoincisal

mL/kg milliliter per kilogram

MLL malignant lymphoma, lymphoblastic (type)

mL/L milliliter per liter

mL/min milliliter per minute

MLNS mucocutaneous lymph node syndrome

MLO
mediolateral oblique
mesiolinguo-occlusal

MLP
left mentoposterior (fetal position) [L. *mento-laeva posterior*] (*See also* LMP)
mesiolinguopulpal

MLR
mean length of response
middle latency response
mixed lymphocyte reaction
multiple logistic regression
myocardial laser revascularization

MLRA multiple linear regression analysis

mlRNA messenger-like RNA

MLS
Maroteaux-Lamy syndrome
middle lobe syndrome
mini lag-screw system
mucolipidoses

mL/sec milliliter per second

MLSI multiple line-scan imaging

MLST multilocus sequence typing

MLT median lethal time

MLU mean length of utterance

MLUm mean length of utterance in morphemes

MLV monitored live voice

mlx millilux

MM
macromolecule
malignant melanoma
Marshall-Marchetti (procedure for urinary incontinence)
meningococcic meningitis
methadone maintenance
micrometastases
minimal medium
mismatch
mucous membrane
multiple myeloma
muscularis mucosae

M0 to M7 FAB classification categories of acute nonlymphoblastic leukemia

M&M morbidity and mortality

Mm mandible mentum

mM millimolar

mμ millimicron (nanometer)

mm
millimeter
muscles

mm^2 square millimeter

mm^3 cubic millimeter (*See also* cu mm)

MMA
  mastitis, metritis, agalactia (syndrome)
  maxillomandibular advancement
  methyl methacrylate
  monocyte monolayer assay
MMAA mini-microaggregated albumin colloid
MMb metmyoglobin
MMC myelomeningocele
mμc millimicrocurie
MMD myotonic muscular dystrophy
MMDG mesial marginal developmental groove
MME M-mode echocardiography
MMF
  magnetomotive force
  mandibulomaxillary fixation
  maxillomandibular fixation
  mean maximal flow
MMG mechanomyography
mμg millimicrogram
mmHg millimeter of mercury
mmH₂O millimeter of water
MMK Marshall-Marchetti-Krantz (cystourethropexy)
MML
  medical markup language
  myelomonocytic leukemia
mmm micromillimeter
MMN
  mismatch negativity
  morbus maculosus neonatorum
  multifocal motor neuropathy
MMO
  maxillomandibular osteotomy
  maximal mouth opening
M-mode motion mode
mmol millimole
mmol/L millimole per liter
MMP
  matrix metalloproteinase
  multiple medical problems
MMPI
  matrix metalloproteinase inhibitor

  Minnesota Multiphasic Personality Inventory
MMR
  maternal mortality rate
  measles-mumps-rubella (vaccine)
  mesial marginal ridge
  mismatch repair
MMS Mohs micrographic surgery
mμs millimicrosecond
MMSE Mini Mental State Examination
mm/sec millimeter per second
MMTV monomorphic ventricular tachycardia
mmu millimass unit
MMV
  mandatory minute ventilation
  mandatory minute volume
MMWR Morbidity and Mortality Weekly Report
MN
  blood group in MNS blood group system
  median nerve
  meganewton
  melena neonatorum
  membranous nephropathy (neuropathy)
  mesenteric node
  mononuclear
  motor neuron
  mucosal neurolysis
  multinodular
  myoneural
M&N morning and night
Mn manganese
mN micronewton
MNA maximal noise area
MNAP mixed nerve action potential
MNCV motor nerve conduction velocity
MND
  modified neck dissection
  motor neuron disease
MNF myelinated nerve fiber
MNG multinodular goiter

MNJ myoneural junction

MN/m² meganewton per square meter

MNPRT mixed neutron and photon radiotherapy

MNS blood group system consisting of groups M, N, and MN

MnSSEP median nerve somatosensory evoked potential

MNTB medial nucleus of trapezoid body

MNX meniscectomy

MO
  medial oblique (x-ray view)
  mesioocclusal
  minute output
  molecular orbital
  morbidly obese
  myositis ossificans

Mo molybdenum

mΩ milliohm

mo month

MOA
  mechanism of action
  monoamine oxidase

MOC
  maximal oxygen consumption
  medial olivocochlear
  mother of child

MOD
  mean optical density
  mesial, occlusal, distal
  mode of death
  moderate
  moment of death
  Multi-Operatory Dentalaser
  multiorgan dysfunction

MOD A moderate assistance (assist)

MOF
  mesial occlusal facial
  multiorgan failure

MOI
  maximal oxygen intake
  mechanism of injury

MOJAC mood, orientation, judgment, affect, content

MOL molecular layer

mol mole

mole per second mole per second

mol/kg mole per kilogram

mol/L mole per liter

mol/m³ mole per cubic meter

mol wt molecular weight

MOM
  Milk of Magnesia
  multiples of median

MONO
  monocyte
  mononucleosis
  Monospot (test)

mono, di monochorionic, diamniotic (twins)

mono, mono monochorionic, monoamniotic (twins)

MORA mandibular orthopedic repositioning appliance

MORD magnetic optical rotatory dispersion

MORFAN mental retardation, pre-and postnatal overgrowth, remarkable face, acanthosis nigricans (syndrome)

morph morphine

morphol morphology

MOS
  medial orbital sulcus
  medical optical spectroscopy
  mirror optical system
  mitral opening snap

MOSF multiple organ system failure

mOsm milliosmole

mOsm/kg milliosmole per kilogram

MOT
  mini object test
  motility (examination)

MOTSA multiple overlapping thin-slab acquisition

MOTT mycobacteria other than *Mycobacteria tuberculosis*

MP
  mean pressure
  mechanical percussion
  medial plantar
  menstrual period

mentum posterior (fetal position)

mesial pit

mesiopulpal

motor potential

mouth pressure

myocardial perfusion

mp melting point

MPA

main pulmonary artery

medial preoptic area

metatarsus primus adductus

MPa megapascal

MPAP

mean pulmonary artery pressure

multipurpose access port

MPAWP mean pulmonary artery wedge pressure

MPB

male pattern baldness

modified piggyback

MPBFV mean pulmonary blood-flow velocity

MPC

maximum permissible concentration

mucopurulent cervicitis

MPCD minimal perceptible color difference

MPCh medial posterior choroidal (ophthalmology)

MPCN microscopically positive, culturally negative

MPCP mean pulmonary capillary pressure

MPCWP mean pulmonary capillary wedge pressure

MPD

maximal permissible dose

minimal peripheral dose

minimal phototoxic dose

myeloproliferative disease

MPDS

mandibular pain dysfunction syndrome

myofascial pain dysfunction syndrome

MPDW mean percentage of desirable weight

MPE

malignant pleural effusion

multiphoton excitation

MPEC

monopolar electrocoagulation

multipolar electrocoagulation

MPED minimal phototoxic erythema dose

MPF mean power frequency

MPFL medial patellofemoral ligament

MPFM mini-Wright peak flow meter

MPG magnetopneumography

MPGN

membranoproliferative glomerulonephritis (type I, II)

mesangiocapillary glomerulonephritis (type I, II)

mesangioproliferative glomerulonephritis

MPGR multiple planar gradient-recalled

MPH

male pseudohermaphroditism

midparental height

mph mile per hour

MP-H mandibular plane to hyoid (craniometric)

M phase phase of mitosis in cell growth cycle

mphot milliphot

MPHR maximum predicted heart rate

MPI myocardial perfusion imaging

MPL mesiopulpolingual

MP-L midpapillary longitudinal

MPLA, MPLa mesiopulpolabial

MPLC medium pressure liquid chromatography

MPM medial pterygoid muscle

MPO

male pattern obesity

M

MPO *(continued)*
  maximum power output
  minimal perceptible odor
MPOA medial preoptic area
MPP
  maximal perfusion pressure
  medial pterygoid plate
  multiple presentation
    phenotype
mppcf millions of particles per
  cubic foot (of air)
MPPG microphotoelectric
  plethysmography
MPPv main portal vein peak
  velocity
MPQ McGill Pain Questionnaire
MPR
  maximal pulse rate
  multiplanar reformatting
    (view)
  myeloproliferative reaction
  myocardial perfusion reserve
MPS
  mean particle size
  movement-produced stimulus
  mucopolysaccharidoses (plural)
  mucopolysaccharidosis
  myocardial perfusion
    scintigraphy
  myofascial pain syndrome
mps meter per second
MP-T midpapillary transverse
MPT
  maximal predicted phonation
    time
  multiple-parameter telemetry
  multipuncture test
MPTAH Mallory
  phosphotungstic acid
  hematoxylin (stain)
MPTh mechanical pain
  threshold
MPTR motor, pain, touch,
  reflex (deficit)
MPTS minocycline periodontal
  therapeutic system
MPV
  mean plasma volume
  mean platelet volume

  metatarsus primus varus
  mitral valve prolapse
mpz millipieze
MQ memory quotient
MQC microbiologic quality
  control
MR
  Maddox rod
  magnetic resonance
  megaroentgen
  methyl red
M&R measure and record
M$_r$
  molecular weight ratio
  relative molecular mass
Mr mandible ramus
mR milliroentgen
MRA
  magnetic resonance
    angiography
  magnetic resonance
    arteriography
mrad millirad
MRAr magnetic resonance
  arthrography
MRBF mean renal blood flow
MRC
  magnetic resonance
    cholangiogram
  magnetic resonance
    colonography
MRCA magnetic resonance
  coronary angiography
MRCP magnetic resonance
  cholangiopancreatography
MRCPs movement-related
  cortical potentials
MRD
  matched related donor
  minimal reacting dose
mRd millirutherford
MRE
  magnetic resonance
    elastography
  manual resistance exercise
  most recent episode
MRELD mixed receptive-
  expressive language disorder
mREM millirem

MRF

magnetic resonance flowmetry
mesencephalic reticular
  formation
midbrain reticular formation
mitral regurgitant flow
MRG murmur, rub, and gallop
MRH

Maddox rod hyperphoria
melanotropin-releasing hormone
MRI magnetic resonance
  imaging
MRIH melanocyte release-
  inhibiting hormone
MRL minimal response level
MRLVD maximum residue
  limits of veterinary drugs
MRM

magnetic resonance
  mammography
modified radical mastectomy
MRN

magnetic resonance
  neurography
medical record number
mRNA messenger ribonucleic
  acid
mRNP messenger
  ribonucleoprotein
MRO

minimal recognizable odor
muscle receptor organ
MRP

magnetic resonance
  pancreatography
mandibular reconstruction
  plate
MRR maximal relaxation rate
MRS magnetic resonance
  spectroscopy
MRSA methicillin-resistant
  Staphylococcus aureus
MRSE methicillin-resistant
  Staphylococcus epidermidis
MRSI magnetic resonance
  spectroscopic imaging

MRT

magnetic resonance
  tomography
milk ring test
MRTA magnetic resonance
  tomographic angiography
MRU

magnetic resonance urography
mass radiography unit
mean relational utterance
MRV

magnetic resonance
  venography
minute respiratory volume
mononuclear Reed variant
  (cell)
MRVP

mean right ventricular
  pressure
methyl red, Voges-Proskauer
  (medium)
MRX *Moraxella catarrhalis*
  vaccine
MR X 1, MRx1 may repeat
  times one (once)
MRXS1–6 X-linked mental
  retardation syndrome 1–6
MRZ measles, rubella and
  zoster (vaccine)
3MS Modified Mini-Mental
  Status (examination)
M&S microculture and
  sensitivity
MS

mass spectrometry
Meckel syndrome
melanonychia striata
menopausal syndrome
mental status
metabolic syndrome
mitral sound
mitral stenosis
mongolian spot
morning stiffness
morphine sulfate (*See also*
  MSO_4)
motile sperm
multiple sclerosis
musculoskeletal

m/s meter per second (*See also* m/sec)

m/s² meter per second squared

ms

manuscript

millisecond (*See also* msec)

MSA

mannitol salt agar

mitotic spindle apparatus

multichannel signal averager

MSAF meconium-stained amniotic fluid

MSAP mean systemic arterial pressure

MSB

mainstem bronchus

martius scarlet blue

MSC midsystolic click

MSCC midstream clean-catch (urine culture)

MSCP, mscp

MSD

male sexual dysfunction

microsurgical diskectomy

midsagittal diameter

midsleep disturbance

most significant digit

MSDBP mean sitting diastolic blood pressure

MSDS material safety data sheet

MSE mental status examination

m/sec meter per second (*See also* m/s)

msec millisecond (*See also* ms)

MSER mean systolic ejection rate

MSET multistage exercise test

MSEV microsurgical epididymovasostomy

MSF Mediterranean spotted fever

MSG monosodium glutamate

MSIS Multiple Severity of Illness System

MSK

medullary sponge kidney

musculoskeletal (*See also* MS)

MSL

mean sentence length

midsternal line

MSLT Multiple Sleep Latency Test

MSM

men (who have) sex with men

midsystolic murmur

mineral salts medium

MSN

medial septal nucleus

mildly subnormal

MSNA muscle sympathetic nerve activity

MSO

medial superior olive

mental status, oriented

MSO₄ morphine sulfate (*See also* MS)

MSP Munchausen syndrome by proxy

MSPS

musculoskeletal pain syndrome

myocardial stress perfusion scintigraphy

MSPv midshunt peak velocity

MSQ mental status questionnaire

MSS-CR mean sac size and crown-rump length

MST

maladies sexuellement transmissible (French for sexually transmitted disease)

maximum stimulation test

mean swell time (botulism test)

medial superior temporal

mental stress test

MSTA mumps skin test antigen

MSTh mesothorium

MSU

memory for symbolic unit

midstream urine (specimen)

MSUA midstream urinalysis

MSUD maple syrup urine disease

MSV
maximal sustained (level of) ventilation
mean scale value

mSv millisievert (radiation unit)

MSVC maximal sustained ventilatory capacity

MSVL maximal spatial vector to left

MSW multiple stab wounds

MT
macular target
maggot therapy
magnetization transfer
maintenance therapy
malaria therapy
Martin-Thayer (plate, medium)
medial temporal
medial thalamus
mediastinal tube
membrana tympani
microtome
microtubule
middle turbinate
multitest (plate)
muscle tone

M/T mass (or) tenderness

MT/AK music therapy/audiokinetics

MTB
methylthymol blue
Mycobacterium tuberculosis

MTBE meningeal tick-borne encephalitis

mTBI mild traumatic brain injury

MTC
magnetization transfer contrast (radiology)
metatarsocuneiform

MTCT mother-to-child transmission

MTD
Monroe tidal drainage
multiple tic disorder
Mycobacterium tuberculosis direct (test)

MTDDA Minnesota Test for Differential Diagnosis of Aphasia

mtDNA mitochondrial deoxyribonucleic acid

MTDT modified tone decay test

MTF
maximal terminal flow
mesial triangular fossa

MTG
middle temporal gyrus (gyri)
midthigh girth

MTI
magnetization transfer imaging
minimal time interval

MTL Metropolitan Life Table (for desirable weight)

MTLE medial (mesial) temporal-lobe epilepsy

MT-M multitest mycology (plate)

MTM
modified Thayer-Martin (agar)
mouth-to-mouth (resuscitation)

MTP
maximal tolerated pressure
medial tibial plateau
medical termination of pregnancy
metatarsophalangeal (joint)
multidisciplinary treatment plan

MTR
magnetization transfer ratio
mass, tenderness, rebound (abdominal examination)
Meinicke turbidity reaction

MTS moderate tactile stimulus

MTSS menstrual toxic shock syndrome

MTT
mammillothalamic tract
maximal treadmill testing
mean transit time
medial tibial torsion

MTV
maximum tolerable volume
metatarsus varus

M

MT-Y multitest yeast (plate)
MU
  megaunit
  million units
  motor unit
  Murphy unit
mu milliunit
MUA
  manipulation under anesthesia
  middle uterine artery
MUAC middle upper arm
  circumference
MUAP motor unit action
  potential
MUCL medial ulnar collateral
  ligament
MUCP maximum urethral
  closure pressure
MUD
  matched unrelated donor
  minimal urticarial dose
MUDDLES miosis, urination,
  diarrhea, diaphoresis,
  lacrimation, excitation (CNS),
  salivation (cholinesterase
  inhibitor effects)
MUDPILES methanol or
  metformin; uremia, diabetic
  ketoacidosis, phenformin,
  paraldehyde, iron or isoniazid
  or ibuprofen, lactic acidosis,
  ethanol or ethylene glycol,
  salicylates or sepsis (causes
  of metabolic acidosis)
MUFA monounsaturated fatty
  acid
MUGA multiple gated
  acquisition
MUGEx multiple gated (blood
  pool scan during) exercise
MUGR multiple gated (blood
  pool image at) rest
MUGS, MUGUS monoclonal
  gammopathy of undetermined
  (unknown) significance
mulibrey muscle, liver, brain,
  eye (disease)
mult multiple
multiorgan dysfunction
multip multiparous

MUP
  maximal urethral pressure
  motor unit potential
MUPIT Martinez universal
  interstitial template
MURD matched unrelated donor
MUSE medicated urethral
  system for erection
mus-lig musculoligamentous
MUST medical unit, self-
  contained and transportable
MV
  measles virus
  mechanical ventilation
  megavolt
  microvillus
  midventricular
  mitral valve
  multivesicular
  multivessel
mV millivolt
MVA
  manual vacuum aspiration
  mechanical ventricular
    assistance
  mevalonic acid
  microvascular angiopathy
  microvillus atrophy
  mitral valve area
  motor vehicle accident
MV·A megavolt-ampere
mV·A millivolt-ampere
MVB
  manual ventilation bag
  mixed venous blood
  multivesicular body
MVC
  maximal vital capacity
  maximal voluntary contraction
  microvessel count
  minute virus of canines
  motor vehicle collision (crash)
  myocardial vascular capacity
MVc mitral valve closure
MVD
  microvascular decompression
  microvessel density
  mitral valve disease
  multivessel (coronary) disease
  myocardial vasodilation

MVE
    mitral valve echo
    mitral valve (leaflet)
        excursion
    Murray Valley encephalitis
MVG, MVgrad mitral valve
    gradient
MVL mitral valve leaflet
MVLS mandibular
    vestibulolingual sulcoplasty
MVM
    medullary venous
        malformation
    microvillous membrane
MVMT movement
MVN
    medial ventromedial nucleus
    medial vestibular nucleus
MVO mitral valve opening
    (orifice)
mVO$_2$ minimal venous oxygen
    (consumption)
MVO2, MVO$_2$
    maximal venous oxygen
        (consumption)
    myocardial ventilation, oxygen
        (rate)
    oxygen content of mixed
        venous blood
MVOA mitral valve orifice area
MVO$_2$S mixed venous oxygen
    saturation
MVP
    mean platelet volume
    mean venous pressure
    microvascular pressure
    mitral valve prolapse
MVPS mitral valve prolapse
    syndrome
MVPT Mertens Visual
    Perception Test
MVR
    massive vitreous retractor
        (blade)
    maximal ventilation rate
    microvitreoretinal
    minimal vascular resistance
    mitral valve regurgitation

MVS
    mitral valve stenosis
    motor, vascular, and sensory
mV-sec millivolt-second
MVU Montevideo units (uterine
    contractions)
MVV
    maximal ventilatory volume
    maximum voluntary ventilation
    mixed vespid venom
MW
    mean weight
    megawatt
mW milliwatt
mw microwave
MWB minimal weight bearing
mWb milliweber
MWC Monod-Wyman-Changeux
    (anesthetics model)
MWD
    maximum walking distance
    microwave diathermy
    molecular weight distribution
M-W-F Monday-Wednesday-
    Friday
MWP mean wedge pressure
MWT
    maintenance of wakefulness
        test
    Mallory-Weiss tear
    malpositioned wisdom teeth
    maximum walking time
6-MWT 6-minute walking test
MX matrix
Mx
    mastectomy
    maxillary
    maxwell (magnetic flux)
    multiple
MX, M0, M1 metastases (TNM
    classification)
My
    myopia
    myxedematous
mycol mycology
MYD mydriatic
myel myelin
myelo myelogram
myg myriagram

M

myL myrialiter
mym myriameter
myo myocardium
MyoD myogenic regulatory protein (family of genes)
myop myopia
MYS medium yellow soft (stools)
MZ monozygotic (twin)
M_z longitudinal magnetization

m:z mass to charge ratio
MZA monozygotic (twins raised) apart
MZL
   mantle zone lymphoma
   marginal zone (cell) lymphoma
   marginal zone lymphocyte
MZT monozygotic (twins raised) together

N

antigenic determinant of erythrocytes
asparagine (*See also* Asn)
inherited blood factor in MNS blood group
nasion
negative (*See also* neg)
neutron number
newton
nitrogen
normality (equivalent/liter)
north
nucleus
number (quantity of)
refractive index (*See also* ref ind, RI)

$\overline{n}$ mean value of n for a number of observations (in statistics)

n
haploid chromosome number
nano- (prefix)
nerve
2n diploid chromosome number
3n triploid chromosome number
4n tetraploid
n_0 Loschmidt number
0.02N fiftieth-normal (solution)
0.1N tenth-normal (solution)
0.5N half-normal (solution)
2N double-normal (solution)
N=1 trial number equal to one; single patient trial
N2O:O2 nitrous oxide to oxygen ratio
N2Or nitrous oxider
NA
Avogadro number (*See also* L)
neurologic age
Nomina Anatomica
normal axis
nosocomially acquired
nuclear antibody
nuclear antigen

nucleic acid
nucleus accumbens (septi)
nucleus ambiguus
N&A normal and active
N/A
no alternative
not applicable
N.A. numerical aperture
Na sodium [L. *natrium*]
nA nanoampere
NAA no apparent abnormalities
NAAC no apparent anesthetic complication
NAAP National Arthritis Action Plan
NAAT nucleic acid amplification techniques (testing)
NAB
nonweightbearing ambulation
not at bedside
NABS normoactive bowel sounds
NABX needle aspiration biopsy
NAC
accessory nucleus (Monakow nucleus)
nerve-approximating clamp
nipple-areola complex
no acute changes
NACD no anatomical cause of death
NaCl sodium chloride (salt)
NaClO sodium hypochlorite
NACT neoadjuvant chemotherapy
NAD
no abnormality demonstrable
no active disease
no acute distress
no apparent distress
no appreciable disease
normal axis deviation
nothing abnormal detected
NaD sodium dialysate

NADA New Animal Drug Application
NAE net acid excretion
Na$_e$ exchangeable body sodium (natrium)
NAF
net acid flux
normal adult female
Notice of Adverse Findings (FDA post-audit letter)
NaF sodium fluoride
NaFl sodium fluorescein
NAG
narrow-angle glaucoma
nonagglutinating
NaHCO$_3$, Na HCO3 sodium bicarbonate
NAI
net acid input (urinary)
no action indicated
no acute inflammation
nonaccidental injury
nonadherence index
NaI sodium iodide
Na&K sodium and potassium (in urine)
NALL null (cell line of) acute lymphocytic leukemia
NALP neuroadenolysis of pituitary
NALS neonatal adjuvant life support
NALT nasopharyngeal-associated lymphoid tissue
NAM
Native American male
normal adult male
NANB non-A, non-B (hepatitis)
NANBNC non-A, non-B, non-C hepatitis
NANSAIDs nonaspirin nonsteroidal antiinflammatory drugs
N ant/post anterior and posterior zones (nerve cell groups—nuclei of hypothalamus)
NAP
narrative, assessment, and plan

nasion pogonion (angle of convexity in craniometrics)
nerve action potential
nosocomial acquired pneumonia
8NAP eighth nerve action potential
NaP sodium phosphate
NAPD no active pulmonary disease
NAPI Neurodevelopmental Assessment (Procedure) for Preterm Infants
NAR
nasal airway resistance
no action required
no adverse reaction
nonambulatory restraint
not at risk
NARC, narc narcotic
NAS
nasal
Neonatal Abstinence Score
neonatal air leak syndrome
no abnormality seen
no added salt
NAS-BA nucleic acid sequence-based amplification
Na-Spt sodium spot (urine test)
NASS Neonatal Abstinence Scoring System
NAT
natal
no action taken
no acute trauma
nucleic acid test (testing)
NATB NonReading Aptitude Test Battery
NATP neonatal alloimmune thrombocytopenic purpura
NAUC normalized area under the curve
NAVEL nerve, artery, vein, empty space, lymphatics (thigh anatomy)
NAW nasal antral window
NAWM normal-appearing white matter
NB
nail bed

needle biopsy
Negri bodies
nervus buccalis
neuroblast
neuroblastoma
neurometric (test) battery
newborn
nitrogen balance
non-B (hepatitis)
normoblast
nuclear bag (certain intrafusal
  muscle fiber nuclei of a
  neuromuscular spindle)
nutrient broth
Nb niobium
n.b. note well [L. *nota bene*]
NBC
nasobiliary catheter
nonbacterial cystitis
nonbattle casualty
nonbed care
nuclear, biologic, chemical
  (weapon, warfare)
NBCC nevoid basal cell
carcinoma
NBD
nasobiliary drain
necrotizing bowel disease
neurogenic bladder dysfunction
neurologic bladder dysfunction
no brain damage
NBF not breastfed
NBH new bag (bottle) hung
NBHH newborn helpful hints
NBI
neutrophil bactericidal index
no bone injury
nonbattle injury
nosocomial bacterial infection
NBIL neonatal bilirubin
nBiPAP nasal bilevel (biphasic)
positive airway pressure
NBM
no bowel movement
normal bone marrow
normal bowel movement
nucleus basalis of Meynert

NBN
narrow band noise
newborn nursery
NBNC CLD non-B, non-C
chronic liver disease
NBP
needle biopsy of prostate
no bone pathology
nonbacterial prostatitis
NBQC narrow-base quad cane
NBR no blood return
NBS
neonatal Bartter syndrome
New Ballard Score
newborn screen (serum
  thyroxine and
  phenylketonuria)
no bacteria seen
normal blood serum
normal bowel sounds
normal brain stem
NBT
nitroblue tetrazolium (test)
normal breast tissue
NBTNF newborn, term, normal,
female
NBTNM newborn, term, normal,
male
NBW normal birth weight
NC
nasal cannula
nasal clearance
nerve conduction
neural crest
neurocirculatory
neurogenic claudication
nevus comedonicus
noise criterion
noncontributory
normocephalic
N:C nuclear to cytoplasmic
ratio
nC nanocoulomb
NCA
neurocirculatory asthenia
neutrophil chemotactic activity
no congenital abnormalities
nuclear cerebral angiogram

N

NCAM, N-CAM nerve-cell
adhesion molecule
N/CAN nasal cannula
NCAP nasal continuous airway
pressure
NCAT, NC/AT normocephalic
and atraumatic
NCB
natural childbirth
needle core biopsy
no code blue
NCC
noncoronary cusp
nucleus caudalis centralis
nursing care card
nursing care continuity
NCCP noncardiac chest pain
NCCT noncontrast helical
computed tomography
NCD
neck-capsule distance
neurocirculatory dystonia
no congenital deformities
normal childhood diseases
not considered disabling
Nursing-Care Dependency
(scale)
NCE
negative contrast
echocardiography
nonconvulsive epilepsy
NCGL nucleus corporis
geniculati lateralis
NCI
nuclear contour index
nucleus colliculi inferioris
nursing care integration
nCi nanocurie
NCIS nursing care information
sheet
NCIT Nursing Care Intervention
Tool
NCJ needle catheter jejunostomy
NCM nailfold capillary
microscope
N/cm^2 newton per square
centimeter
NCNC normochromic,
normocytic

NCP
nonclonogenic proliferating
(cells)
noncollagen protein
noncontrast phase
nursing care plan
NCPAP, n-CPAP nasal
continuous positive airway
pressure
NCPB neurolytic celiac plexus
block
NCPE noncardiogenic pulmonary
edema
NCPF noncirrhotic portal
fibrosis
NCPR no cardiopulmonary
resuscitation
NCRC nonchild-resistant
container
NCS
nasal congestion score
nerve conduction study
not clinically significant
numb chin syndrome
NCT
neoadjuvant chemotherapy
nerve compression test
nerve conduction test
neutron capture therapy
noncontact tonometer
number connection test
NCV
nerve conduction velocity
nuclear venogram
ND
nasoduodenal
nasolacrimal duct
neck dissection
neoplastic disease
neurologic development
neuropsychologic deficit
Newcastle disease (poultry)
new drug
nondiabetic
none detectable
normal dose
nucleus of Darkschewitsch
nurse's diagnosis
N/D no defects
Nd neodymium

NDA New Drug Application
NDC nondifferentiated cell
NDD no-dialysis days
NDE near-death experience
NDF
neutral density filter (test)
no disease found
NDI nephrogenic diabetes insipidus
NDIRS nondispersive infrared spectrometer
NDM neonatal diabetes mellitus
N dm/vm nucleus dorsomedialis-ventromedialis
N/D NHL nodular/diffuse non-Hodgkin lymphoma
NDR
neonatal death rate
normal detrusor reflex
nucleus dorsalis raphe
NDS
Neurologic Disability Score
New Drug Submission
NDST neurodevelopmental screening test
NDT
nasal duodenostomy tube
neurodevelopmental treatment (physical therapy)
noise detection threshold
nondestructive testing
NDx nondiagnostic
Nd:YAG neodymium:yttrium-aluminum-garnet (surgical laser)
Nd:YLF neodymium: yttrium-lithium-fluoride (laser)
NE
national emergency
nausea and emesis
neonatal encephalopathy
nerve excitability (test)
neuroendocrine
neuroepithelium
neurologic examination
not elevated
not enlarged
not equal
not evaluated
not examined
nutcracker esophagus
Ne neon
NEA no evidence of abnormality
NEAA nonessential amino acid
NEAT nonexercise activity thermogenesis
NEB
nebulizer
neuroendocrine body
NEC
Neurologic Examination for Children
no essential change
noise equivalent count
not enough cells
nec necessary
NECT nonenhanced computed tomography
NED
no evidence of disease
normal equivalent deviation
NEEP negative end-expiratory pressure
NEF
negative expiratory force
negative factor
NEFA nonesterified fatty acid
NEFG normal external female genitalia
neg negative (*See also* N)
NEJ neuroeffector junction
NEM no evidence of malignancy
nem nutritional milk unit [Ger. *Nährungs Einheit Milch*]
NEMD nonexudative macular degeneration
NENAR noneosinophilic nonallergic rhinitis
NENT nasal endotracheal tube
neo
neonatal (*See also* neonat)
neovascularity
NEOH neonatal/high (risk)
NEOM neonatal/medium (risk)
neonat neonatal (*See also* neo)

NEP
  needle-exchange program
  negative expiratory pressure
  no evidence of pathology
  noise equivalent power
NEPD no evidence of
  pulmonary disease
neph nephritis
NER
  no evidence of recurrence
  nonionizing electromagnetic
    radiation
NERO noninvasive evaluation
  of radiation output
NES
  nonepileptic seizure
  nonstandard electrolyte
    solution
NET nerve excitability test
NETT nasal endotracheal tube
NETZ needle (diathermy)
  excision of the transformation
  zone
NEV noninvasive extrathoracic
  ventilator
NEX
  nose to ear to xiphoid
  number of excitations
    (radiology)
NEY, NEYA neomycin egg yolk
  (agar)
NF
  National Formulary
  necrotizing fasciitis
  neurofibromatosis
  neurofilament
  neutral fraction
  night frequency (of voiding)
  Nissen fundoplication
  noise factor
  normal flow
nF nanofarad
NFA nerve fiber analyzer (laser
  ophthalmoscope)
NFAR no further action
  required
NFB nonfermenting bacteria
NFCS neonatal facial coding
  system
NFD neurofibrillary degeneration

NFFD not fit for duty
NFH nonfamilial hematuria
NFI
  nerve-function impairment
  no-fault insurance
  no further information
NFP
  natural family planning
  not for publication
NFS neural foraminal stenosis
NFT no further treatment
NFTD normal full-term delivery
NFTSD normal full-term
  spontaneous delivery
NG nasogastric
ng nanogram
NGA nutrient gelatin agar
NGB neurogenic bladder
NGC nucleus (reticularis)
  gigantocellularis
NGF nerve growth factor
NG fdgs nasogastric feedings
NGHD-SS nongrowth hormone-
  deficient short stature
NGI Nurse's Global Impressions
NGJ nasogastrojejunostomy
NGJT nasogastrojejunal tube
ng/mL nanogram per milliliter
NGR narrow gauze roll
NGSF nothing grown so far
NGT
  nasogastric tube
  normal glucose tolerance
NgTD negative to date
NGU nongonococcal urethritis
NGVB nightguard vital
  bleaching
NH
  natriuretic hormone
  neonatal hemochromatosis
  neonatal hepatitis
  neurologically handicapped
  nonhuman
NH3 ammonia
NHA no histologic abnormalities
NHBCD nonheart-beating
  cadaver donor
NHBD nonheart-beating donor
NHC neonatal hypocalcemia
NH4Cl ammonium chloride

NHDL nonhigh-density lipoprotein
NHG normal human globulin
NHH neurohypophyseal hormone
NHI
National Health Insurance
Neisseria-Haemophilus Identification
NHIS Naylor-Harwood Intelligence Scale
NHL non-Hodgkin lymphoma
nHL normalized hearing level
NHM no heroic measures
NHML non-Hodgkin malignant lymphoma
NHP
normal human (pooled) plasma
nursing home placement
NHPA no histopathologic abnormality
NHPP normal human pooled plasma
NHR
net histocompatibility ratio
noise to harmonic ratio
NHS
normal horse serum
normal human serum
NHT
neoadjuvant hormonal therapy
nonpenetrating head trauma
nursing home transfer
NHTR nonhemolytic transfusion reaction
NHW nonhealing wound
NHWM normal human white matter
NI
neurologic improvement
no information
noise index
not identified
nucleus intercalatus
Ni nickel
NIA
nephelometric inhibition assay
neutrophil-inducing activity
no information available

NIAL not in active labor
NIBP noninvasive blood pressure
NIC
neurogenic intermittent claudication
noninvasive carotid (study)
Nursing Interventions Classification
NiCad nickel-cadmium
NICC noninfectious chronic cystitis
NICE noninvasive carotid examination
NICO noninvasive cardiac output (monitor)
NICU
neonatal intensive care unit
neurologic intensive care unit
NID
no identifiable disease
not in distress
NIDA five amphetamines, cocaine, marijuana, opiates, phencyclidine
NIDDM noninsulin-dependent diabetes mellitus
NiF n negative inspiratory force
NIFS noninvasive flow study
NIH-CPSI National Institutes of Health Chronic Prostatitis Symptom Index
NIHD noise-induced hearing damage
NIHF nonimmune hydrops fetalis
NIHL noise-induced hearing loss
NIHSS National Institutes of Health Stroke Scale
NIID neuronal intranuclear inclusion disease
NIL
noise interference level
not in labor
nil. nothing [L. *nihil*]
NIMA noninherited maternal antigen

NIMH-DIS National Institute of Mental Health Diagnostic Interview Schedule

NIMH-OC National Institute of Mental Health-Global Obsessive Compulsive Scale

NIMV noninvasive motion ventilation

NI-NR no infection-no rejection

NINVS noninvasive neurovascular studies

NIOPCs no intraoperative complications

NIP
catnip
negative inspiratory pressure
nipple
no infection (inflammation) present
nonspecific interstitial pneumonitis

NIPA noninherited paternal antigen

NIPD nightly intermittent peritoneal dialysis

NIPH no improvement with pinhole

NIPPV noninvasive positive pressure ventilation

NIPS
Neonatal Infant Pain Scale
noninvasive programmed stimulation

NIPTS noise-induced permanent threshold shift

NIRP near infrared photoplethysmography

NIRS near-infrared spectroscopy

NIS no inflammatory signs

NISD neonatal iron-storage disease

NISH nonradioactive in situ hybridization

NISM (bed) nucleus of stria medullaris

NISs New Injury Severity Score

NIST (bed) nucleus of stria terminalis

NIT
nasointestinal tube

neonatal isoimmune thrombocytopenia

NITD
neuroleptic-induced tardive dyskinesia
noninsulin-treated disease

nit. ox. n nitric oxide (*See also* NO)

nitro nitroglycerin

NITTS noise-induced temporary threshold shift

NIV noninvasive ventilation

NIVA noninvasive vascular assessment

NIVLS noninvasive vascular laboratory studies

NIVS noninvasive ventilatory support

NIW nursing intensity weights

NIZ noninfarct zone

NJ nasojejunal (tube)

NJC needle catheter jejunostomy

NK
natural killer (cell)
not known

N.K. Nomenklatur Kommission

NKA no known allergies

nkat nanokatal

NKC nonketotic coma

NKD no known diseases

NKDA no known drug allergies

NKE needle-knife electrocautery

NKF needle-knife fistulotomy

NKFA no known food allergies

NKH nonketotic hyperglycemia

NKHA nonketotic hyperosmolar acidosis

NKHC nonketotic hyperosmolar coma

NKHG nonketotic hyperglycinemia

NKHHC nonketotic hyperglycemic-hyperosmolar coma

NKHS nonketotic hyperosmolar syndrome

NKMA no known medication allergies

NKP needle-knife papillotomy

NKPP needle-knife precut
papillotomy
NL
  nasolacrimal
  neural lobe
  nodular lymphoma
  nonlatex
  normal libido
  normal limits
  normolipemic
NLA
  neuroleptanalgesia
  neuroleptanesthesia
  normal lactase activity
NLB needle liver biopsy
NLC nasolabial crease
NL ClCl, NLC&C, NL C/Cl
  normal libido, coitus, and
  climax
NLD
  nasolacrimal duct
  necrobiosis lipoidica
  diabeticorum
  no local doctor
NLDL normal low-density
lipoprotein
NLE neonatal lupus
erythematosus
NLEA Nutrition Labeling and
Education Act of 1990
NLF
  nasolabial fold
  neonatal lung fibroblast
NLFGNR nonlactose fermenting
gram-negative rod
NLH nodular lymphoid
hyperplasia
NLM
  noise level monitor
  no limitation of motion
nL n nanoliter
NLO nasolacrimal occlusion
NLOB needle-localized open
biopsy
NLP
  natural language processing
  neurolinguistic programming
  normal luteal phase

NLS
  neonatal lupus syndrome
  nonlinear least squares
  (method)
  nuclear localization signal
  (motif)
NLT
  normal lymphocyte transfer
  (test)
  nucleus lateralis tuberis
NM
  neuromedical
  neuromuscular
  nictitating membrane [L.
  nictitare to wink]
  nonmalignant
  nonmotile (bacteria)
  not measurable
  not motile (sperm)
  nuclear matrix
  nuclear medicine
  nuclear membrane
N&M
  nerves and muscles
  night and morning
N/m newton per meter
N/m² newton per square meter
nM nanomolar
nm
  nanometer
  nonmetallic
NMA neurogenic muscular
atrophy
NMBA neuromuscular blocking
agent
NMC
  neuromuscular control
  nodular, mixed cell
  (lymphoma)
  no malignant cells
  nucleus reticularis
  magnocellularis
NMD
  neuromuscular disorder
  normal muscle development
NMEP neurogenic motor evoked
potential
NMES neuromuscular electrical
stimulation

N

NMF
  neuromuscular facilitation
  nonmigrating fraction (of
    spermatozoa)
NMH neurally mediated
  hypotension
NMI
  no manifest improvement
  no mental illness
  no middle initial
  normal male infant
NMIS nuclear medicine
  information system
NMJ neuromuscular junction
NML nodular mixed lymphoma
NMM
  nevoid malignant melanoma
  nodular malignant melanoma
NMN
  neurotized melanocytic nevus
  no middle name
  Novy-McNeal-Nicolle
    (medium)
NMNKB not married, not
  keeping baby
NMOH no medical ocular
  history
nmol/Lr nanomole per liter
nmolr nanomoler
NMP
  nail matrix phenolization
  neuromuscular pacification
  normal menstrual period
NMR
  neonatal mortality rate
  neonatal mortality risk
  nictitating membrane response
  nuclear magnetic resonance
  nuclear medicine
NMRI nuclear magnetic
  resonance imaging
NMRL normal-mode ruby laser
NMRS nuclear magnetic
  resonance spectroscopy
NMS
  neurally mediated syncope
  neuroleptic malignant
    syndrome
  neuromuscular spindle
N·m/s newton meter per second

NMSIDS near-miss sudden
  infant death syndrome
NMT
  nebulized mist treatment
  neuromuscular tension
  neuromuscular transmission
  no more than
  nuclear medicine technology
NMTB neuromuscular
  transmission blockade
NMTS neuromuscular tension
  state
NMTSS nonmenstrual toxic
  shock syndrome
NMU neuromuscular unit
NMVS neurally mediated
  vasovagal syncope
NN
  narrative notes
  Navajo neuropathy
  neonatal
  neural network
  normally nourished
  normal nursery
N:N azo group (chemical group
  with two nitrogen atoms)
N/N negative/negative
n.n. new name [L. *nomen
  novum*] (*See also* n. nov.,
  nom. nov., nov. n.)
nn nerves
N-N nurse-to-nurse (orders)
NNA normochromic normocytic
  anemia
NNAS neonatal narcotic
  abstinence syndrome
NNB normal newborn
NNBC node negative breast
  cancer
NND
  neonatal death
  New and Nonofficial Drugs
NNE neonatal necrotizing
  enterocolitis
NNI noise and number index
NNL no new laboratory (test
  orders)
NNM neonatal mortality
NNN normal neonatal nursery
NNO no new orders

n. nov. new name [L. *nomen novum*] (*See also* n.n., nom. nov., nov. n.)

NNP
nerve net pulse
nonnociceptive pain

N:NPK grams of nitrogen to nonprotein kilocalories

NNR New and Nonofficial Remedies

NNS
neonatal screen (hematocrit, total bilirubin, and total protein)
nicotine nasal spray
nonneoplastic syndrome
nonnutritive sucking

NNT
neonatally tolerant
number needed to treat

NNWI Neonatal Narcotic Withdrawal Index

NO
nitric oxider (*See also* nit. ox. n)
nitroso-

No nobelium

no. number [L. *numero*] (*See also* N)

N2O nitrous oxide

NO₂ nitrogen dioxide

NOAEL no observed adverse effect level

NOBT nonoperative biopsy technique

noc, noct
nocturia
nocturnal [L. *noctis*, of the night]

NOD notify of death

NOE
nasoorbitoethmoid
nuclear Overhauser effect

NOED no observed effect dose

NOEL no observed effect level (of toxin)

NOF National Osteoporosis Foundation (treatment criteria)

NOFT nonorganic failure to thrive

NOH neurogenic orthostatic hypotension

NOI nature of illness

NOK next of kin

NOL not on label

NOM
nonsuppurative otitis media
normal extraocular movements

nom. dub. doubtful name [L. *nomen dubium*]

NOMI nonocclusive mesenteric infarction (ischemia)

NOMID neonatal-onset multisystem inflammatory disease

nom. nov. new name [L. *nomen novum*] (*See also* n.n., n. nov., nov. n.)

nom. nud. name without designation [L. *nomen nudum*]

NO/N2r nitric oxide/nitrogen

NOND none detected

NONF nonfasting

non pal not palpable

non-Q MI non-Q-wave myocardial infarction (*See also* NQMI)

non reb nonrebreathing (mask)

NONS nonspecific

nonsegs nonsegmented (neutrophils)

non-SSM nonskin-sparing mastectomy

nonvis, nonviz nonvisualized

NOOB not out of bed

N₂O/O₂/opioid nitrous oxide-oxygen-opioid (anesthetic technique)

NOR
nucleolar organizing region (cytogenetics)
nucleolus organizing region

norm normal

NOS
new-onset seizures
no organisms seen
not otherwise specified

N

NOSIE Nurses' Observation
Scale for Inpatient Evaluation

NOSPECS
no (signs or symptoms), only
(signs), soft (tissue
involvement with symptoms
and signs), proptosis,
extraocular (muscle
involvement), corneal
(involvement), sight
(loss/visual acuity)
(mnemonic for Graves
ophthalmopathy)

NOT
nocturnal oxygen therapy
nucleus of optic tract

NOTT nocturnal oxygen therapy
trial

nov. new [L. *novum*]

nov. n. new name [L. *novum
nomen*] (*See also* n.n., n. nov.,
nom. nov.)

nov. sp. new species [L.
novum species]

NP
nasopharyngeal
nasopharynx (*See also* NPhx)
near point (ophthalmology)
neonatal-perinatal
neuropathology
neuropsychiatry
nitrogen-phosphorus (detector
in gas chromatography)
nonpathologic
normal pressure
nosocomial pneumonia
not palpable
not perceptible
nuclear pharmacy
nucleoplasmic (index)
nursed poorly
nursing practice (procedure)

Np
neper (unit for comparing
magnitude of two powers,
usually electrical or
acoustic)
neptunium

n.p. proper name [L. *nomen
proprium*]

NPA
nasopharyngeal airway
nasopharyngeal aspirate
near point of accommodation
nucleus of pretectal area

NPAT nonparoxysmal atrial
tachycardia

NPB
Nellcor Puritan Bennett
(instrumentation)
nodal premature beat
nonprotein bound

NPBC node-positive breast
cancer

NPC
near point of convergence
nodal premature contractions
nonparenchymal (liver) cell
nonproductive cough
no prenatal care
nucleus of posterior
commissure

NPCa nasopharyngeal carcinoma

NPCIS nasopharyngeal
carcinoma in situ

NP-CPAP, NPCPAP nasal prong
continuous positive airway
pressure

NPD
narcissistic personality disorder
negative pressure device
nonprescription drugs
no pathologic diagnosis

NPDL nodular poorly
differentiated lymphocytic
(lymphoma)

NPDR nonproliferative diabetic
retinopathy

NPE
neuropsychologic examination
normal pelvic examination

NPEM nocturnal penile erection
monitoring

NPF
nasopharyngeal fiberscope
no predisposing factor

NPG nonpregnant

NPH
neutral protamine Hagedorn
(insulin)

no previous history
normal-pressure hydrocephalus
nucleus prepositus hypoglossi
nucleus pulposus herniation
NPhx nasopharynx (*See also* NP)
NPI
    neonatal perception inventory
    Neuropsychiatric Inventory
    no present illness
NPII Neonatal Pulmonary Insufficiency Index
NPIS Numeric Pain Intensity Scale
NPL
    nasopharyngolaryngoscopy
    nodular poorly differentiated lymphoma
NPLSM neoplasm
NPN nonprotein nitrogen
NPNT nonpalpable, nontender
NPO nothing by mouth [L. *nil per os*]
NPO/HS nothing by mouth at bedtime [L. *nil per os hora somni*]
NPP
    normally progressing pregnancy
    normal pool plasma
    normal postpartum
NPPB normal perfusion pressure breakthrough
NPPNG non-penicillinase-producing *Neisseria gonorrheae*
NP polio nonparalytic poliomyelitis
NPPV
    nasal positive pressure ventilation
    noninvasive positive-pressure ventilation
NPR
    nasopharyngeal reflux
    net protein ratio
    normal pulse rate
    nothing per rectum

NPRL normal pupillary reaction to light
NPRM notice of proposed rulemaking
NPS nasopharyngeal stenosis
NPSA nonphysician surgical assistant
NPSD nonpotassium-sparing diuretic
NPSG nocturnal polysomnogram
NP-SLE, NPSLE neuropsychiatric systemic lupus erythematosus
NPT
    neuropsychological test
    nocturnal penile tumescence
    normal pressure and temperature
NPV
    negative predictive value
    negative pressure ventilation
    nothing per vagina
    nucleus paraventricularis
NPZ neuropsychological test Z score
NQMI non-Q-wave myocardial infarction (*See also* non-Q MI)
NR
    nerve root
    neutral red
    nonreactive
    nonrebreathing
    normal range
    normal reaction
    normal record
N/R not remarkable
N_R Reynolds number (*See also* R_e)
n.r. do not repeat [L. *non repetatur*]
NRA
    nucleus raphe alatus
    nucleus retroambigualis
NRB
    nonrebreather (oxygen mask)
    nonrejoining (DNA strand) break
NRBC
    normal red blood cell

N

NRBC *(continued)*
nucleated red blood cell (mass)

NRC
noise reduction coefficient
normal retinal correspondence

NRDS neonate respiratory distress syndrome

NREH normal renin essential hypertension

NREM nonrapid eye movement (sleep)

NRF normal renal function

NRFC non-rosette-forming cell

NRGC nucleus reticularis gigantocellularis

NRH nodular regenerative hyperplasia (of liver)

NRI
nerve root irritation
nonrespiratory infection
no recent illnesses

NRL nucleus reticularis lateralis

N-RLX nonrelaxed

NRM
nonrebreathing mask
no regular medicines
normal retinal movement
nucleus raphe magnus
nucleus reticularis magnocellularis

nRNA nuclear ribonucleic acid

NROM normal range of motion

NRP
nonreassuring pattern
nucleus reticularis parvocellularis

NRPC nucleus reticularis pontis caudalis

NRPG nucleus reticularis paragigantocellularis

NRPR nonbreathing pressure relieving

NRR
Noise Reduction Rating
note, record, report

NRS
Neurobehavioral Rating Scale
normal reference serum
numeric rating scale

NRT
neuromuscular reeducation technique
nicotine replacement therapy

NRTI nucleoside reverse transcriptase inhibitor

NRV nucleus reticularis ventralis

NS
nasal steroid
nephrosclerosis
nephrotic syndrome
nervous system
neurologic sign
neurologic surgery
neurosecretory
neurosyphilis
nevus sebaceus
nipple stimulation
nodus sinuatrialis
nonspecific
normal serum
normospermic
no specimen
not sufficient
nuclear sclerosis

N/S normal saline

Ns nasopinale (craniometrics)

NSA
neck-shaft angle
nonspecific arrhythmia
normal serum albumin
no salt added
no significant abnormality
nutritional status assessment

NSAD no signs of acute disease

NSAE nonsupported arm exercise

NSAID nonsteroidal antiinflammatory drug

NSAP nonspecific abdominal pain

NSBGP nonspecific bowel gas pattern

NSBR Nottingham modification of Scarff-Bloom-Richardson (grading, breast cancer)

NSC
neurosecretory cell
no significant change

NSCC   nonsmall cell cancer
NSCD   nonservice-connected disability
NSCLC   nonsmall cell lung cancer
NSCST   nipple stimulation contraction stress test
NSD
nasal septal deviation
neonatal staphylococcal disease
neurosensory deficit
nominal standard dose
normal single dose
normal spontaneous delivery
no significant difference
no significant disease
NSDA   nonsteroid-dependent asthmatic
NSDU   neonatal stepdown unit
NSE   normal saline enema
nsec   nanosecond
NSF   no significant findings
NSFTD   normal spontaneous full-term delivery
NSG   nursing
NSHD   nodular sclerosing Hodgkin disease
NSHL   nonsyndromic hearing loss
NSHPT   neonatal severe hyperparathyroidism
NSI
negative self-image
neurosensory impairment
no sign of infection (inflammation)
NSIDS   near sudden infant death syndrome
NSL   non-salt loser
NSM   nerve sheath myxoma
N·s/m²   newton-second per square meter
NSND   nonsymptomatic, nondisabling
NSO
nonnutritive sucking opportunity
nucleus supraopticus

NSP
neck and shoulder pain
neurotoxic shellfish poisoning
NSPE   no specimen (obtainable)
NSR
nasoseptal reconstruction
normal sinus rhythm
NSRP   nerve-sparing radical prostatectomy
NSRRL   neutral, sidebent right, rotated left
NSRT   nonsurgical septal reduction therapy
NSS
nasal symptom score
neurological signs stable
normal saline solution
normal size and shape
not statistically significant
NSSC   normal size, shape, and consistency
NSSL   normal size, shape, and location
NSSP   normal size, shape, and position
NSSPAVAF   normal size, shape, and position, anteverted and anteflexed (uterus)
NSST   nonspecific ST (wave segment changes on electroencephalogram)
NSSTT   nonspecific ST and T (wave)
NSST-TWCs   nonspecific ST-T wave changes
NST
nonshivering thermogenesis
nonstress test (fetal monitoring)
normal sphincter tone
nutrition support team
NSTD   nonsexually transmitted disease
NSTI   necrotizing soft-tissue infection
NSU
necrotizing sclerocorneal ulceration
nonspecific urethritis

N

NSV nonspecific vaginitis
NSVD normal spontaneous vaginal delivery
NSVT nonsustained ventricular tachycardia
NSX neurosurgical examination
N-T, N&T nose and throat
NT
  nasotracheal
  neurofeedback training
  nontypable
  normotensive
  not tender
  not tested
  numbness and tingling
N:T neck to thigh ratio
N Tachy nodal tachycardia
NTB necrotizing tracheobronchitis
N/TBC nontuberculous
NTCC National Type Culture Collection
NTCS no tumor cells seen
NTD
  negative to date
  neural tube defect
  nitroblue tetrazolium dye
  noise tone difference
NTE
  neutral thermal environment
  nontest ear
  not to exceed
NTF
  nasogastric tube feeding
  normal throat flora
NTG
  nontoxic goiter
  normal-tension glaucoma
NTI
  narrow therapeutic index
  nasotracheal intubation
  no treatment indicated
NTL nectar-thick liquid (diet consistency)
NTLE neocortical temporal-lobe epilepsy
NTM
  nocturnal tumescence monitor
  nontuberculous mycobacteria

NTMI nontransmural myocardial infarction
NTMNG nontoxic multinodular goiter
NTN nephrotoxic nephritis
NTND not tender, not distended (abdomen)
NTNG nontoxic nodular goiter
NTP
  narcotic treatment program
  National Toxicology Program (Department of Health and Human Services)
  nonthrombocytopenic preterm (infant)
  normal temperature and pressure
NTPD nocturnal tidal peritoneal dialysis
NTR
  negative therapeutic reaction
  nutrition
NTS
  nasotracheal suction
  nicotine transdermal system
  nontyphi *Salmonella*
  nucleus of the tractus solitarius
NTT
  nasotracheal tube
  nearly total thyroidectomy
  nonthrombocytopenic term (infant)
  nuchal translucency thickness
NTU nephelometric turbidity units
NTZ normal transformation zone (colposcopy)
NU name unknown
Nu
  nucleolus
  nucleus
nU nanounit
NUC nuclear medicine
Nuc nucleoside
nuc nucleated
nucl nuclear
NUD nonulcer dyspepsia
NUG necrotizing ulcerative gingivitis

nullip nulliparous
num numerator
NuMA nuclear mitotic apparatus
numc number concentration
NUN nonurea nitrogen
NUP necrotizing ulcerative
periodontitis
NURB Neville upper reservoir
buffer
NURD nonuniform rotational
defect
NUV
near-ultraviolet
negative ulnar variance
NV
near vision
negative variation
neovascularization
neurovascular
normal value
normovolemic
not vaccinated
trigeminal nerve (fifth cranial
nerve)
N&V nausea and vomiting
Nv, Nv. naked vision
NVA
near visual acuity
normal visual acuity
NVAF nonvalvular atrial
fibrillation
NVB neurovascular bundle
NVBG nonvascularized bone
graft
NVC
neurovascular checks
nonvalved conduit
normal vital capacity
NVCC neurovascular cross
compression
NVD
nausea, vomiting, diarrhea
neck vein distention
neovascularization (of optic)
disc
nonvalvular (heart) disease
normal vaginal delivery
no venereal disease
no venous distention

NVDC nausea, vomiting,
diarrhea, and constipation
NVE
native valve endocarditis
neovascularization elsewhere
(on retina)
NVFS nuclear ventricular
function study
NVG
neovascular glaucoma
nonventilated group
NVI neovascularization of iris
NVL neurovascular laboratory
NVLD nonverbal learning
disability
NVM
neovascular membrane
nonvolatile matter
NVP
nausea and vomiting of
pregnancy
near visual point
NVR no radiographically visible
recurrence
NVS
nasal vestibular stenosis
neurologic vital signs
neurovascular status
NVSS normal variant short
stature
NW
naked weight
nasal wash
nonwithdrawn
not weighed
NWB
nonweightbearing
no weightbearing
NWC number of words chosen
NWD neuroleptic withdrawal
NWI
Neonatal Withdrawal
Inventory
notch width index
NWm nitrogen washout,
multiple (breath)
NWs nitrogen washout, single
(breath)

N

257

NX
  nephrectomy
  regional lymph nodes cannot
    be addressed (TNM system)
Nx no nodes (TNM
  classification)
NYC New York City (medium)
NYD
  not yet diagnosed
  not yet discovered

NYHA New York Heart
  Association (classification)
NYP not yet published
nyst nystagmus
NZ
  enzyme
  neutral zone

O

absence of sex chromosome
agglutinative reactions
blood type in ABO blood
 group
eye [L. *oculus*]
nonmotile organism
no special preparation
 necessary (for test)
objective (findings)
occlusal
operator
operon (genetics)
respirations (on anesthesia
 chart)

(O)

oral
orally

O₂ oxygen
O₃ ozone
O+ blood type O positive
O- blood type O negative
o- ortho- (chemical symbol)
1O2 singlet oxygen
O2- superoxide
O2EI oxygen extraction index
O2M oxygen mask

OA

obstructive apnea
occipital artery
occipitoanterior (fetal position)
occipitoatlantal
occupational asthma
ocular albinism
old age
ophthalmic artery
opiate analgesia
optic atrophy
oral alimentation
oral appliance
osteoarthritis
ovarian ablation
overall assessment

O&A

observation and assessment
odontectomy and alveoloplasty

O/A on or about
O₂a oxygen availability
OAA

Old Age Assistance
oxaloacetic acid (test)

OAAD ovarian ascorbic acid
 depletion (test)
OAAS, OAA/S Observer
 Assessment of Alertness and
 Sedation
OAB old age benefits
OABP organic anion-binding
 protein
OAC oral anticoagulant
OAD

obstructive airway disease
occlusive arterial disease
organic anionic dye
overall diameter (of contact
 lens)

OADC oleic acid, albumin,
 dextrose, and catalase
 (medium)
OADMT Oliphant Auditory
 Discrimination Memory Test
OAE otoacoustic emission (test)
OAF

off-axis factor
open air factor

OAG open-angle glaucoma
OAI Ostomy Assessment
 Inventory
OAJ open apophyseal joint
OAO ophthalmic artery
 occlusion
OAP

old age pension(er)
ophthalmic artery pressure
osteoarthropathy
oxygen at atmospheric
 pressure

OAR

off-axis ratio
organs at risk

OAR *(continued)*
  orientation/alertness
    remediation
  Ottawa Ankle Rules
OAS
  Oral Analogue Scale
  overall survival
OAST Oliphant Auditory
  Synthesizing Test
OATS
  oligoasthenoteratozoospermia
    syndrome
  osteochondral autograft
    transfer system
OAV oculoauriculovertebral
  (dysplasia, syndrome)
OAW oral airway
OAWO opening abductory
  wedge osteotomy
OB
  obliterative bronchiolitis
  obstetrics
  occult bleeding
  occult blood
  olfactory bulb
  osteoblast
  osteoblastoma
OBA
  office-based anesthesia
  Office of Biotechnology
    Activities (National Institutes
    of Health)
  oral bile acid
OBC operable breast cancer
OBD organic brain disease
OBE out-of-body experience
OB-GYN, OB/GYN
  obstetrician-gynecologist
  obstetrics and gynecology
obj object(ive)
obl oblique
OB marg obtuse marginal
OBN occult blood negative
OBP
  occult blood positive
  office blood pressure
  ova, blood, and parasites
    (stool exam)

OBS
  observation
  organic brain syndrome
obs obsolete
obsd observed
obst
  obstipation
  obstruct
OB-US obstetrical ultrasound
O-C, O&C onset and course (of
  disease)
OC
  obstetrical conjugate
  occlusocervical
  operative cholangiography
  optical chromatography
  oral contraceptive
  organ confined
  organ culture
  outer canthal (distance)
  ovarian cancer
  oxygen consumed
OCA
  oculocutaneous albinism
  olivopontocerebellar atrophy
  operant conditioning
    audiometry
OCAD occlusive carotid artery
  disease
O₂ cap. oxygen capacity
OCB obsessive-compulsive
  behavior
OCC
  oculocerebrocutaneous
  oral cavity cancer
occ
  occipital
  occiput
  occurrence
OCCC open-chest cardiac
  compression
occl occlusion, occlusal
OCCM open-chest cardiac
  massage
OCCPR open-chest
  cardiopulmonary resuscitation
OccTh occupational therapy
  (See also OT)
occup
  occupation(al)

occupies
occupying
OCD obsessive-compulsive disorder
OCG
omnicardiogram
oral cholecystogram
OCI Ophthalmic Confidence Index
OCL Orthopedic Casting Lab (splint)
OCM Odorant Confusion Matrix
OCOR on-call to operating room
OCP
ocular cicatricial pemphigoid
Onchocerciasis Control Program
oral contraceptive pill
ova, cysts, and parasites (stool exam)
OCPD obsessive-compulsive personality disorder
OCR
ocular counterrolling
ocular countertorsion reflex
oculocardiac reflex
oculocephalic reflux
oculocerebrorenal
off-center ratio
optical character recognition
OCS
Ondine's curse syndrome
oral cancer screening
oral contraceptive steroid
outpatient clinic substation
OCT
optical coherence tomography
optimal cutting temperature (medium)
oral cavity tumors
oral contraceptive therapy
outer canthal distance
oxytocin challenge test
O₂CT oxygen content
OCTT orocecal transit time
OCV ordinary conversational voice

OCVM
occult cerebrovascular malformation
occult vascular malformation
oculocerebrovasculometer
OCWO oblique closing wedge osteotomy
OCX oral cancer examination
OD
occipital dysplasia
occupational dermatitis
occupational disease
oocyte donation
open drop (anesthesia)
optical density
optic disk
optimal dose
oral-duodenal
osteochondritis dissecans
outer diameter
out-of-date
outside diameter
ovarian dysgerminoma
O.D., o.d. right eye [L. *oculus dexter*] (*See also* RE)
ODA
osmotic driving agent
right occipitoanterior (fetal position) [L. *occipitodextroanterior*] (*See also* ROA)
ODAC on-demand analgesia computer
ODAT one day at a time
ODB opiate-directed behavior
ODC
oral disease control
oxygen dissociation curve
ODCH ordinary disease of childhood
ODD
oculodentodigital (dysplasia, syndrome)
once-daily dosing
oppositional defiant disorder
osteodental dysplasia
OD'd (drug) overdosed

ODED oculodig-
itoesophagoduodenal
(syndrome)

ODM, ODm
occlusion dose monitor
ophthalmodynamometer

ODOD oculodentoosseous
dysplasia

odont
odontogenic
odontology

ODP
offspring of diabetic parents
right occipitoposterior (fetal
position) [L.
occipitodextroposterior] (*See
also* ROP)

OD/P right eye patched

ODQ
on direct questioning
opponens digiti quinti
(muscle)

ODSG ophthalmic Doppler
sonogram

ODSU
oncology day stay unit
one day surgery unit

ODT
oculodynamic test
orally disintegrating tablet
right occipitotransverse [L.
occipitodextrotransversa] (*See
also* ROT)

ODTS organic dust toxic
syndrome

ODU optical density unit

OE otitis externa

O-E standard observed minus
expected

O&E observation and
examination

O:E ratio of observed to
expected

Oe oersted (centimeter-gram-
second unit of magnetic field
strength)

OEC
outer ear canal
ovarian epithelial cancer

OEE outer enamel epithelium

OEF oxygen extraction fraction

OEI opioid escalation index

OEM
occupational and
environmental medicine
open-end marriage
opposite ear masked

O₂ER
oxygen enhancement ratio
oxygen extraction rate
oxygen extraction ratio

OERP odor event-related
potential

OERR order entry/results-reports
(VA physician computer order
entry system)

OES
optical emission spectroscopy
oral esophageal stethoscope

oesoph oesophagus (British)

OESP orthopedic examination,
special

OET oral esophageal tube

OF
occipitofrontal
optic fundi
orbitofrontal
osmotic fragility (test)
osteitis fibrosa
Ovenstone factor
oxidation-fermentation
(medium)

OFA oncofetal antigen

OFBM oxidation-fermentation
basal medium

OFC
occipitofrontal circumference
orbitofacial cleft

ofc office

OFCD oculofaciocardiodental
(syndrome)

OFD
object-film distance
(radiology)
occipitofrontal diameter
orofaciodigital (dysostosis,
syndrome)

OF-HA occipitofrontal headache

OFI other febrile illness

OFM
    open face mask
    orofacial malformation
    orofacial movement
OFPF optic fundi and
    peripheral fields
OFR oxygen-free radical
OF rad occipitofrontal radiation
OFTT organic failure to thrive
OG
    occlusogingival
    optic ganglion
    oral gastric
    orange green (stain)
    orogastric (tube, feeding)
OGC oculogyric crisis
OGCT oral glucose challenge
    test
OGD old granulomatous disease
OGF oxygen gain factor
OGIMD oculogastrointestinal
    muscular dystrophy
OGM outgrowth medium
OGS oxygenic steroid
OGTT oral glucose tolerance
    test
OH
    obstructive hypopnea
    occipital horn
    occupational health
    occupational history
    ocular history
    open-heart (surgery)
    oral hygiene
    orthostatic hypotension
    out of hospital
    outpatient hospital
OHA oral hypoglycemic agent
OHB$_{12}$ hydroxocobalamin
    (vitamin B$_{12}$)
O$_2$Hb oxyhemoglobin
OHC outer hair cell
OHD
    organic heart disease
    vitamin D
      (hydroxycholecalciferol)
OHF
    old healed fracture

    Omsk hemorrhagic fever
    overhead frame
OHFT overhead frame trapeze
OHG oral hypoglycemic
OHI
    ocular hypertension indicator
    Oral Hygiene Index
    oral hygiene instructions
OHI-S Oral Hygiene Index-
    Simplified
OHL oral hairy leukoplakia
ohm-cm ohm-centimeter
OHNS otolaryngology, head,
    and neck surgery
OHP
    hydroxyproline
    orthogonal-hole test pattern
    oxygen under high pressure
OHS
    obesity hypoventilation
      syndrome
    ocular hypoperfusion
      syndrome
    open heart surgery
    ovarian hyperstimulation
      syndrome
    Overcontrolled Hostility Scale
OHT
    ocular hypertensive (glaucoma
      suspect)
    overhead trapeze
OHTN ocular hypertension
OHTx orthotopic heart
    transplantation
O-I outer-to-inner
OI
    objective improvement
    obturator internus
    opportunistic infection
    orgasmic impairment
    osteogenesis imperfecta (type
      I–IV)
    otitis interna
    oxygenation index
    oxygen income
oi orbitale inferius
OIA
    optical immunoassay
    osmotically induced asthma

OID
optimal immunomodulating dose
organism identification (number)

OIF
observed intrinsic frequency
oil immersion field (microscopy)
orthoiodohippurate

oint ointment

OIP organizing interstitial pneumonia

OIRDA occipital intermittent rhythmic delta activity

OIS
ocular ischemic syndrome
optical intrinsic signal (imaging)
Organ Injury Scaling

OIU optical internal urethrotomy

OK, ok
correct
optokinetic

OKAN optokinetic after nystagmus

OKCE open kinetic chain exercises

OKN optokinetic nystagmus

OKQ Osteoporosis Knowledge Questionnaire

OL
open label (study)
other location

O.L. left eye [L. *oculus laevus*] (*See also* LE, O.S.)

Ol, ol. oil [L. *oleum*]

OLA left occipitoanterior (fetal position) [L. *occipitolaeva anterior*] (*See also* LOA)

OLBI overlapping biphasic impulse

OLD
obstructive lung disease
occupational lung disease

OLIB osmiophilic lamellar inclusion body

OLM
ocular larva migrans

ophthalmic laser microendoscope

OLP left occipitoposterior (fetal position) [L. *occipitolaevposterior*] (*See also* LOP)

OLR
optic labyrinthine righting
otology, laryngology, and rhinology

OLT
left occipitotransverse (fetal position) [L. *occipitolaevaposterior*] (*See also* LOT)
osteochondral lesion of the talus

OLTx orthotopic liver transplant

OLV one-lung ventilation

OM
obtuse marginal (coronary artery)
occipitomental
occupational medicine
ocular melanoma
oculomotor
organomegaly
osteopathic manipulation
otitis media
ovulation method (birth control)

OMA
obtuse marginal artery
older maternal age

OMAS occupational maladjustment syndrome

OMB obtuse marginal branch

OMB$_1$ first obtuse marginal branch

OMB$_2$ second obtuse marginal branch

OMD
ocular muscle dystrophy
oculomandibulodyscephaly
organic mental disorder
oromandibular dystonia

OME otitis media with effusion

OMF oculomandibulofacial (syndrome)

OMFS oral and maxillofacial surgery
OML orbitomeatal line
OMN
 oculomotor nerve
 oculomotor nucleus
OMP oculomotor palsy (third nerve)
OMR operative mortality rate
OMS
 opsoclonus-myoclonus syndrome
 oral and maxillofacial surgery
 organic mental syndrome
 otomandibular syndrome
OM&S osteopathic medicine and surgery
OMT, OM/T
 oral mucosal transudate
 osteomanipulative therapy
 osteopathic manipulation treatment
OMU ostiomeatal unit
ON
 ophthalmia neonatorum
 optic nerve
 optic neuritis
 optic neuropathy
 oronasal
ONC
 oncology
 over-the-needle catheter
OND
 orbitonasal dislocation
 other neurologic disease
ONH
 optic nerve head
 optic nerve hypoplasia
ONM ocular neuromyotonia
ONSD optic nerve sheath decompression
ONSF optic nerve sheath fenestration
OO
 oophorectomy
 ophthalmic ointment
 osteoid osteoma
 out of
O-O outer-to-outer

OOA outer optic anlage
OOC
 onset of contractions
 out of cast
 out of control
OOH&NS ophthalmology, otorhinolaryngology, and head and neck surgery
OOH-SCD out-of-hospital sudden cardiac death
OOL onset of labor
OOP out of plaster (cast)
OOS
 out of sequence
 out of specification (deviation from standard)
 out of splint
OP
 oblique presentation
 occiput posterior
 olfactory peduncle
 opening pressure
 operation
 ophthalmology
 opponens pollicis (muscle)
 osmotic pressure
 osteoporosis
 outpatient
 ovine prolactin
O&P ova and parasites (stool exam)
Op opisthocranion
OPA
 oral pharyngeal airway
 outpatient anesthesia
OPAC opacity (opacification)
OPAT outpatient parenteral antibiotic therapy
OPC
 oculopalatocerebral (syndrome)
 oropharyngeal candidiasis
 outpatient catheterization
OPCA
 (neonatal) olivopontocerebellar atrophy
 (X-linked) olivopontocerebellar ataxia
OPCAB off-pump coronary artery bypass (grafting)

265

OPCD olivopontocerebellar degeneration

op. cit. in the work cited [L. *opere citato*]

OPCS-4 Classification of Surgical Operations and Procedures (4th revision)

OPD
obstetric prediabetes
obstructive pulmonary disease
optical path difference
optical penetration depth
oropharyngeal dysphagia
otopalatodigital (syndrome)

OpDent operative dentistry

OPDG ocular plethysmodynamography

OPE
oral peripheral examination
outpatient evaluation

OPERA outpatient endometrial resection/ablation

OPG
ocular plethysmography
oculoplethysmograph
ophthalmoplethysmography

OPG/CPA oculoplethysmography-/carotid phonoangiography

OphSeg ophthalmic segment

Ophth
ophthalmology
ophthalmoscope

OPI oculoparalytic illusion

OPL
oral premalignant lesion
osmotic pressure (of proteins in) lymph

OPM
occult primary malignancy
ophthalmoplegic migraine
opponens digiti minimi (muscle)

OPMD oculopharyngeal muscular dystrophy

OPN osteopontin

OPO
optical parametric oscillator
organ procurement organization

OPP
ocular perfusion pressure
osmotic pressure of plasma
oxygen partial pressure

OPPG
ocular pneumoplethysmography
oculopneumoplethysmography

OPS
Objective Pain Scores
operations
Orpington prognostic scale
outpatient surgery

OpScan optical scanning

opt.
best [L. *optimus*]
optical
optician
optics
optimal
optimum
optional

OPTN organ procurement and transplant network

OPV
oral (attenuated) poliovirus vaccine
outpatient visit

OR
oblique ridge
odds ratio
oil retention (enema)
open reduction
operating room
optic radiation
oral rehydration
orienting reflex
overrefraction
own recognizance

O-R oxidation-reduction (system)

ORA
occiput right anterior (fetal position)
opiate (opioid) receptor agonist

ORCH
orchiectomy
orchitis

ORD
optical rotary dispersion

optical rotatory dispersion
oral radiation death

Ord orotidine

OREF open reduction and external fixation

ORF open reading frame

OR&F open reduction and fixation

ORIF open reduction and internal fixation

orig

origin

original

ORL

oblique retinacular ligament

otorhinolaryngology

ORMF open reduction metallic fixation

ORN osteoradionecrosis

ORO oil red O

ORP occiput right posterior (fetal position)

ORS

oral rehydration solution

oral surgery (*See also* OS)

ORT

ocular radiation therapy

oestrogen (estrogen)-replacement therapy

oral rehydration therapy

orthodromic reciprocating tachycardia

Orth, ortho orthopedic

orthot orthotonus

OS

occipitosacral (fetal position)

occupational safety

oligospermic

opening snap (heart sound)

ophthalmic solution

oral surgery (*See also* ORS)

orbitale superius

osteogenic sarcoma

osteoid surface

osteosarcoma

osteosclerosis

overall survival

oxidative stress

O.S. left eye [L. *oculus sinister*] (*See also* LE, O.L.)

Os osmium

OSA

obstructive sleep apnea

osteosarcoma

OSAP Office Sterilization and Asepsis Procedures Research

O₂ sat. oxygen saturation

OSCC oral squamous cell carcinoma

OSD-6 Obstructive Sleep Disorders-6 (test)

OSESC opening snap ejection systolic click

OSF

outer spiral fibers (of cochlea)

outlet strut fracture

overgrowth-stimulating factor

OSHA Occupational Safety and Health Act

OSI optical surface imaging

OSL Osgood-Schlatter lesion

OSM

osmolality

oxygen saturation meter

Osm osmole

osM osmolar

Osm/kg osmole per kilogram (osmolality)

Osm/L osmole per liter (osmolarity)

OSP output signal processor

OS/P left eye patched

OSS

occupational stress syndrome

osseous

over-shoulder strap

Osteo osteopathology

osteocart osteocartilaginous

OSTI Optimal Stent Implantation

OT

(Koch) old tuberculin

object test

oblique talus

occiput transverse (fetal position)

267

OT *(continued)*
  occlusion time
  occupational therapy *(See also* OccTh)
  ocular tension
  old terminology (anatomy)
  olfactory threshold
  olfactory tubercle
  optic tract
  orientation test
  orotracheal (tube)
  otology
O/T oral temperature
OTA
  oligoteratoasthenozoospermia
  open to air
OTC over-the-counter (nonprescription drug)
OTD optimal therapeutic dose
OTHS occupational therapy home service
OTO, Oto one-time only
OTR ocular tilt reaction
OT/RT occupational therapy/recreational therapy
OTS
  occipital temporal sulcus
  orotracheal suction
OTT
  orotracheal tube
  overall treatment time
OTW over the wire
O.U.
  both eyes (together) [L. *oculi unitas*]
  each eye [L. *oculi uterque*]
OU/P both eyes patched
OUS
  obstetric ultrasound
  overuse syndrome
oUW original University of Wisconsin (solution)
OV
  oculovestibular
  office visit
  outflow volume
  overventilation

ovulation
ovum
O₂V oxygen ventilation equivalent
Ov
  ovarian
  ovary
OVAL ovalocyte
OVAS ocular vergence and accommodation sensor
OVD occlusal vertical dimension
OVLT organum vasculosum laminae terminalis
OVS obstructive voiding symptom
OVX ovariectomized
OW
  off work
  once weekly
  open wedge (osteotomy)
  oval window
  ova weight
O/W oil in water (emulsion)
O:W oil to water ratio
OWA organics-in-water (analyzer)
OWR ovarian wedge resection
OWS overwear syndrome (contact lens)
OWT zero work tolerance
OX
  optic chiasm
  orthopedic examination
  oximeter
Ox1 oriented to time
Ox2 oriented to time and place
Ox3 oriented to time, place, and person
Ox4 oriented to time, place, person, and objects (watch, pen, book)
Oxi oximetry
OXT oxytocin
OYE old yellow enzyme
OZ optical zone
oz ounce

P

para (parity)

parietal (electrode placement in electroencephalography)

peta-

phon (unit of loudness)

proline (*See also* Pro)

P wave (depolarization wave crossing atria, in electrocardiography)

/P partial lower denture

P/ partial upper denture

P/3 proximal third (of bone)

P₁ first parental generation

P₂ pulmonic second sound

P_Na plasma sodium

p

frequency of the more common allele of a pair

papilla (optic)

para

pico-

proton

short arm of chromosome

p- *para-* (chemical prefix for two symmetrical substitutions in benzene ring)

P=R pupils equal in size and reaction

PA

alveolar partial pressure

paralysis agitans

periodontal abscess

pernicious anemia

phakic-aphakic

pituitary-adrenal

posteroanterior (position for x-ray)

pulmonary artery

pulpoaxial

yearly [L. *per annum*]

P&A, P & A percussion and auscultation

Pa

arterial pressure

pascal (unit of pressure measurement)

protactinium

pA picoampere

PAA premarket approval application (drugs, medical equipment, FDA)

PAAI personal access and alert interface (telemedicine)

PAB

premature atrial beat

purple agar base (medium)

PAC premature atrial contraction

PACG primary angle-closure glaucoma

PaCO2, PaCO₂ partial pressure of arterial carbon dioxide

PAD

peripheral arterial disease

photon absorption densitometry

preoperative autologous donation (blood)

public access defibrillator

PADP-PAWP pulmonary artery diastolic and wedge pressure

PADS Post Anesthesia Discharge Scoring System

PAE progressive assistive exercise

PA&E present, active, equal

paed paediatrics (British) (*See also* Peds)

PAEDP pulmonary artery end-diastolic pressure

PAF

paroxysmal atrial fibrillation

platelet activating/aggregating factor

PA&F percussion, auscultation, and fremitus

PAG

periaqueductal gray (matter)

pulmonary angiography

pAg protein A-gold (technique)

PAH predicted adult height

P

PAIC procedures, alternatives, indications and complications
PAIR puncture, aspiration, injection, reaspiration
PAJ paralysis agitans juvenilis
PAK
    pancreas and kidney
    percutaneous access kit
PAL posterior axillary line
PA&Lat posteroanterior and lateral
palp
    palpable
    palpation
PALS pediatric advanced life support
Palv alveolar pressure
PAM periodic acid-silver methenamine
PAN
    panoral x-ray examination
    periodic alternating nystagmus
PANDAS pediatric autoimmune neuropsychiatric disorders associated with streptococcal infections
PANSS Positive and Negative Stroke Scale
PAO
    peripheral airway obstruction
    peripheral arterial occlusion
PAO$_2$ partial pressure alveolar oxygen
PaO$_2$ partial pressure arterial oxygen
PaOD peripheral arterial occlusive disease
PAOG primary open-angle glaucoma
PAO$_2$–PaO$_2$ alveolar-arterial difference in partial pressure of oxygen
Pap Papanicolaou (smear, test)
PAPP pregnancy-associated plasma protein
PAPV
    partial anomalous pulmonary vein (venous)
    positive airway pressure ventilation

Pa-Pv pulmonary arterial pressure-pulmonary venous pressure
PAR
    pulmonary arteriolar resistance
    pulse amplitude ratio
para 0
    nullipara
    nullipara (no child borne)
para 1, para I
    primipara (given birth for first time) (*See also* primip)
    unipara (having borne one child)
para 2, para II
    bipara (having borne two children)
    secundipara (second pregnancy)
para 3, para III tripara
para 4, para IV quadripara
para
    paraparesis
    paraplegic
    parous (having borne one or more children)
para I (*var. of* para 1)
para II (*var. of* para 2)
para III (*var. of* para 3)
parapsych parapsychology
PARK photoastigmatic refractive keratectomy
PAROM passive assistive range of motion
PARS postanesthesia recovery score
PAS
    periodic acid-Schiff (stain)
    photoacoustic spectroscopy
    pulmonary artery systolic (pressure)
Pa·s pascal-second
PAS-AB periodic acid Schiff-Alcian blue (stain)
Pas Ex passive exercise
PASH periodic acid-Schiff hematoxylin (stain)
PASI psoriasis area and severity index

PASM periodic acid-silver methenamine (stain)

PAT
Pain Apperception Test
paroxysmal atrial tachycardia

PATE pulmonary artery thromboendarterectomy

PATH
pathogen
pathologic
pathologist
pathology

PATI Penetrating Abdominal Trauma Index

PAV percutaneous aortic valvuloplasty

PAVM pulmonary arteriovenous malformation

PAVN paraventricular nucleus

PAW
peak airway pressure
pulmonary artery wedge

Paw mean airway pressure

Pawo pressure at airway opening

PAWP pulmonary artery wedge pressure

PAX periapical x-ray

PB
barometric pressure
Paul-Bunnell (antibody, test)
peroneus brevis
Pharmacopoeia Britannica (British Pharmacopoeia) (*See also* BP)
phonetically balanced (word lists)

P&B pain and burning

Pb
lead [L. *plumbum*]
presbyopia

PBA
percutaneous bladder aspiration
pulpobuccoaxial

Pb-B lead level in blood

PBC
peripheral blood cell

pregnancy and birth complication

PBD
percutaneous biliary drainage
postburn day

PBF
percent body fat
peripheral blood flow
placental blood flow

PB-Fe protein-bound iron

PBH pulling-boat hands (exercise)

PBI
partial bony impaction
protein-bound iodine

PBK pseudophakic bullous keratopathy

PBL peripheral blood leukocyte

PBLI premature birth live infant

PBMC peripheral blood mononuclear cell

PBN paralytic brachial neuritis

PBNS percutaneous bladder neck suspension

PBP
peak blood pressure
pseudobulbar palsy

PBPI penile-brachial pressure/pulse index

PBS
peripheral-blood smear
prune belly syndrome

PBSCT peripheral blood stem cell transplantation

PBSP prognostically bad signs (during) pregnancy

PBT Paul Bunnell test

PBW posterior bite wing

PC
platelet count
postcoital
posterior chamber
premature contractions
pubococcygeus (muscle)
pulp canal
Purkinje cell

P&C prism and (alternative) cover test (crossover test,

P&C *(continued)*
screen and cover test in ophthalmology)

p.c. after a meal [L. *post cibum*]

pc parallax second (parsec)

PCA
patient-controlled analgesia
percutaneous coronary angioplasty
postcardiac arrest
postciliary artery
postconceptional age
posterior cerebral artery
posterior communicating artery

PCB
paracervical block
postcoital bleeding
proximal communicating branch

PcB, Pcb near point of convergence to intercentral baseline [L. *punctum convergens basalis*]

PCC
Pasteur Culture Collection
Poison Control Center
posterior central curve

PCD
pacer cardioverter defibrillator
peritoneal dialysis catheter
pneumatic compression device

PCDAI
Paediatric Crohn Disease Activity Index (British)
Perianal Crohn Disease Activity Index

PCE
physical capacity evaluation
pseudophakic corneal edema
(Smith) physical capacities evaluation

P-cell Purkinje cell

PCF
pharyngoconjunctival fever
prothrombin conversion factor

pcf pound per cubic foot

PCG
phonocardiogram
pneumocardiogram

PCHI permanent childhood hearing impairment

PCHL permanent childhood hearing loss

p.c. & h.s. after meals and at bedtime

PCI
percutaneous coronary intervention
posterior curve intermediate (cornea)
prothrombin consumption index

pCi picocurie

PCIOL, PC-IOL posterior chamber intraocular lens

PCL
persistent corpus luteum
posterior chamber lens
posterior cruciate ligament
proximal collateral ligament

PCLI posterior chamber lens implant

PCM protein-calorie malnutrition

PCMF perceptual cognitive motor function

PC-MRI phase-contrast magnetic resonance imaging

PCN penicillin

PCNV postchemotherapy nausea and vomiting

PCO
polycystic ovary
posterior capsule opacification
predicted cardiac output

PCO$_2$, P$_{CO2}$ partial pressure of carbon dioxide

PCoA posterior communicating artery

PCP
phencyclidine
Pneumocystis carinii pneumonia
primary care physician (provider)

pcpt
perception
precipitate

PCR
  percutaneous coronary
    revascularization
  polymerase chain reaction
PCR-DS polymerase chain
  reaction direct sequencing
PCR-ISH polymerase chain
  reaction in situ hybridization
PCS
  peroral cholangioscopy
  portacaval shunt
  postconcussion syndrome
  pulp canal sealer
PCT
  plasma clotting time
  plasmacrit test (for syphilis)
  porphyria cutanea tarda
  portacaval transposition
  positron computed tomography
  prothrombin consumption time
  proximal convoluted tubule
pct percent
PCTA percutaneous coronary
  transluminal angioplasty
PCU protein-calorie
  undernutrition
PCV
  packed cell volume
  polycythemia vera
  pressure-controlled ventilation
PCVC percutaneous central
  venous catheter
PCWP pulmonary capillary
  wedge pressure
PCXR portable chest x-ray
PD
  (inter)pupillary distance
  panic disorder
  paralyzing dose
  Parkinson disease
  parkinsonian dementia
  pediatric dose
  percutaneous discectomy
  percutaneous drain
  peritoneal dialysis
  pocket depth (dental)
  postural drainage
  pressor dose
  pressure dressing

  probing depth
  provocation dose
  pulpodistal
  pyloric dilator
2PD two-point discrimination
P(D−) probability of not having
  disease
P(D+) probability of having
  disease
PD$_{50}$ median paralyzing dose
Pd palladium
p.d. prism diopter
PDA
  patent ductus arteriosus
  plantar digital artery
  polymorphic delta activity
  posterior descending
    (coronary) artery
PDAI Perianal Disease Activity
  Index
PDB
  Paget disease of bone
  preventive dental (health)
    behavior
PDC
  parkinsonism dementia
    complex
  peritoneal dialysis catheter
PD&C postural drainage and
  clapping
PDD pervasive developmental
  disorder
PDE
  peritoneal dialysis effluent
  progressive dialysis
    encephalopathy
  pulsed Doppler
    echocardiography
PDF peritoneal dialysis fluid
PDG parkinsonism dementia
  (complex of) Guam
PDGF platelet-derived growth
  factor
PDH past dental history
PdHO pediatric hematology-
  oncology
PDI
  Pain Disability Index
  Periodontal Disease Index

PDI *(continued)*
    power Doppler imaging
    Psychomotor Development
      Index

PDL
    periodontal ligament
    polycystic disease of liver
    pulsed-dye laser (therapy)

pdl poundal (force of
    acceleration)

PDLC poorly differentiated lung
    cancer

PDLL poorly differentiated
    lymphocytic lymphoma

PDLN poorly differentiated
    (lymphocytic) lymphoma,
    nodular

PDM predentin matrix

PDMS Peabody Developmental
    Motor Scale

PDN
    Paget disease of the nipple
    prosthetic disc nucleus
      (device)

PDP
    papular dermatitis of
      pregnancy
    peak diastolic pressure

PD&P postural drainage and
    percussion

PDPD prolonged-dwell peritoneal
    dialysis

PDPV postural drainage,
    percussion and vibration

PDQ
    parental development
      questionnaire
    Premenstrual Distress
      Questionnaire
    pretty damn quick (slang)

PDR
    peripheral diabetic retinopathy
    Physician's Desk Reference
    proliferative diabetic
      retinopathy

pdr powder

PDRB Permanent Disability
    Rating Board

PDS polydioxanone suture

PDT
    percutaneous dilational
      tracheostomy
    photodynamic therapy

PDU pulsed Doppler
    ultrasonography

PDUFA Prescription Drug User
    Fee Act (1992)

PDV peak diastolic velocity

PE
    parallel elastic (component of
      muscle)
    pedal edema
    pelvic examination
    penile erection
    phacoemulsification,
      phakoemulsification (British)
    pharyngoesophageal
    physical education (*See also*
      phys ed)
    physical examination (*See also*
      PEx)
    point of entry
    preeclampsia
    preexcitation
    pulmonary embolism

P_E expiratory pressure

PEA pulseless electrical activity

PEC
    pectoralis
    pulmonary ejection click

PECHO prostatic echogram

PECO$_2$ mixed expired carbon
    dioxide tension

PECT positron emission
    computed tomography

PED
    percutaneous external drainage
    pharyngoesophageal
      diverticulum
    postexertional dyspnea
    prenatally exposed to drugs

ped pedestrian

PeDS Pediatric Drug
    Surveillance

Peds pediatrics (*See also* paed)

PEEP positive end-expiratory
    pressure

PEEP/CPAP positive end-expiratory pressure/continuous positive airway pressure

PEEPi intrinsic positive end-expiratory pressure

PEER pronation-eversion-external rotation

PEET Pediatric Extended Examination at Three

PEEX Pediatric Early Elemental Examination

PEF
  peak expiratory flow (rate)
  pharyngoepiglottic fold
  pulmonary edema fluid

%PEF percent predicted peak expiratory flow

PEFSR partial expiratory flow-static recoil (curve)

PEG-ELS polyethylene glycol electrolyte lavage solution

PEG-J percutaneous endoscopic gastrojejunostomy

PEH
  palmoplantar eccrine hidradenitis
  postexercise hypotension

PEI
  percutaneous ethanol injection
  physical efficiency index
  postexercise index

PEJ percutaneous endoscopic jejunostomy

PEK punctate epithelial keratopathy

PELCA percutaneous excimer laser coronary angioplasty

PELD percutaneous endoscopic lumbar discectomy

PELs permissible exposure limits

Pel-V elastic pressure-volume (respiratory system)

PEM
  precordial electrocardiographic mapping
  protein-energy malnutrition

P$_{Emax}$ maximal expiratory mouth pressure

PEMF pulsed electromagnetic field

PEMS
  physical, emotional, mental, and safety
  pulsed electromagnetic stimulator

PEN
  parenteral and enteral nutrition
  Pharmacy Equivalent Name

PENG photoelectronys-tagmography

PENS percutaneous epidural neurostimulator

PEO progressive external ophthalmoplegia

PEP
  positive expiratory pressure
  postexposure prophylaxis
  preejection period
  protein electrophoresis

PEPc corrected preejection period

PEP/LVET preejection period/left ventricular ejection time

PEPS peroral electronic pancreatoscope

PER
  peak ejection rate
  pudendal evoked response

P-ER pronation-external rotation

per
  period(ic)
  through, by [L. *per*]

PERC
  perceptual
  percutaneous

percus percussion

perf perforation

PERG pattern-evoked electroretinogram

peri perineal

periap periapical

Peri Care perineum care

perim perimeter

Perio periodontics

peripad perineal pad

P

275

PERL pupils equal and react to light

PERLA pupils equal, react to light and accommodation

perm permanent

PERR pattern evoked retinal response

PERRL pupils equal, round, and reactive to light

PERRLA pupils equal, round, reactive to light and accommodation

PES
pacing esophageal stethoscope
photoelectron spectroscopy
postextrasystolic
preexcitation syndrome
programmed electrical stimulation

PESA percutaneous epididymal sperm aspiration

Pesend end-expiratory esophageal pressure

PESS powered endoscopic sinus surgery

Pess pessary

Pessniff maximal sniff-induced esophageal pressure

PET
paraffin-embedded tissue
peak ejection time
peritoneal equilibration test
poor exercise tolerance
positron emission tomography
postexposure treatment
preeclamptic toxemia
pressure equalization tube
progressive exercise test

PETCO$_2$ partial pressure of end-tidal CO_2

petr petroleum

PETT positron emission transaxial tomography

PEU plasma equivalent unit

peV peak electron volt

PEVN periventricular nucleus

PEx physical examination (*See also* PE)

PF
parafascicular (nucleus)
pars flaccida
patellofemoral (joint)
peak flow
peripheral field
peritoneal fluid
plantar flexion
platelet factor
prostatic fluid
pterygoid fossa
pulmonary fibrosis
pulmonary function
Purkinje fiber
purpura fulminans
push fluids

pF picofarad

PFA
platelet function analysis
profunda femoris artery

PFAGH penalty, frustration, anxiety, guilt, hostility

PFB pseudofolliculitis barbae

PFC
patient-focused care
pelvic flexion contracture
persistent fetal circulation
prolonged febrile convulsions

PFCPH persistent fetal circulation with pulmonary hypertension

PFD
patellofemoral dysfunction
polyurethane foam dressing

PFE pelvic floor exercise

PFFD proximal focal femoral deficiency

PFG peak-flow gauge

PFGE pulsed-field gel electrophoresis

PFM
peak flow meter
porcelain fused to metal

PFNAB percutaneous fine-needle aspiration biopsy

PFNEI percutaneous fine-needle ethanol injection

PFNP peripheral facial nerve palsy

PFO
patent foramen ovale
plantar fasciitis orthosis

PFP
  patellofemoral pain
  platelet-free plasma
PFR
  peak filling rate
  peak flow rate
  pericardial friction rub
PFRC
  plasma-free red cell
  predicted functional residual
    capacity
PFS
  pelvic floor (electrical)
    stimulation
  penile flow study
  preservative-free solution
    (system)
  pressure-flow study
  progression-free survival
  pulmonary function score
PFSDQ Pulmonary Functional
  Status and Dyspnea
  Questionnaire
PFT
  pancreatic function test
  parafascicular thalamotomy
  placentofetal transfusion
  pulmonary function test
PFU plaque-forming unit
PFUO prolonged fever of
  unknown origin
PFW peak flow whistle
PFWT pain-free walking time
PG
  partial gastrectomy
  percutaneous gastrostomy
  Pharmacopoeia Germanica
    (*See also* PhG)
  pituitary gonadotropin
  placental grade (biophysical
    profile)
  plasma glucose
  plasma triglyceride
  postprandial glucose
  pregnant (*See also* preg)
  prostaglandin
  pyoderma gangrenosum
Pg
  gastric pressure

  nasopharyngeal electrode
    placement in
    electroencephalography
  pogonion
pg picogram
PGA pancreaticogastrostomy
  anastomosis
PGAS polyglandular autoimmune
  syndrome
Pgasniff maximal sniff-induced
  gastric pressure
PGC pontine gaze center
PGD preimplantation genetic
  diagnosis
PGE
  percutaneous gastroenterostomy
  proximal gastric exclusion
PGF paternal grandfather
PGGF paternal great-grandfather
PGGM paternal great-
  grandmother
PGH
  pituitary growth hormone
  placental growth hormone
PGM paternal grandmother
Pg-Ppl gastric-intrapleural
  pressure
PGR
  pelvic girdle relaxation
  percutaneous glycerol
    rhizolysis
P-graph penile plethysmograph
PGS postsurgical gastroparesis
  syndrome
PGSE pulsed-gradient spin echo
PGSRA psychogalvanic skin
  response audiometry
PGTT prednisolone glucose
  tolerance test
PGU postgonococcal urethritis
PGV proximal gastric vagotomy
PGVS postganglionic vagal
  stimulation
PGW person gametocyte week
  (malaria)
PGWBI Psychological General
  Well Being Index
PGYE peptone, glucose, and
  yeast extract (medium)

P

PH
> personal history
> porphyria hepatica
> previous history
> prostatic hypertrophy
> pulmonary hypertension
> pulp horn

Ph
> pharmacopeia
> phosphate

pH hydrogen ion concentration (measure of acid/alkaline)

ph phot (illumination)

Ph1, Ph¹ Philadelphia chromosome

Ph¹ (*var. of* Ph1)

PHA
> phytohemagglutinin antigen
> pseudohypoaldosteronism

PHACO phacoemulsification

phal
> phalanges (plural)
> phalanx (singular)

PHARM pharmacy

PHb pyridoxalated hemoglobin

PHC primary health care

PHCA profound hypothermic circulatory arrest

PHD pulmonary heart disease

Phe phenylalanine (*See also* F)

PhEEM photoemission electron microscopy

pheo pheochromocytoma

PhG *Pharmacopoeia Germanica* (*See also* PG)

PHHI persistent hyperinsulinemic hypoglycemia of infancy

PhI *Pharmacopoeia Internationalis*

PHIQ Philadelphia Head Injury Questionnaire

PHN
> postherpetic neuralgia
> public health nursing

PHO public health official

PH₂O partial pressure of water vapor

PHOB phobic anxiety

phos phosphatase

PHP
> panhypopituitarism
> partial hospitalization program
> pooled human plasma
> pseudohypoparathyroidism
> pyridoxalated hemoglobin-polyoxyethylene

PHR
> peak heart rate
> photoreactivity

PHS
> pooled human serum
> posthypnotic suggestion

PHT peroxide hemolysis test

PHTN
> portal hypertension
> pulmonary hypertension

PHV
> peak height velocity
> persistent hypertrophic vitreous

PHVD posthemorrhagic ventricular dilatation/dilation

PHx past history

Phx pharynx

PHY
> pharyngitis
> physical
> physiology

PhyO physician's orders

PHYS physiology

phyS physiologic saline (solution)

phys dis physical disability

phys ed physical education (*See also* PE)

physio physiotherapy

physiol
> physiologic
> physiology

phys med physical medicine

phys ther physical therapy (*See also* PT)

PI
> international protocol
> pars intermedia
> paternity index
> Pearl Index
> performance index
> Periodontal Index
> peripheral iridectomy

personal injury
plaque index
posteroinferior
premature infant
prematurity index
pulmonary infarction
pulmonic insufficiency
pulsatility index
P of I proof of illness
Pi
 parental generation
 pressure in inspiration
PIAT Peabody Individual
 Achievement Test
PIBC percutaneous intraaortic
 balloon counterpulsation
PIC peripherally inserted
 catheter
PICA
 posterior inferior cerebellar
  artery
 posterior inferior
  communicating artery
PICC peripherally
 (percutaneously) inserted
 central catheter
PICSYMS picture symbols
PICT pancreatic islet cell
 transplantation
PID
 pain intensity difference
  (score)
 pelvic inflammatory disease
PIE
 preimplantation embryo
 prosthetic infectious
  endocarditis
 pulmonary infiltrate with
  eosinophilia
 pulmonary interstitial edema
PIEx posteroinferior external
PIF
 peak inspiratory flow
 prostatic interstitial fluid
PIFG poor intrauterine fetal
 growth
PIFR peak inspiratory flow rate
PIFT platelet
 immunofluorescence test

PIGI pregnancy-induced glucose
 intolerance
pigm pigment(ed)
PIH
 pregnancy-induced hypertension
 pseudointimal hyperplasia
PIIS posterior inferior iliac
 spine
PIM pulse-inversion mode
 (ultrasound)
P_{Imax} maximal inspiratory mouth
 pressure
PIMS
 patient information
  management system
 programmable implantable
  medication system
PIN
 patient information network
 posterior interosseous nerve
 prostatic intraepithelial
  neoplasia
PINN proposed international
 nonproprietary name
PIO_2 partial pressure of
 inspiratory oxygen
PION
 posterior interosseous nerve
 posterior ischemic optic
  neuropathy
PIP
 peak inspiratory pressure
 proximal interphalangeal
  (joint)
PI-PB performance versus
 intensity function for
 phonetically balanced words
PIP/DIP proximal
 interphalangeal and distal
 interphalangeal (joints)
PIS Provisional International
 Standard
PISCES percutaneously inserted
 spinal cord electrical
 stimulation
PISH polymerase chain reaction
 in situ hybridization
PIT pacing-induced tachycardia
Pit patellar inhibition test

pit. pituitary
PIWT partially impacted wisdom teeth
PIXE, PIXIE particle (proton)-induced x-ray emission
PIXI peripheral instantaneous x-ray imaging (dual-energy x-ray bone density)
PJ
  patellar jerk
  porcelain jacket (crown)
PJA pancreaticojejunostomy anastomosis
PJB premature junctional beat
PJC premature junctional contraction
PJS peritoneojugular shunt
PJT paroxysmal junctional tachycardia
PK psychokinesis
pK ionization constant of acid
pK′ negative logarithm of dissociation constant of acid
pKa measure of acid strength
pkat picokatal
PKD polycystic kidney disease
PKN parkinsonism
PKP penetrating keratoplasty
PKPG penetrating keratoplasty and glaucoma
PKU phenylketonuria
pkV peak kilovoltage
pkyrs pack-year of smoking (2 packs a day for 20 years would be 40 pack-years)
PL
  palmaris longus
  perception of light
  plantar
  premature labor
  proboscis lateralis
  pulpolingual
Pl
  plasma
  Poiseuille (law, flow)
pL picoliter
pl plural
PLA
  peripheral laser angioplasty
  posterolateral (coronary) artery

Product License Application
pulpolinguoaxial
PLa pulpolabial
PLAD proximal left anterior descending (artery)
plague bubonic plague
PLAP placental alkaline phosphatase
PLAX parasternal long axis
PLB
  percutaneous liver biopsy
  porous layer bead
  posterolateral branch
PLC personal locus of control
PLD
  partial lower denture
  percutaneous laser discectomy
  peripheral light detection
  posterior latissimus dorsi (muscle)
  pregnancy, labor, and delivery
PLDD percutaneous laser disc decompression
PLE
  panlobular emphysema
  protein-losing enteropathy
PLF prior level of function
PLFD perilunar fracture-dislocation
PLG photoablative laser goniotomy
PLH placental lactogenic hormone
PLIC posterior limb of the internal capsule
PLIF posterior lumbar interbody fusion
PLISSIT permission, limited information, specific suggestions, and intensive therapy
PLL
  peripheral light loss
  posterior longitudinal ligament
PLM polarized light microscopy
PLMD periodic limb movement disorder
PLMV posterior leaf mitral valve

PLND pelvic lymph node dissection
PLOF previous level of functioning
PLP
  partial laryngopharyngectomy
  phantom limb pain
  plasma leukapheresis
PLPH postlumbar puncture headache
PLR
  persistent reactivity to light
  pronation-lateral rotation (fracture)
  pupillary light reflex
PLs premalignant lesions
PLSA posterolateral spinal artery
PLSI Psoriasis Life Stress Inventory
PLSO posterior leafspring orthosis
PLST progressively lowered stress threshold
PLT
  peroneus longus tendinopathy
  platelet
  psittacosis, lymphogranuloma venereum, trachoma
PLTF plaintiff
PLUG plug the lung until it grows (neonatology)
PLUT Plutchik (geriatric rating scale)
PLV posterior left ventricular
plx plexus
PM
  pacemaker
  pagetoid melanocytosis
  papilla mammae (nipple)
  papillary muscle
  partial meniscectomy
  pectoralis major
  perinatal mortality
  periodontal membrane
  petit mal (epilepsy)
  physical medicine
  pneumomediastinum
  polymyositis
  postmortem (*See also* post)
  premamillary nucleus
  premolar
  prostatic massage
  pterygoid muscle
  pulpomesial
P:M parent (drug) to metabolite (of drug) ratio
PM$_{10}$ particulate matter less than 10 microns diameter
Pm promethium
pM picomolar
p.m. afternoon [L. *post meridiem*]
pm picometer
PMA
  papillary, marginal, attached (gingiva)
  paramethoxyamphetamine (hallucinogenic drug)
  primary mental abilities
  Prinzmetal angina
  progressive muscular atrophy
  psychomotor agitation
PMAA Premarket Approval Application (medical devices)
PMB postmenopausal bleeding
PMBC percutaneous mitral balloon commissurotomy
PMBV percutaneous mitral balloon valvotomy/valvuloplasty
PMC
  percutaneous mitral commissurotomy
  peripheral multifocal chorioretinitis
  premature mitral closure
  premotor cortex
  pseudomembranous colitis
PMD
  perceptual motor development
  posterior mandibular depth
  private medical doctor
  progressive muscular dystrophy
PMDD premenstrual dysphoric disorder

P

281

pMDI pressurized metered-dose inhaler

PM-DM polymyositis and dermatomyositis

PME
pelvic muscle exercise
progressive myoclonus epilepsy

PMF, pmf
pterygomaxillary fossa
pupils mid-position, fixed

PMH
past medical history
pure motor hemiparesis

PMHR predicted maximal heart rate

PMI point of maximal impulse

PMID PubMed Unique Identifier (National Library of Medicine)

PMIS postmyocardial infarction syndrome

PML
premature labor
progressive multifocal leukodystrophy
prolapsing mitral leaflet
promyelocytic leukemia

pML posterior mitral valve leaflet

PMMA polymethyl methacrylate

PMMF pectoralis major myocutaneous flap

PMN
polymorphonuclear (leukocyte, neutrophil) (*See also* POLY)
Premarket Notification (medical devices)

PMNC peripheral blood mononuclear cell

PMO postmenopausal osteoporosis

pmol picomole

PMP persistent mentoposterior (fetal position)

PMPO postmenopausal palpable ovary

PMR
pacemaker rhythm

percutaneous myocardial revascularization
perinatal morbidity (mortality) rate
polymyalgia rheumatica
posteromedial release
proton magnetic resonance

PMS
premenstrual syndrome
pulse, motor, and sensory
pureed, mechanical, soft (diet)

PMT
percutaneous mechanical thrombectomy
point of maximum tenderness
Porteus maze test

PMV prolapsed mitral valve

PN
parenteral nutrition
percutaneous nephrostogram
percutaneous nucleotomy
peripheral nerve
peripheral neuropathy
phrenic nerve
polyneuritis
pontine nucleus
poorly nourished
positional nystagmus
postnasal
postnatal
premie nipple
pyelonephritis

P:N positive to negative ratio

P&N psychiatry and neurology

pN positive lymph node (part of TNM classification)

pN0 no regional lymph node metastasis (part of TNM classification)

pN1 poorly differentiated myeloblasts in nodes (part of TNM classification)

pN2 tumor metastases to ipsilateral axillary lymph nodes (part of TNM classification)

pN3 tumor metastases to ipsilateral mammary lymph nodes (part of TNM classification)

PN₂, P_{N2}
 nitrogen partial pressure
 partial pressure of nitrogen
PNA Paris Nomina Anatomica
pN1a tumor micrometastases to
 nodes, none larger than 0.2
 cm
PNAB percutaneous needle
 aspiration biopsy
PNB
 percutaneous needle biopsy
 popliteal nerve block
 premature nodal beat
 prostatic needle biopsy
pN1b tumor metastases to
 lymph nodes, larger than 0.2
 cm (part of TNM
 classification)
pN1bi tumor metastases to 1-3
 lymph nodes, from 0.2 to
 2.0 cm (part of TNM
 classification)
pN1bii tumor metastases to 4
 or more lymph nodes, 0.2 to
 2.0 cm (part of TNM
 classification)
pN1biii tumor metastases
 beyond lymph node capsule,
 none larger than 2.0 cm
pN1biv tumor metastases to
 lymph nodes, larger than 2.0
 cm (part of TNM
 classification)
PNC
 peripheral nerve conduction
 peripheral nucleated cell
 premature nodal contraction
PND
 paroxysmal nocturnal dyspnea
 partial neck dissection
 pregnancy, not delivered
 purulent nasal drainage
PNdB perceived noise level
PNE
 pneumoencephalography
 pseudomembranous necrotizing
 enterocolitis

PNF proprioceptive
 neuromuscular fasciculation
 (reaction)
PNG pneumogram
PNH paroxysmal nocturnal
 hemoglobinuria
PNI
 peripheral nerve injury
 postnatal infection
 prognostic nutritional index
 psychoneuroimmunology
PNL
 percutaneous nephrolithotomy
 percutaneous
 nephrostolithotomy
PNLA percutaneous needle lung
 aspiration
PNM
 perinatal mortality
 pneumonia
 postneonatal mortality
 (syndrome)
PNP
 peak negative pressure
 progressive nuclear palsy
 psychogenic nocturnal
 polydipsia
PNPR positive-negative pressure
 respiration
PNS
 parasympathetic nervous
 system
 peripheral nervous system
 posterior nasal spine
PNSP
 penicillin-nonsusceptible
 Streptococcus pneumoniae
 posterior nasal spine to soft
 palate
PNSS Pediatric Nutrition
 Surveillance System
PNT percutaneous nephrostomy
 tube
pnx pneumonectomy
PNZ posterior necrotic zone
PO
 parietooccipital
 perioperative
 periosteum

P

P&O
    parasites and ova
    prosthesis and orthosis
P:O protein to osmolar ratio
Po
    polonium
    porion
p.o. by mouth, orally [L. *per os*]
PO₂, P$_{O2}$ partial pressure of oxygen
PO4 phosphate
POA
    power of attorney
    preoptic area (of the hypothalamus)
POAD peripheral occlusive arterial disease
POAG primary open-angle glaucoma
POC products of conception
POCT point-of-care testing
POD
    pacing on demand
    place of death
    polycystic ovary disease
    postoperative day
    postovulatory day
PODx preoperative diagnosis
POE
    position of ease
    postoperative exercise
    proof of eligibility
POET pulse oximeter/end tidal (carbon dioxide)
POET2 point of entry, traction and twist
POEx postoperative exercise
POF position of function
POG products of gestation
Pog pogonion
POH
    past ocular history
    personal oral hygiene
    postoperative hemorrhage
POIK
    poikilocyte
    poikilocytosis
polio poliomyelitis

POLY
    polydipsia
    polymorphonuclear (leukocyte, neutrophil) (*See also* PMN)
    polyphagia
    polyuria
POM
    pain on motion
    purulent otitis media
PONV postoperative nausea and vomiting
POO prostatic outlet obstruction
POP
    pain on palpation
    persistent occipitoposterior (fetal position)
    plaster of Paris
    popliteal
    posterior oropharynx
POPS peroral pancreatoscopy
PORH postoperative reactive hyperemia
PORP partial ossicular reconstruction prosthesis
PORT
    perioperative respiratory therapy
    postoperative radiotherapy
    postoperative respiratory therapy
POS
    position
    positive
POSHPATE problem, onset, (associated) symptoms, (previous) history, precipitating (factors), alleviating/aggravating (factors), timing, etiology (prompts for H&P)
pos pr positive pressure
POST peritoneal oocyte and sperm transfer
post
    posterior
    postmortem (*See also* PM)
PostCap posterior capsule
postop, post-op postoperative
post prand. after dinner [L. *post prandium*]

POSTS positive occipital sharp transients of sleep
post tib posterior tibial
PostVD posterior vitreous detachment
POSYC Pain Observation Scale for Young Children
POTS postural orthostatic tachycardia syndrome
POU placenta, ovary, uterus
PoV portal vein
POVT puerperal ovarian vein thrombosis
POW prisoner of war
POZ posterior optical zone
PP
  paradoxical pulse
  partial upper and lower dentures
  pedal pulse
  perfusion pressure
  periodontal pockets
  peripheral pulse
  permanent partial
  per protocol
  Peyer patch
  posterior pituitary
  postpartum
  postprandial
  precocious pubarche
  proximal phalanx
  pulsus paradoxus
  punctum proximum (near point of convergence)
PPA
  postpartum amenorrhea
  pyrophosphate arthritis-pseudogout
PP&A, pp&a palpation, percussion, and auscultation
Ppaw pulmonary artery wedge pressure
PPB
  parts per billion
  platelet-poor blood
  prostate puncture biopsy
PPBS postprandial blood sugar
PPC
  peripheral posterior curve

  plaster of Paris cast
  proximal palmar crease
PPCM postpartum cardiomyopathy
PPD purified protein derivative (of tuberculin)
P and PD, P&PD percussion and postural drainage
PPD-B purified protein derivative–Battey
PPD-S purified protein derivative–standard
PPDS phonologic programming deficit syndrome
PPE partial plasma exchange
Ppeak peak airway pressure
PPF
  percutaneous plantar fasciotomy
  plasma protein fraction
PPG
  phalloplethysmography
  photoplethysmography
  postprandial glucose
  pretragal parotid gland
  pylorus-preserving gastrectomy
ppg picopicogram
PPGA postpill galactorrhea/amenorrhea
PPH
  persistent pulmonary hypertension
  postpartum hemorrhage
PPHM parts per hundred million
PPHN persistent pulmonary hypertension of newborn
PPHP pseudopseudohypoparathyroidism
PPHT parts per hundred thousand
PPHTN portopulmonary hypertension
PPI
  partial permanent impairment
  permanent pacemaker insertion
  proton pump inhibitor
PPID peak pain intensity difference (score)

PPIM postperinatal infant mortality
PPK
palmoplantar keratoderma (keratosis)
partial penetrating keratoplasty
PPL
pars plana lensectomy
postprandial lipemia
Ppl pleural pressure
PPLO pleuropneumonia-like organism
PPM
parts per million
permanent pacemaker
persistent pupillary membrane
posterior papillary muscle
pulse per minute
PPMS primary-progressive multiple sclerosis
PPN
partial parenteral nutrition
pedunculopontine nucleus
peripheral parenteral nutrition
PPNG penicillinase producing *Neisseria gonorrhoeae*
PPO passive prehension orthosis
PPOB postpartum obstetrics
PPoma pancreatic polypeptide-secreting tumor
PPP
Pain Perception Profile
palatopharyngoplasty
passage, power, and passenger (progress of labor)
patient prepped and positioned
pearly penile papules
pedal pulse present
peripheral pulse palpable
platelet-poor plasma
postpartum psychosis
pustulosis palmaris et plantaris
PP&P posterior pole and periphery
PPPD pylorus-preserving pancreatoduodenectomy
PPPH purified placental protein, human

PPPPP pain, pallor, pulse loss, paresthesia, and paralysis
PPPPPP pain, pallor, paresthesia, pulselessness, paralysis, prostration
PPQ Postoperative Pain Questionnaire
PPR
photopalpebral reflex
pitch period perturbation
Price precipitation reaction
PPr
paraprosthetic
periodontal prophylactics
PPRF
paramedian pontine reticular formation
postpartum renal failure
PPROM
preterm premature rupture of membranes
prolonged premature rupture of membranes
PPS
Pap plus speculoscopy
parapharyngeal space
postpartum sterilization
postpolio syndrome
postpump syndrome
pulse per second
PPSEQ Postpartum Self-Evaluation Questionnaire
PPT
partial prothrombin time
parts per trillion
peak-to-peak threshold
person, place, and time
Physical Performance Test
posterior pelvic tilt
pressure pain threshold
PPTL
postpartum tubal ligation
pressure pain tolerance level
PPU perforated peptic ulcer
PPV
pars plana vitrectomy
patent processus vaginalis
pneumococcal polysaccharide vaccine
positive-pressure ventilation

Ppv pulmonary vein pressure
PPW

plantar puncture wound
pylorus-preserving Whipple
modification

PQ

permeability quotient
pronator quadratus

pQCT peripheral quantitative
computed tomography
PQNS protein, quantity not
sufficient
PQOL perceived quality of life
PQRST

palliation, quality, radiation,
severity, time
position, quality, radiation,
severity, time

PR

far point (of accommodation)
[L. *punctum remotum*]
palindromic rheumatism
Panama red (variety of
marijuana)
parallax (and) refraction
pars recta
peer review
pelvic rock
percentile rank
per rectum
phenol red
photoreaction
physical rehabilitation
pityriasis rosea
pregnancy rate
pressoreceptor
progesterone receptor
progressive relaxation
prone
prosthion
public relations
pulse rate
pyramidal response

P&R

pelvic and rectal
(examination)
pulse and respiration

P–R time between P wave and
beginning of QRS complex
in electrocardiography
P:R productivity to respiration
ratio
Pr praseodymium
PRA

panel of reactive antibodies
phonation, respiration,
articulation, resonance
progesterone receptor assay

PRAFO pressure-relief ankle-foot
orthosis
PRAGMATIC pregnancy,
rheumatoid arthritis,
acromegaly, glucose
metabolism disorder,
mechanical injury, amyloid,
thyroid disease, infectious
disease, crystals of gout or
pseudogout (disorders
associated with carpal tunnel
syndrome)
prand. dinner [L. *prandium*]
PRBC packed red blood cells
PRE

passive resistance exercise
physical reconditioning
exercise
progressive resistance exercise

preemie premature (*See also*
prem, preemie)
preg, pregn

pregnancy
pregnant (*See also* PG)

PREM Prematurity Risk
Evaluation Measure
prem

premature (*See also* preemie,
premie)
prematurity

premie premature (*See also*
preemie, prem)
preop, pre-op preoperative
prep prepare (for surgery)
prev

prevention
preventive
previous

287

PREZ posterior root entry zone
PRF
   percutaneous radiofrequency
      rhizolysis
   pontine reticular formation
PRFD percutaneous
   radiofrequency denervation
PRFNB percutaneous
   radiofrequency facet nerve
   block
PRFR pressure-retaining flow-
   relieving
PRG
   phleborheography
   purge
PRGI percutaneous
   retrogasserian glycerol
   injection
PRI
   Pain Rating Index
   plexus rectales inferiores
      (venous plexus)
   Prescriptive Reading Inventory
PRICE protection, restricted
   activity, ice, compression,
   elevation
PRICES protection, rest, ice,
   compression, elevation,
   support (first aid)
primip primipara (given birth
   for first time) (*See also* para
   1)
PRINS primed in situ labeling
PR interval onset of ventricular
   depolarization
PRISM Pediatric Risk of
   Mortality (Score)
PRIST paper
   radioimmunosorbent technique
PRK
   photorefractive keratectomy
   photorefractive keratoplasty
PRL, Prl preferred retinal locus
PRLA pupils react to light and
   accommodation
PRM
   partial rebreathing mask
   Primary Reference Material
PrM preventive medicine

PRN, p.r.n. as needed [L. *pro
   re nata*]
Pro proline (*See also* P)
proct, procto
   proctology
   proctoscopy
PROG
   prognathism
   program
PROM
   passive range of motion
   premature rupture of (fetal)
      membranes
proph, prophy
   prophylactic
   prophylaxis
pros, prostat
   prostate
   prostatic
PROST pronucleate stage
   (embryo, tubal) transfer
prosth
   prosthesis
   prosthetic
protime prothrombin time (*See
   also* PT)
PROT REL protrusive
   relationship
prox proximal
PRP
   physiologic rest position
   platelet-rich plasma
   poor progression of R wave
      in precordial leads
   postural rest position
   proliferative retinopathy
      photocoagulation
   pulse repetition frequency
PrP prion protein
PRP-T polysaccharide tetanus
   conjugate vaccine
PRS
   photon-radiosurgical therapy
   positive rolandic spike
   prolonged respiratory support
PRT
   percutaneous rotational
      thrombectomy
   photoradiation therapy
   photostress recovery time

physiologic reflux test
progressive relaxation training
psychotic trigger reaction
PRTCA percutaneous rotational
transluminal coronary
angioplasty
PRV polycythemia rubra vera
PRVC pressure-regulated volume
control
PRVEP pattern reversal visual
evoked potential
PRVR peak-to-resting-velocity
ratio
Prx prognosis
PS
pacemaker syndrome
paradoxical sleep
parasympathetic (division of
autonomic nervous system)
pathologic stage
peripheral smear
photosynthesis
phrenic (nerve) stimulation
physical status (patient
surgical classification)
point of symmetry
posterior synechiae
postmaturity syndrome
P&S
pain and suffering
paracentesis and suction
permanent and stationary
P:S polyunsaturated to saturated
fat ratio
PSA
polysubstance abuse
power spectral analysis
procedural sedation and
analgesia
prostate-specific antigen
PsA psoriatic arthritis
PSAD psychoactive substance
abuse and dependence
PSAP peak systolic aortic
pressure
PSAX parasternal short axis
PSB
patellar stabilizing brace
protected specimen brushing

PSC
Pediatric Symptom Checklist
percutaneous suprapubic
cystostomy
pluripotential stem cell
posterior semicircular canal
posterior subcapsular cataract
pubosacrococcygeal (diameter)
pulse-synchronized contractions
PSC Cat posterior subcapsular
cataract
PSCH peripheral stem cell
harvest
PSCT peripheral stem cell
transplant
PSD
percutaneous stricture
dilatation
periodic synchronous discharge
photon-stimulated desorption
posterior sagittal diameter
psychosomatic disease
PSE
Pidgin Sign English
portosystemic encephalopathy
postshunt encephalopathy
preparticipation sports
examination
Present State Examination
psec picosecond
PSF posterior spinal fusion
psf pound per square foot
PSG
polysomnogram
presystolic gallop
PSGN poststreptococcal
glomerulonephritis
PSH
past surgical history
postspinal (anesthetic)
headache
P&SH personal and social
history
PSI
Pediatric Speech Intelligibility
Test
pelvic support index
Pneumonia Severity Index
posterior sagittal index

P

PSI *(continued)*
>posterior superior iliac (spine)
>Predictive Salvage Index
>prostate seed implant

p.s.i. pound per square inch

PSIL
>percentage signal intensity loss
>preferred frequency speech interference level

PSIS posterior sacroiliac spine

PSM
>polysomnogram
>presystolic murmur

PSMA proximal spinal muscular atrophy

PSMS Physical Self Maintenance Scale

PSNS parasympathetic nervous system

PSO pelvic stabilization orthosis

pSO2 arterial oxygen saturation (*See also* SaO_2)

Psol partly soluble

PSP
>paralytic shellfish poisoning
>periodic short pulse
>photostimulable phosphor dental radiography
>postsynaptic potential
>professional simulated patient
>pseudopregnancy

PSR
>percutaneous stereotactic radiofrequency (rhizotomy)
>proliferative sickle retinopathy
>Psychiatric Status Rating (scale)

PSROM preterm spontaneous rupture of membranes

PSS
>Peritonitis Severity Score
>physiologic saline solution
>portosystemic shunting
>psoriasis severity scale

PSS-HN performance status scale for head and neck cancer

PSS:NICU Parental Stressor Scale: Neonatal Intensive Care Unit

PST
>phonemic segmentation test
>poststimulus time
>postural stimulation test
>postural stress test
>prefrontal sonic treatment
>promontory stimulation test
>protein-sparing therapy
>proximal straight tubule

PSUD psychoactive substance use disorder

PSV
>pressure support ventilation
>psychological, social, and vocational (adjustment factors)

PSWL peroral shock wave lithotripsy

psych
>psychiatry
>psychology

PT
>pertussis toxin
>pertussis toxoid
>phonation time
>physical therapy (*See also* phys ther)
>physiotherapy
>posttransplantation
>pronator teres
>prothrombin time (*See also* protime)
>proximal tubule
>pulmonary toilet
>pure tone (audiometry)

P&T
>paracentesis and tubing (of ears)
>peak and trough
>permanent and total (disability)

P_T total pressure

Pt platinum

pt
>patient
>pint
>point

PTA
  percutaneous transluminal angioplasty
  posttraumatic amnesia
  pure tone acuity
PT(A) pure tone average
PTAB popliteal-tibial artery bypass
PTAH phosphotungstic acid-hematoxylin (stain)
PTAP purified (diphtheria) toxoid (precipitated by) aluminum phosphate
PTAS percutaneous transluminal angioplasty with stent placement
PTB
  patellar tendon-bearing (cast prosthesis)
  pretibial buttress
  prior to birth
  pulmonary tuberculosis
PTBA percutaneous transluminal balloon angioplasty
PTBD
  percutaneous transhepatic biliary drainage
  percutaneous transluminal balloon dilatation
PTBS posttraumatic brain syndrome
PTB-SC-SP patellar tendon-bearing–supracondylar-suprapatellar (prosthesis)
PTC
  percutaneous transhepatic cholangiogram
  post-tetanic count
  pseudotumor cerebri
PTCA percutaneous transluminal coronary angioplasty
PTCC percutaneous transhepatic cholecystoscopy
PTCR percutaneous transluminal coronary revascularization
PTCRA
  percutaneous transluminal coronary rotational ablation

  percutaneous transluminal coronary rotational atherectomy
PTCS percutaneous transhepatic cholangioscopy
PTCSL percutaneous transhepatic cholangioscopic lithotomy
PTD
  percutaneous transhepatic drainage
  percutaneous transluminal dilatation
  percutaneous transpedicular discectomy
  permanent total disability
  photodynamic therapy
PTDP permanent transvenous demand pacemaker
PTE pretibial edema
PTE-4 pediatric trace elements (four elements, injection)
PTE-5 pediatric trace elements (five elements, injection)
PTEF peak tidal expiratory flow
PTFL posterior talofibular ligament
PTG photoplethysmogram
PTGBD percutaneous transhepatic gallbladder drainage
PTI pressure time index
PT-INR prothrombin time international normalized ratio
PTL
  pharyngotracheal lumen (airway)
  posterior tricuspid (valve) leaflet
  preterm labor
  pudding-thick liquid (diet consistency)
PTLD, PTLPD, PT-LPD posttransplantation lymphoproliferative disease
PTLR percutaneous transmyocardial laser revascularization

P

PTM
    pressure time per minute
    preterm milk
Ptm
    pterygomaxillary (fissure)
    transmural pressure (airway,
        blood vessel)
PTMDF pupils, tension, media,
    disc, and fundus (eye exam)
PTN posterior tibial nerve
PTNB preterm newborn
pTNM pathological tumor,
    nodes, metastases (pathological
    part of TNM classification
    system)
PTO
    part-time occlusion (eye
        patch)
    percutaneous transhepatic
        obliteration
PTP
    percutaneous transhepatic
        portography
    Physical Tolerance Profile
    posterior tibial pulse
Ptp transpulmonary pressure
PTPN peripheral (vein) total
    parenteral nutrition
PT-PTT prothrombin time and
    partial thromboplastin time
PTR
    patella tendon reflex
    psychotic trigger reaction
PTRA
    percutaneous transluminal
        renal angioplasty
    percutaneous transluminal
        rotational atherectomy
Ptrx pelvic traction
PTS Pediatric Trauma Scale
    (Score)
PTSD posttraumatic stress
    disorder
PTSMA percutaneous
    transluminal septal myocardial
    ablation
PTT
    partial thromboplastin time
    pure tone threshold

PTU pregnancy, term,
    uncomplicated
PTUCA percutaneous
    transluminal ultrasonic
    coronary angioplasty
PTV
    percutaneous transtracheal jet
        ventilation
    posterior terminal vein
    posterior tibial vein
PTX
    pancreas transplant
    parathyroidectomy
    pelvic traction
    pneumothorax
PU
    posterior urethra
    pregnancy urine
    by way of urethra [L. *per
        urethra*]
Pu plutonium
PUA pelvic (examination) under
    anesthesia
PUB pubic
PUC pediatric urine collector
PUD
    partial upper denture
    peptic ulcer disease
PUL, pul
    percutaneous ultrasonic
        lithotripsy
    pubourethral ligament
PULHES (general) physical,
    upper extremities, lower
    extremities, hearing, eyes,
    psychiatric (exam)
pulm
    pulmonary
    pulmonic
PULP pulpotomy
PULSE OX, pulsox pulse
    oximetry
PULSES (general) physical,
    upper extremities, lower
    extremities, sensory, excretory,
    social support (physical
    profile)
PUND pregnancy, uterine, not
    delivered

PUNL percutaneous ultrasonic nephrolithotripsy
PUP percutaneous ultrasonic pyelolithotomy
PU/PL partial upper and lower dentures
PUPPP pruritic urticarial papules and plaques of pregnancy
purg purgative
PUSH Pressure Ulcer Scale for Healing
PUVA pulsed ultraviolet actinotherapy
PUW pick-up walker
PV
   papillomavirus
   parvovirus
   per vagina
   phonation volume
   photovoltaic
   plasma volume
   pneumococcus vaccine
   polio vaccine
   popliteal vein
   portal vein
   postvoiding
   pressure-volume
   projectile vomiting
   pulmonary vein
   by way of vagina [L. *per vaginam*]
P&V
   peak and valley
   percuss and vibrate
   pyloroplasty and vagotomy
P:V pressure to volume ratio
Pv venous pressure
PVA Prinzmetal variant angina
PVB
   paravertebral block
   porcelain veneer bridge
   premature ventricular beat
PVC
   porcelain veneer crown
   postvoiding cystogram
   predicted vital capacity

   premature ventricular contraction
   primary visual cortex
Pvco2 partial pressure of carbon dioxide in mixed venous blood
PVD
   percussion, vibration, and drainage
   peripheral vascular disease
   posterior vitreous detachment
PVE
   periventricular echogenicity
   prosthetic valve endocarditis
PVEP pattern visual evoked potential
PVER pattern visual evoked response
PVF peripheral visual field
PVG periventricular gray matter
PVL plasma viral load
PVM paravertebral muscle
PVMT Primary Visual Motor Test
PVN predictive value of a negative (test)
PVO
   peripheral vascular occlusion
   portal vein occlusion
PVo pulmonary valve opening
PvO2, Pvo2 partial venous gas tension of oxygen
PVOD peripheral vascular occlusive disease
PVP
   portal venous pressure
   posteroventral pallidotomy
PVR
   postvoid residual
   prosthetic valve regurgitation
   pulmonary vascular resistance
PVS
   percussion, vibration, and suction
   peripheral vascular system
   peritoneovenous shunt
   persistent vegetative state
   prosthetic valve stenosis

P

PVT

paroxysmal ventricular tachycardia

portal vein thrombosis

pressure, volume, temperature

PVW posterior vaginal wall

PW

pacing wire

peristaltic wave

plantar wart

posterior wall (of heart)

psychological warfare

pulsed wave

pulse width

puncture wound

PWA person(s) with AIDS

P wave part of the electrocardiographic cycle representing atrial depolarization

PWB partial weightbearing

PWC physical work capacity

PWD

person(s) with a disability

pulsed-wave Doppler

PWI perfusion-weighted (magnetic resonance) imaging

PWMI posterior wall myocardial infarction

PWOS post workout syncope

PWS port-wine stain

PWV pulse wave velocity

Px prophylaxis

PXM projection x-ray microscopy

PXS dental prophylaxis (cleaning)

PY, P/Y

pack-year (cigarettes)

person year

PYR person-year rad

Pz parietal midline (zero) electrode placement in electroencephalography

pz pieze (unit of pressure)

PZP pregnancy zone protein

Q

Q
electrocardiographic wave
glutamine (*See also* Gln)
quantity (of heat)
quaternary
quotient

q
each, every [L. *quaque*]
four [L. *quattuor*]
frequency of rarer allele of a gene pair
long arm of chromosome
quintal

q.2h. every two hours [L. *quaque secunda hora*]

q.3h. every three hours [L. *quaque tertia hora*]

q.4h. every four hours [L. *quaque quarta hora*]

QA quality assessment (assurance)

QAC
before every meal
quaternary ammonium compound

QALE quality-adjusted life expectancy

QALY quality-adjusted life-years

QAM quality assurance monitor

q.a.m. every morning [L. *quaque ante meridiem*]

Q angle
quadriceps angle
Quatrefages angle (parietal angle)

QAP quality assurance program

QAR
quality assurance reagent
quantitative autoradiographic

QA/RM quality assurance/risk management

QAS
quality-adjusted survival
quality assurance standards

QAT quality assurance technical (material)

QAUR quality assurance and utilization review

QB Quantitative (Electrophysiological) Battery

Q$_B$ blood flow

QBCA quantitative buffy-coat analysis

QBV whole blood volume

QC
quad cane
quality control

Qc pulmonary capillary blood flow (perfusion)

QCA
quantitative coronary angiography
quantitative coronary arteriography

QC-PCR quantitative competitive polymerase chain reaction

QCT quantitative computed tomography

QCU qualitative coronary ultrasound

QD, q.d. every day [L. *quaque die*]

QDAM, q.d.a.m. once daily in the morning

QDPM, q.d.p.m. once daily in the evening

QDR quantitative digital radiography

q.e.d. that which is to be demonstrated [L. *quod erat demonstrandum*]

QEE quadriceps extension exercise

QEEG quantitative electroencephalogram

QET Quality Extinction Test

QF
quadratus femoris
quality factor (relative biologic effectiveness)
quick freeze

Qf rate of fluid filtration

295

Q fever Queensland (Australian) fever

q.h. every hour [L. *quaque hora*]

QHS, q.h.s. at bedtime [L. *hora somni hour of sleep*]

QID, q.i.d. four times daily [L. *quater in die*]

QIg quantitative immunoglobulin

QJ quadriceps jerk

QLI Quality of Life Index

QLQ Quality of Life Questionnaire

QLS
Quality of Life Scale
quasielastic laser light-scattering spectroscope

QM Quénu-Muret (sign)

QMB qualified Medicare beneficiary

QMI Q-wave myocardial infarction

QMV quadricusp mitral valve

QNA quadriceps neutral angle

QNS, q.n.s. quantity not sufficient

QO₂
oxygen consumption
oxygen quotient
oxygen utilization

QOD, q.o.d. every other day [L. *quaque altera die*]

QOL quality of life

QOM quality of movement

QP
quadrant pain
quanti-Pirquet (reaction)

Qp pulmonary blood flow

Qpc pulmonary capillary blood flow

QPCR, Q-PCR quantitative polymerase chain reaction

QPEEG quantitative pharmacoelectroencephalography

QPM, q.p.m. each evening [L. *quaque post meridiem*]

QPOS Quality Point of Service

QP:QS, Qp:Qs pulmonary to systemic flow ratio

QPT Quick prothrombin time

QQH, q.q.h. (*See also* q.4h.) every four hours [L. *quaque quarta hora*]

QR quieting response

qr quadriradial

QRC qualitative radiocardiography

QRNG quinolone-resistant *Neisseria gonorrhoeae*

QRS electrocardiographic wave (complex or interval)

QRS-ST electrocardiographic junction between QRS complex and ST segment

QRS-T electrocardiographic angle between QRS and T vectors

QS
Q-switched
quadriceps set
quantitation standard
quantity sufficient
quiet sleep

QS2 total electromechanical systole

Qs systemic blood flow

QSAR quantitative structure-activity relationship

Q-SART Quantitative Sudomotor Axon Reflex Test

QSC quasistatic compliance

QS₂I shortened electrochemical systole

Q sign Quant sign

Qsp physiologic shunt flow

QSRL Q-switched ruby laser

Q-S test Queckenstedt-Stookey test

QSYAG Q-switched YAG laser

QT
electrocardiographic interval from the beginning of QRS complex to end of the T wave
Quick test (prothrombin, liver function)

qt
quart
quiet

QTc, QT_c QT corrected for heart rate
QTd QT dispersion
QTL quantitative trait locus
Q-TWIST, Q-TWiST quality-adjusted time without symptoms (of disease) and toxicity
qty quantity
quad
quadrant
quadriceps
quadriplegia
quadruplet
quad ex quadriceps exercise
qual
qualitative
quality
qual anal qualitative analysis
QUALY quality adjusted life-year
quant
quantitative
quantity
quar quarantine
QUART quadrantectomy, axillary dissection, radiation therapy
quart.
fourth [L. *quartus*]
quarterly
quats quaternary ammonium compounds
QUEST
Quality of Upper Extremities Test
Quality, Utilization, Effectiveness, Statistically Tabulated
quest.
question
questionable
quint quintuplet
QUS quantitative ultrasound
q.v. which see (literature citation) [L. *quod vide*]
QW every week
QWE every weekend
q. 4 wk. every four weeks
q. wk once a week

R
arginine (*See also* Arg)
electrocardiographic wave in QRS complex
metabolic respiratory quotient
organic radical
rad
Rankine (scale)
ratio
recessive
rectal
red (indicator color)
remote point of convergence
roentgen (*See also* roent)
side chain in amino acid formula

R1 longitudinal relaxivity
R2 transverse relaxivity
+R Rinne (hearing) test positive
-R Rinne (hearing) test negative
r
angle of refraction
correlation coefficient
product moment
recombinant
ring chromosome 1–22
r. far point [L. *remotum*]
RA
radioactive
radiographic absorptiometry
radionuclide angiography
ragweed antigen
reading age
reciprocal asymmetrical
regional anesthesia
renal artery
renin-angiotensin
repeat action (drugs)
residual air
right angle
right arm
right atrium
Rokitansky-Aschoff (sinus)
rotational atherectomy
rrheumatoid arthritis
Ra radium

RAA renin-angiotensin-aldosterone (system)
RAAPI resting ankle-arm pressure index
RABA radioantigen-binding assay
RABP retinoic acid-binding protein
RAC radial artery catheter
rac
racemate
racemic
RACAT rapid acquisition computed axial tomography
RACCO right anterior caudocranial oblique (portography position)
RAD
ionizing radiation unit
radiation absorbed dose
radical
reactive airways disease
right anterior descending (coronary artery)
right axis deviation
roentgen administered dose
RADA right acromiodorsoanterior (fetal position)
RADP right acromiodorsoposterior (fetal position)
RADS retrospective assessment of drug safety
rad/s radian per second
RADT rapid antigen-detection test
RAE right atrial enlargement
RAFF rectus abdominis free flap
RAG
ragweed
room air gas
RAH
radioactive Hippuran (test)
right atrial hypertrophy

RAHB right anterior hemiblock
rAHF antihemophilic factor (recombinant)
RAI
radioactive iodine
resting ankle index
RAID radiolabeled antibody imaging
RAIS reflection-absorption infrared spectroscopy
RAIT radioimmunotherapy
RALT routine admission laboratory test
RAM
radioactive material
rapid alternating movements
rectus abdominis muscle
rectus abdominis musculocutaneous (flap)
RAMI Risk-Adjusted Mortality Index
RAMP
Rate Modulated Pacing
right atrial mean pressure
RANA rheumatoid arthritis nuclear antigen
RAO
right anterior oblique
right anterior occipital
RAP
relative average perturbation
remote access perfusion
renal artery pressure
rheumatoid arthritis preciptin
right abdominal pain
right atrial pressure
RAPD
random amplified polymorphic DNA
relative afferent pupillary defect
RAQ right anterior quadrant
RAR right arm recumbent (reclining)
RARE rapid acquisition with resolution enhancement
RAS
renal artery stenosis
renin-angiotensin system
reticular activating system

right arm, sitting
Rokitansky-Aschoff sinus
rotational atherectomy system
RASE rapid-acquisition spin echo
RASP Rapidly Alternating Speech Perception (Test)
RAST radioallergosorbent assay test
RAT
right anterior thigh
rotating aspiration thromboembolectomy
RATx radiation therapy
RAU radioactive uptake
RAUC raw area under curve
RAVLT Rey Auditory Verbal Learning Test
RAW, R (AW), R$_{AW}$
airway resistance
RB
rebreathing
Renaut body
respiratory burst
reticulate body
retinoblastoma
retrobulbar
R&B right and below
Rb rubidium
RBA
rescue breathing apparatus
risks, benefits, and alternatives (discussion with patient)
rose bengal antigen
RBAP repetitive bursts of action potential
RBB right bundle branch
RBBB right bundle branch block
RBC red blood cell
RBC frag red blood cell fragility
RBCM red blood cell mass
RBC:P red blood cell to plasma ratio
RBC s/f red blood cell spun filtration
RBCV red blood cell volume

RBD
 right border of dullness
  (percussion of heart)
 right brain damage
RBE
 radiobiologic equivalent
 relative biologic effectiveness
RBF
 regional blood flow
 renal blood flow
RBG
 random blood glucose
 red blue green (Doppler)
RBL
 radiographic baseline
 Reid baseline
 rubber band ligation
RBON retrobulbar optic neuritis
RBOW rupture(d) of bag of
 waters
RBP resting blood pressure
Rb-82 PET rubidium-82
 positron emission tomography
RBR radiation bowel reaction
RBRVS resource-based relative
 value scale
RBS
 random blood sugar
 rutherford backscattering
RBSI radiographic bone strength
 index
RBSP ramus, body, symphysis,
 palate
RBV right brachial vein
RB-V right bundle ventricular
RBW relative body weight
RC
 radiocarpal
 red corpuscle
 reflection coefficient
 rehabilitation counseling
 resistance and capacitance
 respiratory care
 response criteria
 rest cure
 retrograde cystogram
 retruded contact (position)
 rib cage
 right coronary

 right (ear), cold (stimulus)
 root canal
 rotator cuff
 routine cholecystectomy
R & C reasonable and
 customary
Rc
 receptor
 response, conditioned
RCA
 radiographic contrast agent
 radionuclide cerebral
  angiogram
 Raji cell assay
 red (blood) cell agglutination
 renal carcinoma
 retained cortical activity
 right carotid artery
 right coronary angiography
 right coronary artery
 rotational coronary
  atherectomy
RCBF renal cortical blood flow
rCBF regional cerebral blood
 flow
RCC
 radiographic coronary
  calcification
 radiologic control center
 red (blood) cell cast
 red (blood) cell concentrate
 red (blood) cell count
 renal cell carcinoma
 right common carotid
 right coronary cusp
Rcc radiochemical
RCCA right common carotid
 artery
RCCT randomized controlled
 clinical trial
RCD relative (area of) cardiac
 dullness
RCE right carotid
 endarterectomy
RCF
 red (blood) cell folate
 Reiter complement fixation
 relative centrifugal force

RCF *(continued)*
　　Ross carbohydrate free
　　　(formula)
RCFA
　　right common femoral
　　　angioplasty
　　right common femoral artery
RCHF right-sided congestive
heart failure
RCI
　　rate change induced
　　respiratory control index
RCIT, RCITR red (blood) cell
iron turnover rate
RCL
　　radial collateral ligament
　　range of comfortable loudness
　　renal clearance
RCM
　　radiocontrast material
　　radiographic contrast medium
　　restrictive cardiomyopathy
　　right costal margin
　　Roux conditioned medium
RCMI red cell morphology
index
RCP retrograde cerebral
perfusion
RCR
　　relative consumption rate
　　replication-competent retrovirus
　　　(assay)
　　respiratory control ratio
　　rotator cuff repair
RCS
　　red (blood) cell suspension
　　red color sign
　　repeat cesarean section
　　right coronary sinus
RCT
　　randomized clinical trial
　　retrograde conduction time
　　root canal therapy
　　Rorschach content test
RCV
　　red cell volume
　　right colic vein
RCX ramus circumflexus
RD
　　radial deviation

Raynaud disease
reaction of degeneration
Reiter disease
respiratory distress
restricted duty
retinal detachment
Reye disease
right dorsoanterior
ruptured disc
R&D research and development
Rd rutherford (unit of
radioactivity)
RDA
　　recommended daily allowance
　　right dorsoanterior (fetal
　　　position)
　　right ductus arteriosus
RdA reading age
RDB
　　randomized double-blind (trial)
　　Rosai-Dorfman disease
RDFS ratio of decayed and
filled surfaces
RDFT ratio of decayed and
filled teeth
RDG retrograde
duodenogastroscopy
RDI
　　recommended daily intake
　　relative dose intensity
　　respiratory distress index
　　rupture-delivery interval
　　　(obstetrics)
RDM rod disc membrane
rDNA ribosomal
deoxyribonucleic acid
RDOD retinal detachment,
oculus dexter (right eye)
RDOS retinal detachment,
oculus sinister (left eye)
RDP
　　radiopharmaceutical drug
　　　product
　　random-donor platelet
　　right dorsoposterior (fetal
　　　position)
RDPase ribonucleic acid-
dependent deoxyribonucleic
acid polymerase

RDS · Refl

RDS respiratory distress
syndrome (of newborn)
RDT
regular (hemo)dialysis
treatment
routine dialysis therapy
RDTD referral, diagnosis,
treatment, and discharge
RDU recreational drug use
RDW
red (blood cell) distribution
width (index)
reticulocyte distribution width
RE
concerning (regarding)
racemic epinephrine
Rasmussen encephalitis
rectal examination
renal excretion
resting energy
reticuloendothelial
right ear (*See also* A.D.)
right eye (*See also* O.D.)
rostral end
R&E
rest and exercise
round and equal
R$_e$ Reynolds number (*See also*
N$_R$)
RE√ recheck
R↑E right upper extremity (*See
also* RUX, RUE)
Re rhenium
REA
radiation emergency area
radioenzymatic assay
restriction endonuclease
analysis
restriction enzyme analysis
right ear advantage
readm readmission
REAL Revised European-
American Lymphoma
(classification)
REB roentgen-equivalent biologic
REC
radioelectrocomplexing
recommendation
record

recovery
recreation
recur
right external carotid
RECA right external carotid
artery
recd, rec'd received
RECG radioelectrocardiography
recom smallest unit of DNA
capable of recombination
recond recondition
RecOS reconstruction occlusal
surface
rect
rectal
rectum
rectus (muscle)
recur
recurrence
recurrent
RED radiation experience data
red. reduce
redn reduction
redox oxidation-reduction
REE
rapid extinction effect
rare earth element
resting energy expenditure
re-ed reeducation
REEDS retention of tears,
ectrodactyly, ectodermal
dysplasia, strange hair, skin
and teeth (syndrome)
REEG radioelectroencepha-
lography
R-EEG resting
electroencephalogram
REF
ejection fraction at rest
referred
refused
REFI regional ejection fraction
image
ref ind refractive index (*See
also* N, RI)
Refl
reflect
reflection
reflex

303

REFRAD released from active duty

REG
radiation exposure guide
radioencephalogram
regression (analysis)
rheoencephalography

reg
regarding
region
regular
regulation

reg block regional block anesthesia

regen regenerate

reg rhy regular rhythm

reg. umb. umbilical region [L. *regio umbilici*]

regurg regurgitation

REHAB, rehab rehabilitation

REL
rate of energy loss
recommended exposure level
relative
religion
resting expiratory level

RELE resistive exercises, lower extremities

REM
radiation-equivalent-man
rapid eye movement (sleep)
recent event memory
remission

REMAB radiation-equivalent-manikin absorption

REMCAL radiation-equivalent-manikin calibration

REMP roentgen-equivalent-man period

REN renal

REO respiratory enteric orphan (virus)

REP
rapid electrophoresis
repair
repetition
report
resistive exercise product
rest-exercise program

roentgen equivalent-physical (surgical) repair

rep replication

rep. let it be repeated [L. *repetatur*]

rep B&S repetitive bending and stooping

REP CK rapid electrophoresis creatine kinase

repol repolarization

reprep re-preparation

REPS repetitions

req
requested
required

RER
renal excretion rate
respiratory exchange ratio
rough endoplasmic reticulum

RER+ replication error positive

RER- replication error negative

RES
radionuclide esophageal scintigraphy
resection
resident
reticuloendothelial system

res
research
reserve
residue

resist. ex. resistive exercise

resp
respective
respiration
respiratory

RESP-A respiratory battery, acute

REST
regressive electroshock treatment
restoration
restriction of environmental stimulation therapy

resus resuscitation

RET
rearranged during transfection
retention
retina

retired
return
ret rad equivalent therapeutic
RETA rete testis aspiration
ret cath retention catheter
ret detach retinal detachment
RETHINK recognize, empathize, think, hear, integrate, notice, keep
RETIC reticulocyte
retro pyelo retrograde pyelogram
RETRX retraction
Re-Tx retransplantation
REU rectal endoscopic ultrasonography
reu radiation effect unit
REUE resistive exercises to upper extremities
REUS rectal endoscopic ultrasonography
REV, rev
reversal
reverse
review
revolution
rev/min revolution per minute
Rev of Sys review of systems (*See also* ROS)
re-x reexamination
REZ root exit zone
RF
radial fiber (of cochlea)
rapid filling
receptive field (of visual cortex)
recognition factor
reduction fixation
Reitland-Franklin (unit)
relative flow
renal failure
resistance factor
respiratory failure
restricted fluids
reticular formation
retroflexed
rheumatic fever
rheumatoid factor
risk factor

root (canal) filling
rosette formation
R&F radiographic and fluoroscopic
R$_F$ rate of flow
Rf rutherfordium
RFA
radiofluorescent antibody
radiofrequency ablation
right frontoanterior (fetal position)
RFB
radial flow chromatography
retained foreign body
RFC
radiofrequency coil
radiofrequency current
retrograde femoral catheter
right frontal craniotomy
RFCA radiofrequency catheter ablation
RFD residue-free diet
RFDT Reach in Four Directions Test
RFE return flow enema
RFI
recurrence-free interval
renal failure index
RFL
radionuclide functional lymphoscintigraphy
right frontolateral (fetal position)
RFLF retained fetal lung fluid
RFLP restriction fragment length polymorphism
RFP
rapid filling period
renal function panel
right frontoposterior (fetal position)
RFR
rapid filling rate
refraction
RFS
rapid frozen section
refeeding syndrome
relapse-free survival
renal function study

305

RFT
> right frontotransverse (fetal position)
> rod-and-frame test

RFTA radiofrequency thermal ablation

RFTC radiofrequency thermocoagulation

RFV right femoral vein

RFW rapid filling wave

RG
> regurgitated (infant feeding)
> retrograde

R/G red/green

RGAS retained gastric antrum syndrome

RGC radio-gas chromatography

RGD range-gated Doppler

RGE
> relative gas expansion
> respiratory gas equation

RGO reciprocating gait orthosis

RGP rigid gas-permeable (contact lens)

RH
> radial hemolysis
> radiant heat
> reactive hyperemia
> regulatory hormone
> releasing hormone
> retinal hemorrhage
> rheumatoid

Rh
> rhesus (blood factor)
> rhinion (craniometric point)
> rhodium

Rh– rhesus negative

Rh+ rhesus positive

r/h roentgen per hour

rHA recombinant human albumin

RHB
> raise head of bed
> right heart border
> right heart bypass

RH/BSO radical hysterectomy and bilateral salpingo-oophorectomy

RHBV right heart blood volume

RHC
> resin hemoperfusion column
> respiration has ceased
> right heart catheterization
> routine health care

RhC rhesus C antigen

RhCE rhesus gene CE

RHCT renal helical computed tomography

RHD
> radial head dislocation
> radiologic health data
> renal hypertensive disease
> rheumatic heart disease
> right-hand dominant
> right hemisphere (brain) damage

RhD
> rhesus D antigen
> rhesus gene D
> rhesus (hemolytic) disease

RHE respiratory heat exchange

RhE rhesus E antigen

rheum rheumatic

RHF right heart failure

RHG
> radial hemolysis in gel
> right hand grip

rhGH recombinant human growth hormone

RHH right homonymous hemianopia (hemianopsia)

RhIG, RhIg rhesus immune globulin

rhIGF recombinant human insulinlike growth factor

RhIGIV Rh immune globulin intravenous

rhIL recombinant human interleukin

rhin rhinitis

rhino rhinoplasty

RHINOS fiberoptic rhinoscopy

r-hirudin recombinant hirudin

RHM routine health management

Rhm roentgen per hour at one meter

RhMK, RhMk, RhMkK rhesus monkey kidney

RHN Rockwell hardness number
Rh$_{null}$ rhesus factor null (all Rh factors are lacking)
RHO right heeloff
Rho(D) immunoglobulin G anti-Rho(D)(given to Rh-negative individuals exposed to Rh-positive blood)
rhom rhomboid (muscle)
RHP resting head pressure
RHR resting heart rate
R/hr roentgen per hour
RHS
  radial head subluxation
  reciprocal hindlimb-scratching (syndrome)
  right heel strike
RHT
  renal homotransplantation
  right hypertropia
rHuEPO recombinant human erythropoietin
RI
  radioimmunology
  radioisotope
  ramus intermedius (coronary artery)
  reference interval
  refractive index (*See also* N, ref ind)
  relative intensity
  renal insufficiency
  resistance index
  respiratory index
R/I rule in
RIA
  radioimmunoassay
  right iliac artery
RIBA radioimmunoblot assay
RICE rest, ice, compression, elevation
RID
  radioimmunodetection
  radioimmunodiffusion
RIE radiation induced emesis
RIG rabies immune globulin
RIGH rabies immune globulin, human

RIGS radioimmunoguided surgery
RIM
  radioisotope medicine
  rapid identification method
  relative-intensity measure
RIMA right internal mammary artery
RIMS resonance ionization mass spectrometry
RIN radiation-induced neoplasm
RIND reversible ischemic neurologic deficit
RINN recommended international nonproprietary name
R$_{int}$ intrinsic flow resistance
RINV radiation-induced nausea and vomiting
RIP
  radioimmunoprecipitation (test)
  rapid infusion pump
  respiratory inductance plethysmograph
  rhythmic inhibitory pattern
RIPA radioimmunoprecipitation assay
RIRB radioiodinated rose bengal (dye)
RIS
  radiographic imaging system
  radioimmunoglobulin scintigraphy
  rapid immunofluorescence staining
  respiratory index score
RIs Rehabilitation Indicators
RISA
  radioimmunosorbent assay
  radioiodinated serum albumin
RIST radioimmunosorbent test
RIT
  radioimmunoglobulin therapy
  radioimmunotherapy
  Rorschach Inkblot Test (*See also* Ror)
RIU radioiodine uptake
RIV
  ramus interventricularis
  right innominate vein

RIVC
　　radionuclide (imaging of)
　　　inferior vena cava
　　right inferior vena cava
RIX　radiation-induced xerostomia
RJ
　　radial jerk (reflex)
　　right jugular
RJI　radionuclide joint imaging
RK
　　radial keratotomy
　　right kidney
RKG　radio(electro)cardiogram
RKS　retrograde kidney study
RKW　renal kalium (potassium)
　　wasting
RKY　roentgen kymography
R or L　right or left
RL
　　reticular lamina
　　right lateral (*See also* RT
　　　LAT)
　　right leg
　　right lower
　　right lung
　　Ringer lactate (solution)
　　rotation left
R_L　pulmonary resistance (*See
　　also* $R_L R_P$, R_p)
R L, R→L, R/L, R-light-to-left
　　(shunt)
RLA
　　radiographic lung area
　　right lower arm
RLB　right lateral bending
RLC　residual lung capacity
RLD
　　related living donor
　　resistive load detection
　　right lateral decubitus
　　　(position)
　　ruptured lumbar disc
RLE
　　recent life event
　　right lower extremity
RLF　right lateral femoral
RLG　right lateral gaze
RLL
　　right lower limb
　　right lower lobe

RLN
　　recurrent laryngeal nerve
　　regional lymph node
RLND
　　regional lymph node
　　　dissection
　　retroperitoneal lymph node
　　　dissection
RLO　Right-Left Orientation Test
RLQ　right lower quadrant
RLR　right lateral rectus
　　(muscle)
$R_L R_P$　pulmonary resistance (*See
　　also* R_L, R_p)
RLS
　　person who stammers having
　　　difficulty enunciating R, L,
　　　and S
　　restless legs syndrome
RLSB
　　right lower scapular border
　　right lower sternal border
RLT　red light therapy
RLTCS　repeat low transverse
　　cesarean section
RLUs　relative light units
RM
　　radical mastectomy
　　rehabilitation medicine
　　repetition maximum
　　resistive movement
　　rhabdomyosarcoma
　　right median
　　room
　　ruptured membranes
1-RM　one-repetition maximum
R&M　routine and microscopic
Rm
　　relative mobility
　　remission
RMA
　　right mentoanterior (fetal
　　　position) (*See also* MDA)
　　Rivermead motor assessment
RMB　right main-stem bronchus
RMBF　regional myocardial
　　blood flow
RMCA, R-MCA
　　right main coronary artery
　　right middle cerebral artery

RME
  resting metabolic expenditure
  right mediolateral episiotomy
R meter roentgen meter
RMI Rivermead Mobility Index
RML
  right mediolateral
  right mentolateral (fetal position)
  right middle lobe (of lung)
RMLB right middle lobe bronchus
RMP
  resting membrane potential
  right mentoposterior (fetal position) (*See also* MDP)
RMR
  resting metabolic rate
  right medial rectus (muscle)
RMS
  red-man syndrome
  repetitive motion syndrome
  Rocky Mountain spotted fever vaccine
rms root-mean-square
RMSF Rocky Mountain spotted fever
RMT
  retromolar trigone
  right mentotransverse (fetal position) (*See also* MDT)
RMV respiratory minute volume
RN
  radionucleotide (scanning)
  radionuclide
  red nucleus
  reticular nucleus
Rn radon
RNA
  radionuclide angiogram
  ribonucleic acid
  rough, noncapsulated, avirulent (bacterial culture)
RNAse, RNase ribonuclease
RND radical neck dissection
RNFL retinal nerve fiber layer
RNG radionuclide angiography
RNP ribonucleoprotein

RNS
  reference normal serum
  repetitive nerve stimulation
RNST reactive nonstress test
RNV
  radionuclide venography
  radionuclide ventriculogram
RO
  reality orientation
  relative odds
  reverse osmosis
  Ritter-Oleson (technique)
  routine order
R/O rule out
ROA
  regurgitant orifice area
  reversal of antagonist
  right occipitoanterior (fetal position) (*See also* ODA)
ROAD reversible obstructive airways disease
ROAM roaming optical access multiscope
rob. robertsonian (translocation)
ROC
  receiver operating characteristic
  record of contact
roc reciprocal ohm centimeter
Roch-Ochs Rochester-Ochsner (forceps)
RODA rapid opiate detoxification under anesthesia
RODAC replicate organism detection and counting
RODAC-TM replicate organism direct agar contact
RODEO rotating delivery of excitation off resonance
ROE
  report of event
  right otitis externa
roent
  roentgen (*See also* R)
  roentgenology
ROF review outside films
ROI
  reactive oxygen intermediate

ROI (*continued*)
   region of interest
   release of information
ROIDS hemorrhoids
ROJM range of joint motion
ROL right occipitolateral (fetal position)
ROM
   range of motion
   rupture of membranes
Rom, Romb Romberg (sign)
rom reciprocal ohm meter
ROMI rule out myocardial infarction
romied ruled out for myocardial infarction
RON radiation optic neuropathy
ROP
   regional organ procurement
   retinopathy of prematurity
   right occipitoposterior (fetal position) (*See also* ODP)
ROPE respiratory ordered phase encoding
ROR French acronym for measles-mumps-rubella vaccine
Ror Rorschach (Inkblot Test) (*See also* RIT)
RoRx roentgen therapy
ROS
   reactive oxygen species
   review of systems (*See also* Rev of Sys)
RoS rostral sulcus
ROSC return of spontaneous circulation
ROT
   remedial occupational therapy
   right occipitotransverse (fetal position) (*See also* ODT)
   rotating
   rotator
   rule of thumb
rot. ny rotatory nystagmus
ROUL
   rouleau
   rouleaux (plural)
rout. routine
RP
   radial pulse

   radical prostatectomy
   radiographic planimetry
   radiopharmaceutical
   Raynaud phenomenon
   rectal prolapse
   reentrant pathway
   refractory period
   resting potential
   resting pressure
   retinitis pigmentosa
   retrograde pyelogram
   retroperitoneal
   reverse phase
   root plane
R:P respiratory (rate) to pulse (rate) (index)
R_p pulmonary resistance (*See also* R_L, $R_L R_P$)
RPA right pulmonary artery
rPBF regional pulmonary blood flow
RPC
   retained products of conception
   root planing and curettage
RPCV retropubic cystourethropexy
RPD removable partial denture
RPE
   rating of perceived exertion
   retinal pigment epithelial (cell)
RPEP rabies postexposure prophylaxis
RPF relaxed pelvic floor
RPF[a] arterial renal plasma flow
RPF[v] venous renal plasma flow
RPG rheoplethysmography
RPGR retinitis pigmentosa GTPase regulator gene
RPHA reversed passive hemagglutination
RPI
   resting pressure index
   reticulocyte production index
RPICCE round pupil intracapsular cataract extraction

RPM, rpm
    revolution per minute
    rotation per minute
RPN resident's progress note
RPO right posterior oblique
    (radiologic view)
RPP
    radical perineal prostatectomy
    rate-pressure product
    retropubic prostatectomy
RPPI role perception picture
    inventory
RPR rapid plasma reagin
R Pr retinitis proliferans
RPRCT rapid plasma reagin
    card test
RPS, rps
    reverse pivot shift
    revolution per second
RPT rapid pull-through
    (technique)
rpt report
rptd ruptured
RPU retropubic urethropexy
RPV
    right portal vein
    right pulmonary vein
RQ
    recovery quotient
    respiratory quotient
RQS repeated quick stretch
RQS-E repeated quick stretch
    from elongation
RQS-SEC repeated quick stretch
    superimposed upon an
    existing contraction
RR
    radial rate
    radiation reaction
    radiation response
    rate ratio
    recovery room
    red reflex
    respiratory rate
    response rate
    retinal reflex
    risk ratio
    road rash
    rotation right

R/R rales/rhonchi
R&R
    rate and rhythm
    recess-resect
    rest and recuperation
RRA
    right radial artery
    right renal artery
RRAM rapid rhythmic
    alternating movements
RRE regressive resistive
    exercise
RR&E round, regular, and
    equal (pupils)
RREF resting radionuclide
    ejection fraction
RREID rapid rabies enzyme
    immunodiagnosis
RRF
    ragged red fiber
    right rectus femoris
RRI
    reflex relaxation index
    relative response index
RR-IOL remove and replace
    intraocular lens
RRM right radical mastectomy
RRMS relapsing-remitting
    multiple sclerosis
rRNA ribosomal ribonucleic
    acid
RROM resistive range of
    motion
R rot right rotation
RRP
    radical retropubic
      prostatectomy
    relative refractory period
RRQG right rostral quarter
    ganglion
RRR regular rate and rhythm
RRRN round, regular, react
    normally (pupils)
RRS retrorectal space
R_{rs} respiratory system resistance
RRV right renal vein
RRVN retrolabyrinthine/retrosig-
    moid vestibular neurectomy

RRVS recovery room vital signs

RRW rales, rhonchi or wheezes

RS
random sample
reading of standard
rectosigmoid
Reed-Sternberg (cell)
respiratory symptom
respiratory system
response to stimulus ratio
rhythm strip
right side
Ringer solution
Ritchie sedimentation (technique, stool examination)
rumination syndrome

R&S restraint and seclusion

R/S
reschedule
rest stress
rupture (of membranes) spontaneous

R/s roentgen per second

Rs
respond
response

r_s rank correlation coefficient

RSA
regular spiking activity
right sacroanterior (fetal position) (*See also* SDA)

RSBI Rapid Shallow Breathing Index

RSBT rhythmic sensory bombardment therapy

RSC
radioscaphocapitate
rectosigmoid neocolpopoiesis
rested state contraction

RScA right scapuloanterior (fetal position)

RSCL Rotterdam Symptom Check List

RScP right scapuloposterior (fetal position)

RSCS respiratory system compliance score

RSD
rad surface dose
reflex sympathetic dystrophy

RSG Reitan Strength of Grip

RSI
rapid-sequence induction (of anesthesia)
rapid sequence intubation
repetitive strain (stress) injury

RSIVP rapid-sequence intravenous pyelography

RSL
renal solute load
right sacrolateral (fetal position)

R SL brace right short leg brace

RSLT reduced-size liver transplantation

RSLTx right single lung transplant

RSNI round spermatid nuclear injection

RSO
right salpingo-oophorectomy
right superior oblique (muscle)

rSO2, rSO_2 regional oxygen saturation

RSP
rapid straight pacing
removable silicone plug
rhinoseptoplasty
right sacroposterior (fetal position) (*See also* SDP)

RSR
regular sinus rhythm
response-stimulus ratio

RSRI renal:systemic renin index

RSS
rearfoot stability system
rectosigmoidoscope
repetitive stress syndrome
representative sample
sectioned

RSSE Russian spring-summer encephalitis

RST
rapid simple tests
rapid surfactant test

reagin screen test
right sacrotransverse (fetal position) (*See also* SDT)
rubrospinal tract
RSV
regurgitant stroke volume
respiratory syncytial virus
right subclavian vein
RSVC right superior vena cava
RSV-IGIV, RSV-IVIG respiratory syncytial virus intravenous immunoglobulin
RSW right-sided weakness
RT
radiotelemetry
reading task
reciprocating tachycardia
recovery time
recreational therapy
relaxation time
renal transplant
repetition time
resistance training
respiratory therapy
room temperature
R_T total pulmonary resistance
R/T
rectal temperature
related to
Rt right
RTA renal tubular acidosis
RTC
(a)round the clock
residential treatment center
return to clinic
RTD
repetitive trauma disorder
residual thermal damage
routine test dilution
rtd retired
RtH right-handed
RTI
respiratory tract infection
reverse transcriptase inhibitor
RTKP radiothermokeratoplasty
RTL reactive to light (pupils)
RT LAT right lateral (*See also* RL)

RTN
renal tubular necrosis
routine
rtn return
RTO right toe-off (gait evaluation)
RTP
radiation treatment planning
return to play
RTR retention time ratio
RTS
real-time scan
Revised Trauma Score
right toe strike (gait evaluation)
RTSW Repeated Test of Sustained Wakefulness
RTU relative time unit
RTUS real-time ultrasonography
RTW return to work
RTWD return to work determination
RTx radiation therapy
RU
radioactive uptake
radioulnar
rectourethral
residual urine
resin uptake
retrograde urogram
retroverted uterus
right upper
Ru ruthenium
RUA routine urine analysis
RUE right upper extremity (*See also* RUX, R↑E)
RUG
resource utilization group
retrograde urethrogram
RUL
right upper (eye)lid
right upper lateral
right upper limb
right upper lobe
right upper lung
RUM right upper medial
RUQ right upper quadrant
RUR resin uptake ratio
RUS real-time ultrasonography

RUT rapid urease test

RUTF ready to use therapeutic food

RUV residual urine volume

RUX right upper extremity (*See also* R↑E, RUE)

RV
  random variable
  rectal vault
  rectovaginal
  reference value
  reserve volume
  residual volume
  respiratory volume
  retrovaginal
  retroversion
  right ventricle
  rubella vaccine
  rubella virus

R_V radius of view

Rv rotavirus

RVA reentrant ventricular arrhythmia

RVAD right ventricular assist device

RVC respond to verbal command

RVCB right ventricular copulsation balloon

RVD right ventricular dimension

RVDP right ventricular diastolic pressure

RVDT retinal venous dilation and tortuosity

RVEDD right ventricular end-diastolic diameter

RVEDP right ventricular end-diastolic pressure

RVEDV right ventricular end-diastolic volume

RVEDVI right ventricular end-diastolic volume index

RVEF
  right ventricular ejection fraction
  right ventricular end-flow

RVESV right ventricular end-systolic volume

RVESVI right ventricular end-systolic volume index

RVF
  renal vascular failure
  Rift Valley fever
  right ventricular failure
  right ventricular function
  right visual field

RVFP right ventricular filling pressure

RVG
  radionuclide ventriculogram
  radiovisiography
  right ventrogluteal

RVH
  renal vascular hypertension
  right ventricular hypertrophy

RVHD rheumatic valvular heart disease

RVI relative value index

RVID right ventricular internal diameter

RVIT right ventricular inflow tract (view)

RVL right vastus lateralis

RVLG right ventrolateral gluteal

RVLM rostral ventrolateral medulla

RVM right ventricular mass

RVN
  radionuclide ventriculogram
  retrolabyrinthine vestibular neurectomy

RVO
  relaxed vaginal outlet
  retinal vein occlusion
  right ventricular outflow

RVol regurgitant volume

RVOT right ventricular outflow tract

RVP
  red veterinary petrolatum
  renovascular pressure
  resting venous pressure

RVR rapid ventricular response

RV:RA renal vein to renal activity ratio

RVRC renal vein renin concentration

RV/RF retroverted/retroflexed

RVRI renal vascular resistance index

RVS

relative value schedule

retrovaginal space

RVSO right ventricle stroke output

RVSP right ventricular systolic pressure

RVSW right ventricular stroke work

RVSWI right ventricular stroke work index

RVT renal vein thrombosis

RV:TLC residual volume to total lung capacity ratio

RVU relative value unit

RVV Russell's viper venom

RVVT Russell's viper venom time

RW

radiologic warfare

ragweed

respiratory work

right (ear), warm (stimulus)

round window

R-W Rideal-Walker (coefficient)

RWECochG round window electrocochleography

RWIS restraint and water immersion stress

RWM regional wall motion

RWP R-wave progression (electrocardiography)

RWT

Roche-Wainer-Thissen method of height prediction

R-wave threshold (electrocardiography)

RX rapid exchange

Rx

medication

pharmacy

prescription (*See also* script)

take [L. *recipe*]

Rxd prescribed

RXN reaction

Rx Phys treating physician

RXT

radiation therapy

right exotropia

R-Y Roux-en-Y (anastomosis)

RZ reserve zone

S

entropy (in thermodynamics)
midpoint of sella turcica
  (point)
serine (*See also* Ser)
siemens
smooth (bacterial colony)
sone (unit of loudness)
south
sulfur
synthesis (phase in cell
  cycle)
systole
S7 summation gallop
S/β sickle cell beta
/S/ signature (prescription)
s

sample standard deviation
satellite (chromosome)
7's serial sevens test
S1–S4

first through fourth heart
  sounds
suicide risk classification
S1–S5

first to fifth sacral nerves
first to fifth sacral vertebrae
SA

sacroanterior
serratus anterior
siblings (raised) apart
sinoatrial (node)
sinus arrhythmia
skeletal age
sleep apnea
social age
subarachnoid
substance abuse
Sa

most anterior point of
  anterior contour of the sella
  turcica (point)
samarium
SAARD slow-acting
antirheumatic drug

SAB

short-acting block
sinoatrial block
spontaneous abortion
subarachnoid bleed
SAC seasonal allergic
conjunctivitis
SAD

seasonal affective disorder
separation anxiety disorder
SADDAN severe achondroplasia
with developmental delay and
acanthosis nigricans
SAE supported arm exercise
SAFE

sexual assault forensic
  evidence
stationary attachment flexible
  endoskeleton (foot
  prosthesis)
SAFHS sonic accelerated
fracture healing system
SAH

subarachnoid hemorrhage
systemic arterial hypertension
SAHS

sleep apnea-hypersomnolence
  syndrome
sleep apnea-hypopnea
  syndrome
SAIDS simian acquired
immunodeficiency syndrome
SAL

saline
suction-assisted lipectomy
sal

salicylic
saliva
salt
SALT-P Slosson Articulation
Language Test with
Phonology
SAM

scanning acoustic microscope
subcutaneous augmentation
  material

SAMPLE symptoms/signs, allergies, medications, past medical history, last oral intake, events prior to arrival (EMT mnemonic)

SANS sympathetic autonomic nervous system

SAO
small airway obstruction
Southeast Asian ovalocytosis
splanchnic artery occlusion

SaO₂, S$_{Ao2}$
arterial oxygen saturation (*See also* pSO2)
oxygen saturation (*See also* O₂ sat., SO₂)

SAP
sensory action potential
stable angina pectoris
systolic arterial pressure

SAPS II Simplified Acute Physiology Score version II

SAQLI Sleep Apnea Quality of Life Index

SARA
sexually acquired reactive arthritis
SQUID array for reproductive assessment

SART sinoatrial recovery time

SAS
saline, agent, and saline
short arm splint
sleep apnea syndrome
subaortic stenosis
subarachnoid space
supravalvular aortic stenosis
synthetic absorbable suture

SASH saline, agent, saline, and heparin

SAT
saturation
speech awareness threshold
spermatogenic activity test

SATA spatial average-temporal average

SATS oxygen saturation level

sat. sol., sat. soln. saturated solution

SAVD spontaneous assisted vaginal delivery

SB
scleral buckle
sick bay (military)
side bend
sinus bradycardia
Southern blot
spina bifida
sternal border
suction biopsy

+SB wearing seat belt

SB- not wearing seat belt

Sb antimony [L. *stibium*]

SBA spina bifida aperta

SBB
stereotactic breast biopsy
Sudan Black B

SBDX scanning-beam digital x-ray

SBE
saturated base excess
self-breast examination
short below-elbow (cast)
subacute bacterial endocarditis

SBEP somatosensory brainstem evoked potential

SBF systemic blood flow

SBI
silent brain infarction
silicone (gel-containing) breast implant
systemic bacterial infection

SBJ skin, bones, joints

SBK spinnbarkeit (cervical mucus)

SBO
small-bowel obstruction
spina bifida occulta

SBOD scleral buckle, right eye (oculus dexter)

SBOH State Board of Health

SBOS scleral buckle, left eye (oculus sinister)

SBP
scleral buckling procedure
systolic blood pressure (*See also* SYS BP)

SBQC small-base quad cane

SBR Scarff-Bloom-Richardson
(breast cancer grade)
SBS shaken baby syndrome
SBT single-breath test
SBV single binocular vision
SC
  sacrococcygeal
  Schwann cell
  Sciana (blood group)
  self-care
  self-control
  sex chromatin
  sickle cell
  Snellen chart
  spinal cord
  squamous carcinoma
  stem cell
  sternoclavicular
  subclavian catheter
  subcostal (view)
  superior colliculus
  surface colony
  systolic click
S&C
  sclera and conjunctiva
    (singular)
  sclerae and conjunctivae
    (plural)
  singly and consensually
Sc
  scandium
  scapula
s̅c without correction (without
  glasses) [L. *sine correctione*]
  (*See also* s̅ gl)
SCA
  sickle cell anemia
  spinocerebellar ataxia
  superior cerebellar artery
SCa, S$_{Ca}$ serum calcium
ScA scapuloanterior
SCAN Screening (Test for
  Identifying) Central Auditory
  Disorder
SCAP
  scapulae (plural)
  scapula (singular)
SCAT sickle cell anemia test

SCBA self-contained breathing
  apparatus
SCC
  sequential combination
    chemotherapy
  sickle cell crisis
  small cell cancer (carcinoma)
  spinal cord compression
  squamous cell cancer
    (carcinoma)
SCD
  sequential compression device
  service-connected disability
  sudden cardiac death
ScDA right scapuloanterior (fetal
  position) [L.
  scapulodextroanterior]
ScDP right scapuloposterior
  (fetal position) [L.
  scapulodextroposterior]
SCHISTO, SCHIZ schizocyte
schiz schizophrenia
SCI
  Science Citation Index
  Sertoli cell index
  spinal cord injury
SCIDS severe combined
  immunodeficiency syndrome
SCIWORA, SCIWOA spinal
  cord injury without
  radiographic abnormality
SCJ
  squamocolumnar junction
  sternoclavicular joint
SCL
  scaphocapitolunate
  soft contact lens
SCL-90 Symptoms Checklist 90
  (items)
ScLA left scapuloposterior (fetal
  position) [L. *scapulolaeva
  anterior*]
SCLC small-cell lung cancer
ScLP left scapuloposterior (fetal
  position) [L. *scapulolaeva
  posterior*]
SCM
  sensation, circulation, motion
  sternocleidomastoid

SCN suprachiasmatic nucleus
SCOP, scop
    scopolamine
    Structural Classification of Proteins
SCOPE
    Surveillance and Control of Pathogens of Epidemiologic Importance
    systematic, complete, objective, practical, empirical
scope
    arthroscopy
    perform endoscopy
ScP scapuloposterior (fetal position)
script prescription (*See also* Rx)
SC/RP scaling and root planing
SCS
    spinal cord stimulation
    systolic click syndrome
SCSP, SC-SP supracondylar-suprapatellar
SCT
    Sertoli-cell tumor
    sickle cell trait
    stem cell transplantation
SCV
    smooth, capsulated, virulent (bacteria)
    subcutaneous vaginal (block)
SD
    seborrheic dermatitis
    senile dementia
    sensory deficit
    shallow distance (aquatic therapy)
    shoulder dislocation
    skin dose
    spasmodic dysphonia
    speech discrimination
    spontaneous delivery
    sudden death
    suicide-depression
S:D systolic to diastolic ratio
SDA
    right sacroanterior (fetal position) [L.

sacrodextroanterior] (*See also* RSA)
    Sabouraud dextrose agar
SDE subdural empyema
SDEEG stereotactic depth electroencephalogram
SDH
    spinal dorsal horn
    subdural hematoma
    systolic-diastolic hypertension
SDL
    self-directed learning
    speech discrimination loss
SD:N signal-difference to noise ratio
SDP
    right sacroposterior (fetal position) [L. *sacrodextroposterior*] (*See also* RSP)
    stomach, duodenum, and pancreas
SDS sudden death syndrome
SDT
    right sacrotransverse (fetal position) [L. *sacrodextrotransverse* (*See also* RST)
    speech detection threshold
SDU Standard Deviation Unit
SE
    Seeing Eye
    self-examination
    side effect
    Signed English
    spin-echo
    squamous epithelium
    status epilepticus
    surgical excision
Se selenium
SEA spontaneous electrical activity
SEBI stereotactic external-beam irradiation
SEC
    series elastic component (of muscles)
    size exclusion chromatography
    squamous epithelial cell
sec second

SECG
    scalp electrocardiogram (fetal)
    stress electrocardiography
SECRET stiffness of joints,
    elderly, constitutional
    (symptoms), arthritis, elevated
    ESR, temporal arthritis
    (polymyalgia rheumatica)
SED
    serious emotional disturbance
    skin erythema dose
sed rate, sed rt sedimentation
    rate
SEE₁ Seeing Essential English
SEE₂ Signing Exact English
SEER Surveillance,
    Epidemiology, and End
    Results (network, program)
seg segmented neutrophil
SELD slow expressive language
    development
SELI specific expressive
    language impairment
SEM
    scanning electron microscope
    semen
    slow eye movement
    standard error of mean
    systolic ejection murmur
SEMG, sEMG surface
    electromyography
semid half a dram
SEP
    (French) multiple sclerosis [F.
    sclerose en plaques]
    sensory evoked potential
    spinal evoked potential
    Stroke Education Program
SEPA superficial external
    pudendal artery
sept. seven [L. *septem*]
SER
    somatosensory evoked
    response
    systolic ejection rate
Ser serine (*See also* S)
SERI Spondee Error Index

SERPACWA skin exposure
    reduction paste against
    chemical warfare agents
SEWHO shoulder, elbow, wrist,
    hand orthosis
SF-36 Short Form-36 General
    Health Survey
S$_f$, Sf Svedberg flotation (unit)
SFA
    saturated fatty acid
    superficial femoral artery
SFD
    skin-film distance
    small for dates (gestational
    age)
SFF speaking fundamental
    frequency
SFHb stroma-free hemoglobin
    pyridoxalated
SFo speaking phonation
SFTR sagittal, frontal,
    transverse, rotation
SFV superficial femoral vein
SG
    salivary gland
    scrotography
    stent graft
    stratum granulosum
    substantia gelatinosa
    Swan-Ganz (catheter)
SGA
    small for gestational age
    substantial gainful activity
    (employment)
$\bar{s}$ **gl** without correction/without
    glasses (*See also* SC)
SGOT serum glutamic-
    oxaloacetic transaminase
SGPT serum glutamic-pyruvic
    transaminase
SGTX surugatoxin (mollusc
    toxin)
SGtx1 *Scodra griseipes* toxin
    (spider)
SH
    Salter-Harris (fracture)
    Schönlein-Henoch (purpura)
    sex hormone

SH *(continued)*
  sitting height
  social history *(See also* SoHx)
SHAFT sad, hostile, anxious, frustrated, tenacious (patient)
SHAS Supplement to HIV/AIDS Surveillance
SHAV superior hemiazygos vein
SHb, S-Hb sulfhemoglobin
sHBO2T systemic hyperbaric oxygen therapy
SHEENT skin, head, eyes, ears, nose, and throat
shf super high frequency
SHG sonohysterography
Shig *Shigella*
short-FRAME short stature, facial anomalies, Rieger anomaly, midline anomalies, enamel defects
SHORT, S-H-O-R-T short statue, hyperextensibility (joints) or hernia or both, ocular depression, Rieger anomaly, teething delayed
SHRC shortened, held, resisted, contracted
SHx social history
SI
  International System of Units [Fr. *Systeme International d'Unites*]
  sacroiliac
  saline infusion
  self-inflicted
  sexual intercourse
  stroke index
  systolic index
S&I suction and irrigation
S/I superior/inferior
Si
  most anterior point on lower contour of sella turcica (point)
  silicon
SIADH syndrome of inappropriate (excretion) of antidiuretic hormone
sib, sibs sibling(s)

SIBDQ Short Inflammatory Bowel Disease Questionnaire
SIC Standard Industrial Classification
SiC silicon carbide
SICD
  Sequenced Inventory of Communication Development
  sudden infant crib death
SID source-to-image (receptor) distance
SIDA French and Spanish abbreviation for AIDS
SIDER siderocyte
SIDS sudden infant death syndrome
SIESTA snooze-induced excitation of sympathetic triggered activity
SIFT sperm intrafallopian transfer
sig.
  label, write [L. *signa*]
  let it be written, labeled [L. *signetur*]
Siglish Signed English
SIJ, SI jt sacroiliac joint
SIL
  sister-in-law
  speech interference level
  squamous intraepithelial lesion
SILD Sequenced Inventory of Language Development
SILV simultaneous independent lung ventilation
SIMA single internal mammary artery
SIMV synchronized intermittent mandatory ventilation
sin. without [L. *sine*]
sing. singular
SIO sacroiliac orthosis
SiO₂ silica
SIP
  Sickness Impact Profile
  stroke in progression
SIPT Sensory Integration and Praxis Tests
SIQ sick in quarters (military)

SIS
Second International Standard
Stroke Impact Scale
SISI short increment sensitivity
index
SIT
Slosson Intelligence Test
sperm immobilization test
supraspinatus, infraspinatus,
teres (muscle insertions)
SITx small-intestine
transplantation
SIV simian immunodeficiency
virus
SIW self-inflicted wound
SjO₂, SjVO₂ jugular venous
oxygen saturation
SK
senile keratosis
solar keratosis
striae keratopathy
SKA, SKAO supracondylar knee-
ankle orthosis
SKPT simultaneous kidney-
pancreas transplantation
SL
scapholunate
sensation level (of hearing)
side-lying
slit lamp
sublingual(ly)
SLA left sacroanterior (fetal
position) [L. *sacrolaeva
anterior*] (*See also* LSA)
SLAM
scanning laser acoustic
microscope
Systemic Lupus Activity
Measure
SLC-90 Symptom Checklist 90
SLCT Sertoli-Leydig cell tumor
SLD specific language disorder
SLE systemic lupus
erythematosus
SLEM slow lateral eye
movement
SLEX slit-lamp examination
(ophthalmology,
biomicroscopy)

SLFVD sterile low forceps
vaginal delivery
SLI speech and language
impaired
SLK, SLKC superior limbic
keratoconjunctivitis
SLL second-look laparotomy
SLMFD, SLMFVD sterile low
midforceps (vaginal) delivery
SLN
sentinel lymph node
sublentiform nucleus
superior laryngeal nerve
SLO
scanning laser ophthalmoscope
second-look operation
S-LOST sulfur mustard,
Lommel and Steinkopf
(chemical weapon)
SLP
left sacroposterior (fetal
position) [L. *sacrolaeva
posterior*] (*See also* LSP)
single-limb progression
subluxation of patella
SLR
single lens reflex
straight-leg raising
SLT
left sacrotransverse (fetal
position) [L. *sacrolaeva
transversa*] (*See also* LST)
scanning laser tomography
Shiga-like toxin
sl.tr. slight trace
SLUD salivation, lacrimation,
urination, and defecation
SLUDGE salivation, lacrimation,
urination, defecation,
gastrointestinal distress and
emesis
SLWB severely low birth
weight
SM
self-monitoring
self-mutilation
splenomegaly
sports medicine
submandibular

323

SM *(continued)*
    supramamillary (nucleus)
    systolic murmur
S&M sadomasochism
Sm
    samarium
    Smith (antigen)
SMA
    sequential multichannel
      autoanalyzer
    spinal muscular atrophy
SMA-60 Sequential Multiple
    Analysis—sixty chemical
    constituents of blood
SMAC Sequential Multiple
    Analyzer Computer
SMART
    simultaneous multiple-angle
      reconstruction technique
    sperm microaspiration retrieval
      technique
SMAS
    submucosal aponeurotic
      system (flap)
    superficial musculoaponeurotic
      system
SMC sensorimotor cortex
SMD senile macular
    degeneration
SMDA Safe Medical Device
    Act
SMI
    severely mentally impaired
    silent myocardial infarction
SMILE
    safety, monitoring,
      intervention, length of stay,
      and evaluation
    subperiosteal minimally
      invasive laser endoscopic
      (facelift)
    sustained maximal inspiratory
      lung exercise
SML single major locus
SMM scintimammography
SMO supramalleolar orthosis
SMP standard medical practice
SMR
    sensorimotor rhythm
    standardized metabolic rate

SMRR submucous resection and
    rhinoplasty
SMS scalded mouth syndrome
SMT
    spinal manipulative therapy
    stereotactic mesencephalic
      tractotomy
SMV
    submental vertex (view)
    superior mesenteric vein
SN
    sciatic notch
    scrub nurse
    sensorineural
    seronegative
    sinus node
    substantia nigra
S-N sella to nasion
    (cephalometrics)
S:N
    sample to negative control
      ratio
    signal to noise ratio
    speech to noise ratio
SN_A, S-N-A sella-nasion-subspinale
    (point A, in cephalometrics)
Sn
    subnasale
    tin [L. *stannum*]
SNA
    superior nasal artery
    sympathetic nerve activity
SNa serum sodium
    (concentration)
SNAI Standard Nomenclature of
    Athletic Injuries
SNAP Score for Neonatal Acute
    Physiology
SNAP-PE Score for Neonatal
    Acute Physiology-Perinatal
    Extension
SNB sentinel (lymph) node
    biopsy
SN_B, S-N-B sella-nasion-
    supramentale (point B, in
    cephalometrics)
SNc, Snc substantia nigra pars
    compacta
SND selective neck dissection

SNDA Supplemental New Drug Application

SNDO, SNODO Standard Nomenclature of Diseases and Operations

SNF skilled nursing facility

SnF2 stannous fluoride

SNHL sensorineural hearing loss

SN-N sternal notch to nipple

SNODO (*var. of* SNDO)

SNOMED Systematized Nomenclature of Medicine

SNOMED CT Systematized Nomenclature of Medicine Clinical Terms

SNOMED RT Systematized Nomenclature of Medicine Reference Terminology

SNOP Systematized Nomenclature of Pathology

SNOT-16 Sinonasal Outcome Test-16

SNQ superior nasal quadrant

SNR
    substantia nigra zona reticulata
    supernumerary rib

Snr substantia nigra pars reticulata

SNRB selective nerve root block

SNS
    sterile normal saline
    surgical navigation system
    sympathetic nervous system

SNT sinuses, nose, throat

SNV Sin Nombre virus

SO
    salpingo-oophorectomy
    shoulder orthosis
    sphenooccipital (synchondrosis)
    sphincter of Oddi
    superior oblique
    sutures out

SO$_2$ sulfur dioxide

SO3 sulfite

SO4 sulfate

SOA
    supraorbital artery
    swelling of ankles

SOAP subjective (data), objective (data), assessment, and plan (problem-oriented record)

SOAPIE subjective (data), objective (data), assessment, plan, implementation, and evaluation (problem-oriented record

SOAPS suction, oxygen, apparatus, pharmaceuticals, saline (anesthesia equipment)

SOB shortness of breath

SOC
    sequential oral contraceptive
    standard of care
    state of consciousness

SOD sphincter of Oddi dysfunction

SODAS spheroidal oral drug absorption system

SOF superior orbital fissure

SOFA sequential organ failure assessment

SOHN supraoptic hypothalamic nucleus

SoHx social history (*See also* SH)

SOI surgical orthotopic implantation (implant)

SOL space-occupying lesion

soln. solution

solu solute

solv
    dissolve [L. *solve*]
    solvent

SOM serous otitis media

SOMA subjective, objective, management, and analytic

SOMI sternooccipital-mandibular immobilization (brace, orthosis)

SON supraoptic nucleus (of the hypothalamus)

S

sono
> sonogram
> sonography

SOOL spontaneous onset of labor

SOP standard operating procedure

SOr supraorbitale (craniometric)

SOS
> save our ship (universal call for emergency)
> son of sevenless (gene)

SOT
> Sensory Organization Test
> solid organ transplant

SP
> sacroposterior
> sacrum posterior
> septum pellucidum
> seropositive
> spastic paraplegia
> speech pathology
> status post
> summation potential
> suprapatellar
> symphysis pubis
> systolic pressure

Sp
> sacropubic
> speech
> spine

sp.
> species (singular)
> spirit, alcohol [L. *spiritus*] (*See also* spir.)

SPA
> single-photon absorptiometry
> speech pathology and audiology
> sperm penetration assay
> sphenopalatine artery
> suprapubic aspiration

SpA spondyloarthropathy

SPC
> scaphopisocapitate
> simultaneous prism (and) cover test
> single palmar crease
> Summary of Product Characteristics

SPD synpolydactyly

SPE serum protein electrophoresis

Spec Ed special education

SPECT single-photon emission computed tomography

SPEEP spontaneous positive end expiratory pressure

SPF
> semipermeable film
> spectrophotofluorometer
> sun protective factor

SPGR spoiled gradient recalled

sp gr specific gravity

Sph
> sphenoidale
> spherical (lens)

SPI
> Standards for Pediatric Immunization
> structured pain interview
> surgical peripheral iridectomy

SPIA solid-phase immunoabsorbent assay

SPIF solid-phase immunoassay fluorescence

SPIO superparamagnetic iron oxide (imaging agent)

spir. spirit, alcohol [L. *spiritus*] (*See also* sp.)

spiss.
> dried [L. *spissus*]
> inspissated, thickened by evaporation [L. *spissatus*]

SPK simultaneous pancreas-kidney (transplant)

SPLATT split anterior tibial tendon (transfer)

Splx splenectomy

SPM
> scanning probe microscopy
> shocks per minute
> syllables per minute

SPMA spinal progressive muscular atrophy

sp. n. new species [L. *species novum*]

SPO
> sphincter-preserving operation
> status postoperative

SpO₂ oxygen saturation as measured using pulse oximetry
SPP suprapubic prostatectomy
Spp, spp. species (plural)
SPR
 scan projection radiography
 superior peroneal retinaculum
SPRIA solid phase radioimmunoassay
SPROM spontaneous premature rupture of membranes
SPS
 simple partial seizure
 status post surgery
 systemic progressive sclerosis
SpS sphenoid sinus
SPT
 skin prick test
 slow pull-through
 Spondee Picture Test
 standing pivotal transfer
Sp tap spinal tap
SPXv smallpox vaccine (vaccinia virus)
SQ
 social quotient
 subcutaneous (*See also* subcu, subq)
SQ3R survey, question, read, review, recite (study system)
SQUID superconducting quantum interference device (array for reproductive assessment)
SR
 sarcoplasmic reticulum
 senior
 sinus rhythm
 smooth-rough (bacterial colony)
 superior rectus
 suture removal
 systems review
S&R seclusion and restraints
Sr strontium
sr steradian (unit of sphere measurement)
SRA steroid resistant asthma
SR_AW specific airway resistance

SRBC sickle red blood cell
SRBOW spontaneous rupture of bag of waters
SRCS (FDA Division of) Surveillance, Research, and Communication Support
SRD
 service-related disability
 sodium-restricted diet
SRF semirigid fiberglass cast
SRH somatotropin-releasing hormone
SRK smooth-rod Kaneda (thoracolumbar implant)
SRM
 Standard Reference Material
 subretinal membrane
 superior rectus muscle
SRN superficial radial nerve
SRNV subretinal neovascularization
SROM
 spinal range of motion
 spontaneous rupture of membranes
SRP scaling and root planing (dental)
SRS
 sex reassignment surgery
 stereotactic radiosurgery
 suicide risk screen
 Symptom Rating Scale
SRSA, SRS-A slow-reacting substance of anaphylaxis
SRSH self-reported self-harm
SRT
 sleep-related tumescence
 speech reception test
 speech recognition threshold
 surfactant replacement therapy
SRV superior radicular vein
SRY sex-determining region Y (chromosome)
SS
 septic shock
 serum sickness
 short stature
 siblings
 side-to-side

SS *(continued)*
  sliding scale
  Social Security
  systemic sclerosis
Ss subjects
ss
  half [L. *semis*]
  single stranded
  steady state
  subspinale
S&S
  signs and symptoms
  sling and swathe
  soft and smooth (prostate)
  support and stimulation
  swish and spit
  swish and swallow
SSA
  sagittal split advancement
  Salmonella-Shigella agar
  sickle cell anemia
  subsegmental atelectasis
SSAER steady-state auditory
  evoked response
SSB short spike burst
SSC
  somatosensory cortex
  superior semicircular canal
SSCr stainless steel crown
SSD
  serosanguineous drainage
  sickle cell disease
  source-to-skin distance
  speech-sound discrimination
  syndrome of sudden death
SSDI Social Security Disability
  Insurance
SS-DNA, ssDNA single-stranded
  deoxyribonucleic acid
SSFP steady-state free
  precession
SSFSE single shot fast spin
  echo
SSI
  segmental sequential
    irradiation
  segmental spinal
    instrumentation
  sliding scale insulin

  stuttering severity instrument
  Supplemental Security Income
SSIDS sibling of sudden infant
  death syndrome (victim)
SSIT subscapularis,
  supraspinatus, infraspinatus,
  and teres minor (muscles)
SSKI saturated solution of
  potassium iodide
SSM skin-sparing mastectomy
SSO
  sagittal split osteotomy
  special sense organs (animals)
SSP
  subclavian steal syndrome
  supersensitivity perception
Ssp, ssp. subspecies (singular)
SSPE subacute sclerosing
  panencephalitis
SSPL saturation sound pressure
  level
sspp. subspecies (plural)
SS-QOL stroke-specific quality
  of life
SSRI selective serotonin
  reuptake inhibitor
SSRO sagittal split ramus
  osteotomy
SSS
  sick sinus syndrome
  Stanford Sleepiness Scale
SSSB sagittal split setback
  (procedure)
SST
  simple shoulder test
  somatostatin (receptor)
SSU Saybolt seconds universal
S/SX signs/symptoms
st
  stage (of disease)
  stomion (median point of
    oral slit when lips are
    closed)
  subtype
ST
  electrocardiographic wave
    segment
  esotropia
  (heat-)stable (entero)toxin
  sacrotransverse

sacrum transverse
scala tympani
scapulothoracic
semitendinosus (muscle)
siblings (raised) together
sinus tachycardia
split thickness
sternothyroid (muscle)
stokes (kinematic viscosity)
surface tension

St. saint

sT tumor surgery (component of TNM classification)

sT0 tumor surgery not done (component of TNM classification)

sT1 tumor complete resection (component of TNM classification)

sT2 tumor resection, 50%-90% (component of TNM classification)

sT3 tumor resection 5% to 50% (component of TNM classification)

sT4 tumor biopsy (component of TNM classification)

sT5 tumor shunting (component of TNM classification)

STA
superficial temporal artery
superior temporal artery

Sta staphylion (craniometric)

stab, band neutrophil

STAG split thickness autogenous graft

staph staphylococcus

STAR staged abdominal repair

STARS Short-Term Auditory Retrieval and Storage (Test)

START, StaRT stereotactic-assisted radiation therapy

STAT at once [L.*statim*]

STD
sexually transmitted disease
skin-to-tumor distance
standard density (reference)

STEL short-term exposure limit

STEM scanning transmission electron microscope

stereo
stereogram
stereophonic

STET single photon emission tomography

STETH stethoscope

STG
split-thickness graft
superior temporal gyrus

STh, S-Thal sickle cell thalassemia

STIP (basophilic) stippling

STIR short T1 inversion recovery

STM
scanning tunneling microscope
short-term memory

STN (computer assisted) surgical tool navigator

STP
serenity, tranquility, peace (user's term for dimethoxymethylamphetamine)
standard temperature and pressure

STR
skin test reactivity
subtotal resection

strab strabismus

strep streptococcus

STS serologic test for syphilis

STSG split-thickness skin graft

STT
scaphoid, trapezium, trapezoid
spinothalamic tract

STT #1,#2 Schirmer tear test #1,#2

STV superior temporal vein

Stx Shiga toxin

SUA single umbilical artery

SUB Skene, urethral and Bartholin (glands)

subcu, subq subcutaneous (*See also* SQ, subq)

subcut subcutaneous

subling sublingual

subQ subcutaneous (ly)
subq (*var. of* subcu)
SUCC succinylcholine (*See also* SUX)
SUD
    skin unit dose
    sudden unexplained death
SUI
    stress urinary incontinence
    suicide
SUN
    serum urea nitrogen
    Standard Units and Nomenclature
SUNCT short lasting unilateral neuralgiform (headache with) conjunctival injection (and) tearing
SUND sudden unexplained death
SURG
    surgeon
    surgery
    surgical
susp
    suspended
    suspension
SUV standard uptake value
SUX succinylcholine (*See also* SUCC)
SUZI subzonal insemination
SV
    saphenous vein
    seminal vesicle
    simian virus
    snake venom
    spoken voice
    subclavian vein
S:V surface to volume ratio
Sv sievert (unit)
sv. serovar
SVBG saphenous vein bypass graft
SVC superior vena cava
SVC-PA superior vena cava-pulmonary artery (shunt)
SVC-RPA superior vena cava and right pulmonary artery (shunt)
SVCS superior vena cava syndrome

SVD
    single vessel disease
    small vessel disease
    spontaneous vaginal delivery
SVE slow volume encephalography
SVG
    saphenous vein graft
    seminal vesiculography
SvO$_2$, S$_{VO2}$ venous oxygen saturation
SVP selective vagotomy with pyloroplasty
SVR supraventricular rhythm
SW
    short wave
    slow wave
    spike wave
    stab wound
SWAP short wavelength automated perimetry
SWAT skin wound assessment and treatment
SWE slow-wave encephalography
SWI sterile water for injection
SWIM sperm-washing insemination method
SWIORA spinal cord injury without radiologic abnormality
SWL shock wave lithotripsy
SWMA segmental wall motion abnormality
SWR surface wrinkling retinopathy
SWS
    slow-wave sleep
    spike-wave stupor
SWT shock-wave therapy
Sx
    signs
    symptom
SXA single-energy x-ray absorptiometer
SXPL strictureplasty
SXR skull x-ray
sync synchronous
syph
    syphilis
    syphilitic

SYS BP systolic blood pressure
(*See also* SBP)

T
electrocardiographic wave corresponding to repolarization of ventricles
tablespoon (*See also* TBS)
temporal (electrode placement in electroencephalography)
tension (intraocular pressure) (*See also* TEN)
tera-
terminal (banding of chromosomes)
tesla (unit of measure)
tetra
threonine (*See also* Thr)
transformation (zone)

t ton (metric)

T+ increased tension (pressure)

T- decreased tension (pressure)

t$_m$, *t*$_m$ temperature midpoint (Celsius)

T1 spin-lattice or longitudinal relaxation time (MRI scan)

T$_1$ tricuspid first heart sound

t½elim elimination half-life

T1–T12
first to twelfth thoracic nerves
first to twelfth thoracic vertebrae (*See also* D1–D12)

T$_2$
second stage of decreased intraocular tension
tricuspid second heart sound

T3
transurethral thermoablation therapy
Tylenol with codeine (30 mg)

T$_3$ triiodothyronine

T$_3$RIA, T$_3$(RIA) triiodothyronine radioimmunoassay

T$_4$ tetraiodothyronine (thyroxine)

T$_4$RIA, T$_4$(RIA) tetraiodothyronine (thyroxine) radioimmunoassay

T7 free thyroxine factor

TA
Takayasu arteritis
temporal arteritis
tendon of Achilles
tension by applanation
Terminologia Anatomica
thoracoabdominal
tibialis anterior
transantral
tricuspid atresia
truncus arteriosus
tumor antigen

T of A transposition of aorta

T&A tonsillectomy and adenoidectomy

Ta tantalum

TAA
thoracic aortic aneurysm
total ankle arthroplasty
transcoronary alcohol ablation
transverse aortic arch

TAB
tablet
therapeutic abortion

TACC thoracic aortic cross-clamping

TACE transcatheter arterial chemoembolization

tach, tachy tachycardia

TACL-R Tests for Auditory Comprehension of Language-Revised

TAD Test of Auditory Discrimination

TADAC therapeutic abortion, dilation, aspiration, and curettage

TAE
total abdominal evisceration
transcatheter arterial embolization

TA-GVHD transfusion-associated graft-versus-host disease

TAH
total abdominal hysterectomy
total artificial heart

333

TAHBSO total abdominal hysterectomy and bilateral salpingo-oophorectomy

TAHIV transfusion associated human immunodeficiency virus

TAL
tendo Achillis lengthening
total arm length

TALH thick ascending limb of Henle (loop)

TALL, T-ALL T-cell acute lymphoblastic leukemia

TAM
teenage mother
total active motion
transtelephonic ambulatory monitoring (system)

TAML, t-AML therapy-related acute myelogenous (myeloid) leukemia

TAN Treatment Authorization Number

TAO
thromboangiitis obliterans
thyroid-associated ophthalmopathy
turning against object

TAP
tone and positioning
tonometry by applanation (*See also* AT)
transvaginal amniotic puncture

TAPC total anomalous pulmonary circulation

TAP-D Test of Articulation Performance-Diagnostic

TAPP transabdominal preperitoneal polypropylene (hernioplasty)

TAP-S Test of Articulation Performance-Screen

TAPVC total anomalous pulmonary venous connection

TAPVD total anomalous pulmonary venous drainage

TAPVR total anomalous pulmonary venous return

TAR
total ankle replacement

total anorectal reconstruction
treatment authorization request

TART
tenderness, asymmetry, restricted (motion), and tissue (texture changes)
tumorectomy, axillary (dissection), radiotherapy

TAS tetanus antitoxin serum

TASH transcoronary ablation of septal hypertrophy

T-ASI Teen Addiction Severity Index

TAS/TVS transabdominal/trans-vaginal ultrasound

TAT
tetanus antitoxin
thematic apperception test
thrombin-antithrombin
toxin-antitoxin
transverse axial tomography
treponemal antibody test
triple advancement transposition

TAUC target area under the curve

TAV transcutaneous (transvenous) aortovelography

TAWF Test of Adolescent/Adult Word Finding

TB
Tapes for the Blind
thymol blue
toluidine blue
tracheobronchitis
tuberculosis

T-B Thomas-Binetti (test)

Tb terbium

TBA total body (surface) area

TBAGA term birth appropriate for gestational age

T-bar tracheotomy bar (device used in respiratory therapy)

TBB transbronchial biopsy

TBC total-blood cholesterol

TBD
to be determined
total body density
Toxicology Data Base

TBE tick-borne encephalitis

TBFV tidal breathing flow-volume
TBG
tracheobronchogram
tris-buffered Grey (solution)
TBI
thrombotic brain infarction
tooth-brushing instruction
traumatic brain injury
TBILI total bilirubin
TBLB transbronchial lung biopsy
TBLF term birth, living female
TBLM term birth, living male
TBM
total body mass
tuberculous meningitis
TBNA transbronchial needle aspiration
TBR total bed rest
TBS
tablespoon (*See also* T)
The Bethesda System
tracheobronchoscopy
tris-buffered saline
TBSA total body (burn) surface area
TBT
tracheobronchial toilet
tracheobronchial tree
TC
talocalcaneal
teratocarcinoma
tissue culture
tonsillar coblation
tracheal collar
transcutaneous
transhepatic cholangiography
transverse colon
true conjugate
T:C tumor to cerebellum ratio
T&C
turn and cough
type and crossmatch
T$_c$ generation time of cell cycle
Tc
core temperature
technetium

TC$_{50}$ median toxic concentration
TCA
transluminal coronary angioplasty
tricuspid atresia
tricyclic antidepressant
TCB
transcatheter biopsy
transconjunctival blepharoplasty
TCBS thiosulfate-citrate-bile salts-sucrose (agar)
TCC
total contact casting
transcatheter closure
transitional cell carcinoma
TCCL T-cell chronic lymphocytic (leukemia)
TCCS transcranial color-coded sonography
TCD
transcranial Doppler (sonography, ultrasound)
transverse cardiac diameter
TCD$_{50}$ median tissue culture dose
TCE transcatheter embolotherapy
T cell thymus-derived lymphocyte
TCES transcutaneous cranial electrical stimulation
TCET transcerebral electrotherapy
TCGF T-cell growth factor
TCI tricuspid insufficiency
TCi teracurie
TCID$_{50}$ median tissue culture infective dose
TCL
tibial collateral ligament
transverse carpal ligament
T-CLL T-cell chronic lymphatic leukemia
TCM
tissue culture medium
traditional Chinese medicine
transcutaneous monitor
TCMA transcortical motor aphasia

335

TCN
    talocalcaneonavicular (joint)
    terminal capillary network
TCO total contact orthosis
TCP
    teacher-child-parent
    thrombocytopenia
    transcutaneous pacing
$TCPCO_2$, $tcPCO_2$ transcutaneous carbon dioxide pressure
$TCPO_2$, $tcPO_2$
    transcutaneous oxygen pressure (measurement)
    transcutaneous (partial) pressure of oxygen
TCS
    tethered-cord syndrome
    tonic-clonic seizure
TCT
    transcatheter therapy
    Trunk Control Test
TD
    tardive dyskinesia
    temperature differential
    test dose
    tetrodotoxin
    thermodilution
    thoracic duct
    tolerance dose
    tone decay
    toxic dose
    tracking dye
    transdermal
TD_{50} median toxic dose
T_D time required to double number of cells in given population
T_d diffusion time
Td tetanus-diphtheria (toxoid; adult type)
TDB Toxicology Data Bank
TDC thermal dilution catheter
TDD telecommunication device (for the) deaf
TDEE total daily energy expenditure
TDF
    time-dose fractionation (factor)
    tumor dose fractionation
TDH toxic dose, high

TDI
    therapeutic donor insemination
    three-dimensional interlocking (hip)
    tissue Doppler imaging
TDL toxic dose, low
TDM therapeutic drug monitoring
T1DM type 1 diabetes mellitus
T2DM type 2 diabetes mellitus
tDNA transfer deoxyribonucleic acid
TDNWB touchdown nonweightbearing
TDP torsade de pointes
TDPWB touchdown partial weightbearing
TDS temperature, depth, and salinity
TDSP time domain signal processor
TDT
    thermal death time
    tone decay test
TDU time domain ultrasound
TDW target dry weight
TDWB touchdown weightbearing
TE
    tennis elbow
    test ear
    thyrotoxic exophthalmos
    tooth extracted
    tracheoesophageal
T_E expiratory time
Te tellurium
TEA
    thromboendarterectomy
    transluminal extraction atherectomy
TEACCH treatment and education of autistic and related communications handicapped children
TEAP transesophageal atrial pacing
TEC
    transluminal endarterectomy catheter
    transpapillary endoscopic cholecystotomy

T&EC trauma and emergency center

TECAB totally endoscopic (off-pump) coronary artery bypass

TED
threshold erythema dose
thromboembolic disease (hose, stockings)

TEDD total end-diastolic diameter

TEE
transesophageal echocardiography
transnasal endoscopic ethmoidectomy

TEF
tracheoesophageal fistula
trunk extension-flexion (unit)

TEF$_{25}$ tidal expiratory flow at 25% of tidal volume

TEF$_{25}$/PTEF ratio of tidal expiratory flow at 25% of tidal volume and peak tidal expiratory flow

TEF$_{50}$/TIF$_{50}$ ratio of tidal expiratory and inspiratory flow at 50% of tidal volume

teff effective half-life (radioactivity)

TEK total exchangeable potassium

TELD-2 Test of Early Language Development, Second Edition

tele telemetry

TEM transmission electron microscope

temp
temperature
temple
temporal
temporary

TEN
tension (intraocular pressure) (*See also* T)
total enteral nutrition

TENa total exchangeable sodium

TENS transcutaneous electrical nerve stimulator

TENVAD Test of Nonverbal Auditory Discrimination

TEOAE transient evoked otoacoustic emission

TEP
thromboendophlebectomy
tracheoesophageal prosthesis
trigeminal evoked potential
tubal ectopic pregnancy

TeP tender point

TEQ toxic equivalents

TER
therapeutic external radiation
total elbow replacement
transurethral electroresection

ter ternary (threefold)

TERM temporary endodontic restorative material

TES transmural electrical stimulation

TESA testicular sperm aspiration

TESD total end-systolic diameter

TESE testicular sperm extraction

TET
tetanus
tetralogy (of Fallot)
treadmill exercise test
tubal embryo transfer

TETE too early to evaluate

tE/tTOT ratio of expiration time and total time of breathing cycle

tet tox tetanus toxoid (*See also* TT)

TEV talipes equinovarus

TEVAP transurethral electrovaporization of the prostate

TEVG tissue engineered vascular graft

TEVP transesophageal ventricular pacing

TF
tactile fremitus
tail flick (reflex)
testicular feminization

TF *(continued)*
   transfrontal
   tube feeding
   tuning fork
TFA
   thigh-foot angle
   tibiofemoral angle
   trans fatty acids
TFC
   threaded fusion cage
   time to following commands
TFCQ Toronto Functional
   Capacity Questionnaire
TFD
   target-film distance
   thin film dressing
TFEV timed forced expiratory
   volume
TFI tubular-fertility index
TFL
   tensor fasciae latae
   transnasal fiberoptic
    laryngoplasty
TFP treponemal false positive
TFT thyroid function test
TF:UF tubular fluid to
   ultrafiltrate ratio
TG
   tendon graft
   thioglycolate (broth)
   thyroglobulin
   total gastrectomy
   toxic goiter
   Toxoplasma gondii
   trigeminal (neuralgia)
TGA
   transient global amnesia
   transposition of great arteries
TGC time-gain compensation
TGD thyroglossal duct
TGL triglyceride
TGR tenderness, guarding,
   rigidity (abdominal exam)
TGS tincture of green soap
TGY, TGYA tryptone glucose
   yeast (agar)
TH
   thrill
   thyrohyoid
   thyroid hormone

T&H type and hold
Th T-helper (cell)
THA total hip arthroplasty
ThA thoracic aorta
THAN transient
   hyperammonemia of newborn
THC
   tetrahydrocannabinol
   thigh circumference
   transhepatic cholangiogram
THC:YAG thulium-holmium-
   chromium:YAG (laser)
THD transverse heart diameter
THE
   transhepatic embolization
   transhiatal esophagectomy
THI
   therapeutic husband-
    insemination
   transient
    hypogammaglobulinemia of
    infancy
THKAFO trunk-hip-knee-ankle-
   foot orthosis
THORP titanium hollow-screw
   osseointegrating reconstruction
   plate
THP total hip prosthesis
THR
   target heart rate
   total hip replacement
   training heart rate
Thr threonine *(See also* T)
THz terahertz
TI
   terminal ileum
   therapeutic index
   thoracic index
   transverse inlet
   tricuspid
    incompetence/insufficiency
T$_I$
   duration of inspiration
   inspiratory time
Ti titanium
TIA transient ischemic attack
TIBC total iron-binding capacity
tib-fib tibia and fibula
tic (diver)tic(ulum)

TID, t.i.d. three times a day [L. *ter in die*]

TIF$_{50}$ tidal inspiratory flow at 50% of tidal volume

TIg tetanus immune globulin

TIMP Test of Infant Motor Performance

TIN
Tone in Noise (test)
tubulointerstitial nephropathy

TIND Treatment Investigational New Drug (application)

TIP
time to pregnancy
Toxicology Information Program
tubularized incised plate (urethroplasty)

TIPP The Injury Prevention Program

TIPS transjugular intrahepatic portosystemic shunt

TIS
telemedicine information system
tumor in situ

TISS therapeutic intervention scoring system

tI:tTOT ratio of inspiration time and total time of breathing cycle

TIVC thoracic inferior vena cava

TIW three times a week

TJ terajoule

TJA total joint arthroplasty

TJR total joint replacement

TK
through knee
toxicokinetics

TKA
total knee arthroplasty
trochanter-knee-ankle (line)

TKG tocodynagraph

TKO to keep open (vein for IV)

TKP
thermokeratoplasty
total knee prosthesis

TKR total knee replacement

TL
temporal lobe
terminal limen
thermolabile
thermoluminescence
thoracolumbar
total laryngectomy
tubal ligation

Tl thallium

TLA thigh-leg angle

TLC
telephone-linked care
Test of Language Competence
thin-layer chromatography
triple-lumen catheter

TLD
thermoluminescent dosimeter
thoracic lymphatic duct
tumor lethal dose

TLE
temporal lobe epilepsy
thin-layer electrophoresis

TLI
total lymphoid irradiation
translaryngeal intubation

TLK thermal laser keratoplasty

TLP total laryngopharyngectomy

TLS
thoracolumbosacral strain
tight lens syndrome

TLSO
thoracolumbosacral orthosis

TM
temporalis muscle
teres major (muscle)
Thayer-Martin (medium)
transverse myelitis
tympanic membrane

Tm thulium

TMA
transmetatarsal amputation
true metatarsus adductus

T-MAX, T-max maximum temperature

TMB transient monocular blindness

t-MDS therapy-related myelodysplastic syndrome

339

TME total mesorectal excision
TMH trainable mentally handicapped
TMJ, TMJD temporomandibular joint (dysfunction)
TMLR transmyocardial laser revascularization
TMR
    trainable mentally retarded
    transmyocardial revascularization
TMS
    thallium myocardial scintigraphy
    transcranial magnetic stimulation
TMT treadmill test
TN
    (intraocular) tension, normal
    temperature normal
    trigeminal neuralgia
    true negative
Tn
    thoron
    troponin
TNB transthoracic needle biopsy
TNC turbid, no creamy (layer)
TND term normal delivery
TNDM transient neonatal diabetes mellitus
TNE transnasal esophagoscopy
TNF tumor necrosis factor
TNG
    toxic nodular goiter
    training
TnI troponin I
T/NK T/natural killer (cell)
TNM (primary) tumor, (regional lymph) node, (remote) metastases (classification, staging)
TnT troponin T
TNTC too numerous to count
TNVAD Test of Nonverbal Auditory Discrimination
TO
    temperature, oral
    thoracic orthosis
    tincture of opium
    total obstruction

    tracheoesophageal
    tuboovarian
T&O tubes and ovaries
TO₂ oxygen transport
TOAL Test of Adolescent Language
TOBE tests of basic experience
TOCE transcatheter oily chemoembolization
TOD
    tail-on detector (genetics)
    tension oculus dexter (tension of right eye)
    time of death
    Time-Oriented Data (Bank)
    tubal occlusion device
TOE tracheoesophageal
TOF
    time of flight (radiology)
    train-of-four
TOFA time-of-flight and absorbance
TOFMS time-of-flight mass spectometry
TOL trial of labor
TOM transcutaneous oxygen monitor
TOP
    temporal, occipital, parietal
    termination of pregnancy
TOS
    tension oculus sinister (tension of left eye)
    thoracic outlet syndrome
    toxic oil syndrome
TOT
    tincture of time
    tip-of-the-tongue
TOV trial of void
TOWER testing, orientation, work, evaluation, rehabilitation
tox
    toxic
    toxicity
    toxoid
TOXICON Toxicology Information Conversational On-Line Network
TOXLINE Toxicology Information On-Line

TOXO toxoplasmosis

TP

temperature and pressure
temporoparietal
tender point
terminal phalanx
tetanus-pertussis
thought process
thrombophlebitis
total protein
transpyloric
true positive

T&P, T+P

temperature and pulse
turn and position

T:P trough to peak ratio

Tp tampon

TPA

temporopolar artery
total parenteral alimentation
Treponema pallidum
agglutination

tPA tissue plasminogen activator

TPAL term (infants), premature
(infants), abortions, living
(children) (obstetric history)

TPBS three phase bone
scintigraphy

TPD

temporary partial disability
tidal peritoneal dialysis

TPE therapeutic plasma
exchange

TPF temporoparietal fascial flap

TPGYT trypticase-peptone-
glucose-yeast extract-trypsin
(medium)

TPH

transplacental hemorrhage
treponemal hemagglutination

TPI

Treatment Priority Index
trigger point injection

tpk time to peak

T plasty tympanoplasty

T-PLL T-cell prolymphocytic
leukemia

TPM

thrombophlebitis migrans

total particulate matter
total passive motion

TPN total parenteral nutrition

TPO

temporoparietooccipital
thrombopoietin

TPP

thrust plate prosthesis
tubal perfusion pressure

TP&P time, place, and person

TPPD thoracic-pelvic-phalangeal
dystrophy

TPPS Toddler-Preschooler
Postoperative Pain Scale

TPPV trans pars plana
vitrectomy

TPR

temperature, pulse, respiration
Thompson-Parkridge-Richards
(ankle orthosis)
transsphenoidal pituitary
resection

T-PRK tracker-assisted
photorefractive keratectomy

TPS titanium plasma sprayed

TPT

treadmill performance test
trigger point therapy

TPTX thyroparathyroidectomy

TR

rectal temperature
repetition time
therapeutic radiology
transplant recipient
tricuspid regurgitation
tumor registry

T&R tenderness and rebound

T:R thickness to radius ratio

Tr

tragion
trypsin

TRAC traction

trach

trachea
tracheostomy
tracheotomy

TRAFO tone-reducing ankle-foot
orthosis

341

TRAM transverse rectus abdominis myocutaneous (breast reconstruction)

TRAMP transverse rectus abdominis musculoperitoneal (flap, breast reconstruction)

TRAP
telomere repeat amplification protocol
twin reverse arterial perfusion

TRASHES tuberculosis, radiotherapy, ankylosing spondylitis, histoplasmosis, extrinsic allergic alveolitis, silicosis (chest x-ray findings)

TRD
tongue-retaining device
total retinal detachment

TRE true radiation emission

TRG tumor regression grade

TRH thyrotropin-releasing hormone

TRI transient response imaging

TRIC trachoma (and) inclusion conjunctivitis

TRICKS time-resolved imaging contrast kinetics

TRISS Trauma and Injury Severity Scores

TRM
transplant-related mortality
treatment-related mortality

tRNA transfer ribonucleic acid

TROCA tangible reinforcement of operant conditioned audiometry

Trp tryptophan (*See also* W)

TrPs trigger points

TrS trauma surgery

TRT
thermoradiotherapy
thoracic radiation therapy

TRUS transrectal ultrasound-guided sextant (biopsy)

TRUSP transrectal ultrasound of prostate

TS
thoracic spine (*See also* T-spine)
thoracic surgery
transsexual
Trauma Score
tricuspid stenosis

Ts
skin temperature
tension by Schiotz (tonometer)
T suppressor (cell)

TSA
Test of Syntactic Ability
Total Severity Assessment

TSC
transverse spinal sclerosis
tuberous sclerosis complex

TSCA Toxic Substance Control Act

TSD target-skin distance

TSE
testicular self-examination
transmissible spongiform encephalopathy
turbo spin echo

TSF triceps skin fold

TSFS transseptal frontal sinusotomy

TSH thyroid stimulating hormone

TSH-RH thyroid-stimulating hormone releasing hormone

TSIA triple sugar iron agar

TSL terminal sensory latency

T-spine thoracic spine (*See also* TS)

TSS
toxic shock syndrome
transverse spinal sclerosis

TS/SS transverse/sigmoid sinus

TST
treadmill stress test
tuberculin skin test

TSU triple sugar urea (agar)

TT
talar tilt
tetanus toxin
tetanus toxoid (*See also* tet tox)
therapeutic touch
thrombolytic therapy
tibial tuberosity
tine test

total thyroidectomy
transfusion transmitted (virus)
transthoracic
transtracheal
triple therapy
tuberculin test
T&T time and temperature
T/T trace of/trace of (different substances on tests)
TTA transtracheal aspiration
TTBS Tween-TRIS-buffered saline solution
TTC transtracheal catheter
TTD
  tarsal tunnel decompression
  temporary total disability
  total tumor dose
  transverse thoracic diameter
TTDP time-to-disease progression
TTE transthoracic echocardiogram
TTI
  tissue thromboplastin inhibition (test)
  total time to intubation
TTM
  transtelephonic monitoring
  trichotillomania
TTN transient tachypnea of newborn
TTNA transthoracic needle aspiration
TTO transtracheal oxygen
TTP thrombotic thrombocytopenic purpura
TTP-HUS thrombotic thrombocytopenic purpura and hemolytic uremic syndrome
TTR trauma triage rule
TTS
  through the skin
  through-the-scope
  transdermal therapeutic system
TTT
  thymol turbidity test
  tibial talar tilt, tibiotalar tilt
  tilt-table test

TTTS twin-to-twin transfusion syndrome
TTWB touch-toe weightbearing
TTx thrombolytic therapy
TU
  toxic (toxin) unit
  tuberculin unit
  turbidity unit
TUBA transumbilical breast augmentation
TUG timed up and go
TUIP transurethral incision of prostate
TUL transurethral ureterolithotripsy
TULIP transurethral ultrasound-guided laser-induced prostatectomy
TULIPS touch-up and loop incorporated primers (PCR method)
TUMT transurethral microwave thermotherapy
TUNA transurethral needle ablation
TURB transurethral resection of bladder (tumor)
turb turbid(ity)
TURBN transurethral resection of bladder neck
TURM transurethral microwave
TURP transurethral resection of prostate
TURV transurethral resection of valves
TURVN transurethral resection of vesical neck
TUU transureteroureterostomy
TUV transurethral valve
TUVRP transurethral vaporization-resection of prostate
TV
  talipes varus
  thoracic vertebra
  tricuspid valve
  truncal vagotomy
  tuberculin volutin

TVC
    timed vital capacity
    true vocal cord
TV-CDS transvaginal color
    Doppler sonography
TVF
    tactile vocal fremitus
    true vocal fold
TVH total vaginal hysterectomy
TVL tenth value layer
    (radiation)
TVR
    target vessel revascularization
    tonic vibration reflex
    tricuspid valve replacement
TVS transvaginal sonography
TVT
    tension-free vaginal tape
    tunica vaginalis testis
TVUS transvaginal ultrasound
TW2 Tanner-Whitehouse mark 2
    (bone-age assessment)
TWA
    time-weighted average
    T-wave alternans
TWAR Taiwan acute respiratory
    (agent)
T wave electrocardiographic
    wave corresponding to
    repolarization of the ventricles

TWE
    tap water enema
    tepid water enema
TWHW toe walking and heel
    walking
T1WI T1-weighted image
T2WI T2-weighted image
TWOC trial without catheter
TWR total wrist replacement
TWSTRS Toronto Western
    Spasmodic Torticollis Rating
    Scale
T&X type and crossmatch
Tx
    therapy
    traction
    transplant
    treatment
TxCAD transplant coronary
    artery disease
Ty thyroxine
TYMP tympanogram
TYR Tyrode (solution)
Tyr tyrosine (*See also* Y)
TZ transition zone

U

unerupted
unit
upper
uranium
wave on electrocardiogram

1/U one fingerbreadth above umbilicus

U/ at umbilicus

U/3 upper third (of long bone)

U/1 one fingerbreadth below umbilicus

24U 24 hour urine (collection)

UA

ultraaudible (sound)
ultrasonic arteriogram
umbilical artery
unauthorized absence
unit of analysis
unrelated (children raised) apart
unstable angina
upper airway
upper arm
urinalysis

UAC umbilical artery catheter

UA:C

uric acid to creatinine ratio
urinary albumin to creatinine ratio

UAD upper airways disease

UADT upper aerodigestive tract

UAE

unsupported arm exercise
uterine artery embolization

UAGA Uniform Anatomical Gift Act

UAL

ultrasonic-assisted liposuction
umbilical artery line

UA&M urinalysis and microscopy

UAO upper airways obstruction

UAP

unstable angina pectoris
upper abdominal pain

UAR upper airways resistance

UAU uterine activity unit

UB urinary bladder

UBC

University of British Columbia (brace)
unsaturated binding capacity

UBD universal blood donor

UBE

uniaxial balance evaluation
upper body ergometer

UBF uterine blood flow

U-BFP urinary basic fetoprotein

UBG urobilinogen

UBI ultraviolet blood irradiation

UBL undifferentiated B-cell lymphoma

UBM

ultrasound backscatter microscopy
ultrasound biomicroscopy

UBO unidentified bright object

UBP

Universal Bone Plate
ureteral back pressure

UBT

urea breath test
uterine balloon therapy

UBW usual body weight

UC

ulcerative colitis
ultracentrifugal
umbilical cord
undifferentiated carcinoma
unfixed cryostat
unsatisfactory condition
urethral catheterization
urinary catheter
urine concentrate
urine culture (*See also* UCX)
uterine contraction

U:C umbilical artery to middle cerebral artery (pulsatility index ratio)

U

U&C
  urethral and cervical (cultures)
  usual and customary
UCA ultrasound contrast agent
UcA urothelial carcinoma
UCAC uterine cornual access
  catheter
UCB
  umbilical cord blood
  unconjugated bilirubin
  unilateral calcaneal brace
UCBC umbilical cord blood
  culture
UCBT unrelated cord-blood
  transplant
UCD urine collection device
UCE upper completely
  edentulous
UCF urinary free cortisol
UCG
  ultrasonic cardiogram
  urinary chorionic gonadotropin
UCHI usual childhood illnesses
UCHS uncontrolled hemorrhagic
  shock
UCI
  umbilical coiling index
  urethral (urinary) catheter in
UCL
  ulnar collateral ligament
  uncomfortable level
  upper confidence limit
  urea clearance
UCLL uncomfortable listening
  level
UCLP unilateral cleft of lip
  and palate
UCO
  urethral catheter out
  urinary catheter out
UCP
  ultrasound catheter probe
  umbilical cord prolapse
  urethral closure pressure
UCPs urine collection pads
UCR usual, customary, and
  reasonable (fees)
UCS
  unconscious

unicoronal synostosis
uterine compression syndrome
UC&S urine culture and
  sensitivity
UCT ultrasound computed
  tomography
UCTD undifferentiated
  connective tissue disease
UCV uncontrolled variable
UCVA uncorrected visual acuity
UCX urine culture (See also
  UC)
UD
  ulnar deviation
  underdeveloped
  undesirable discharge
    (military)
  unipolar depression
  unit dose
  urethral dilatation
  urethral discharge
  urodynamics
  uterine distention
UDA under direct vision
UDC uninhibited detrusor
  (muscle) capacity
UDI
  urinary diagnostic index
  Urogenital Distress Inventory
UDO undetermined origin
UDP
  unassisted diastolic pressure
  urine drug panel
UDS
  ultra–Doppler sonography
  urine drug screen
UE
  undetermined etiology
  upper esophagus
  upper extremity
UEA upper extremity arterial
UEC uterine endometrial
  carcinoma
UEDs unilateral epileptiform
  discharges
UEG ultrasonic encephalography
UEM universal electron
  microscope
UEP urinary excretion of
  protein

UES upper esophageal sphincter
UESP upper esophageal sphincter pressure
UESR upper esophageal sphincter relaxation
UF
  ultrafiltrate
  ultrafine
  ultrasonic frequency
  unflexed
  unknown factor
UFA unesterified fatty acid
UFC urinary free cortisol
UFCT ultrafast computed tomography
UFD ultrasonic flow detector
UFF unusual facial features
UFH unfractionated heparin
UFO unidentified foreign object
UFOV useful field of view
UFR
  ultrafiltration rate
  urine filtration rate
uFSH urinary follicle-stimulating hormone
UFV ultrafiltration volume
UG
  urinary glucose
  urogenital
UGA
  under general anesthesia
  urogenital atrophy
UGCR ultrasound-guided compression repair
UGD urogenital diaphragm
UGF
  unidentified growth factor
  urinary gonadotropin fragment
UGH uveitis, glaucoma, hyphema (syndrome)
UGH+ uveitis, glaucoma, hyphema plus (vitreous hemorrhage)
UGI upper gastrointestinal (tract, series)
UGI w/SBFT upper gastrointestinal (series) with small bowel follow through

UGK urine glucose (and) ketone
UGNB ultrasonically guided needle biopsy
UGS urogenital sinus
UGVA ultrasound-guided vascular access
UH
  umbilical hernia
  upper half
UHBI upper hemibody irradiation
UHD unstable hemoglobin disease
UHDDS Uniform Hospital Discharge Data Set
UHF ultrahigh frequency
UHFV ultrahigh-frequency ventilation
UHL universal hypertrichosis lanuginosa
UHMM ultrahigh magnification mammography
UHMW ultrahigh molecular weight
UHT ultrahigh temperature
UHV
  ultrahigh vacuum
  ultrahigh voltage
UI
  Ulcer Index
  urinary incontinence
  uteroplacental insufficiency
U/I unidentified
UIBC
  unbound iron-binding capacity
  unsaturated iron-binding capacity
UID/S unilateral interfacetal dislocation or subluxation
UIEP urine immunoelectrophoresis
UIFE urine immunofixation electrophoresis
UIP usual interstitial pneumonia (of Liebow)
UIQ upper inner quadrant

U

UK
    United Kingdom
    urine potassium
UKA unicompartmental knee arthroplasty
UKO unknown origin
U$_k$V urinary potassium volume (excretion rate)
UL
    upper left
    upper lid
    upper limb
    upper limit
    upper lobe
    utterance length
U/L unit per liter
U:L upper body segment to lower body segment ratio
ULBW ultralow birth weight
ULDR ultralow dose rate
uLH urinary luteinizing hormone
ULL uncomfortable loudness level
ULLE upper lid left eye
ULN upper limits of normal
ULO upper limb orthosis
ULP
    ultralow profile
    upper limb prosthesis
ULPA ultralow particulate air
ULPE upper lobe pulmonary edema
ULQ upper left quadrant
ULRE upper lid right eye
ULSB upper left sternal border
ULT ultralow temperature
ULTT1 upper limb tension test 1 (median nerve)
ULTT2a upper limb tension test 2a (medial nerve)
ULTT2b upper limb tension test 2b (radial nerve)
ULTT3 upper limb tension test 3 (ulnar nerve)
ULV ultralow volume
ULYTES urine electrolytes
Umax maximal urinary osmolality

UMB
    umbilical
    umbilicus
umb V line umbilical venous line
UMCL upper midclavicular line
UMI uterine manipulator/injector
UMLS Unified Medical Language System
UMN upper motor neuron
UMS
    upper (fossa active), medial (knee pain), and short (leg on the side ipsilateral to the weak fossa)
    urethral manipulation syndrome
UMT unit of medical time
UN
    ulnar nerve
    undernourished
    unilateral neglect
    urea nitrogen
    urinary nitrogen
U$_{Na}$, UNa urinary sodium
unacc unaccompanied
UNaV urinary sodium excretion
UNC uncrossed
uncovertebral
UNCV ulnar nerve conduction velocity
UNCVA uncorrected visual acuity
UNDEL undelivered
UNHS, UNHSP Universal Neonatal Hearing Screening
UNK unknown
UNL upper normal limit
UNOS United Network for Organ Sharing
UN/P unpatched (eye)
UNX uninephrectomy
UO
    under observation
    undetermined origin
    ureteral orifice
    urinary output
UOAC uterine ostial access catheter
UOQ upper outer quadrant

UOsm urinary osmolality
UOV unit of variance
UOZ upper outer zone (quadrant)
UP
  unipolar
  Unna-Pappenheim (stain)
  ureteropelvic
  uteroplacental
U:P urine to plasma ratio
uPA, u-PA urokinase plasminogen activator
UPD uniparental disomy
UPDRS Unified Parkinson Disease Rating Scale
UPE upper partially edentulous
UPEP urine protein electrophoresis
UPF universal proximal femur (prosthesis)
UPI
  uteroplacental insufficiency
  uteroplacental ischemia
UPJ ureteropelvic junction
UPL unusual position of limbs
UPLIF unilateral posterior lumbar interbody fusion
UPLIFT uterine positioning via ligament investment fixation truncation
UPO (metastatic carcinoma of) unknown primary origin
UPOR usual place of residence
UPP
  urethral pressure profile
  uvulopalatoplasty
UPPP uvulopalatopharyngoplasty
UPS ultraviolet photoelectron spectroscopy
UPSIT University of Pennsylvania Smell Identification Test
UPT urine pregnancy test
UQ upper quadrant
UR
  unconditioned reflex
  unrelated
  upper respiratory
  upper right

  urinary retention
  urology
  utilization review
URA, Ura unilateral renal agenesis
URC
  upper rib cage
  utilization review committee
URC SP uric acid (urine) spot (test)
URD
  unrelated donor
  upper respiratory disease
UREA-S urea nitrogen (urine) spot (test)
URED unable to read (lab result)
URF
  unidentified reading frame
  uterine-relaxing factor
URI upper respiratory (tract) infection (illness) (*See also* URTI)
UR&M urinalysis, routine and microscopic
UROB, UROBIL urobilinogen
UROD ultra-rapid opiate detoxification [under anesthesia]
URO-GEN urogenital
URQ upper right quadrant (of abdomen)
URR
  upstream regulatory region
  urea reduction ratio
URS
  transurethral ureterorenoscopy
  ultrasonic renal scanning
URSB upper right sternal border
URT
  upper respiratory tract
  uterine resting tone
URTI upper respiratory tract illness (infection) (*See also* URI)
US
  ultrasonography
  unconditioned stimulus

U

349

US *(continued)*
　United States
　upper segment
USAMRIID United States Army Medical Research Institute of Infectious Diseases
USB upper sternal border
US-CNB, USCNB ultrasound-guided core-needle biopsy
U-SCOPE ureteroscopy
USCVD unsterile controlled vaginal delivery
USE ultrasonic echography
US-FNAB ultrasound-guided fine-needle aspiration biopsy
USI urinary stress incontinence
US:LS upper strength to lower strength ratio
USM ultrasonic mist
USN
　ultrasonic nebulizer
　unilateral spatial neglect
USO unilateral salpingo-oophorectomy
USOH usual state of health
USP
　unassisted systolic pressure
　United States Pharmacopeia
　upper sternal border
　uterine-stimulating potency
USPDI United States Pharmacopeia Drug Information
USS ultrasound scanning
UST upper single tooth
USUCVD unsterile uncontrolled vaginal delivery
USW ultrashort wave
UT
　unrelated (children raised) together
　untested
　untreated
　upper thoracic
　urea transporter
　urinary tract
uT unbound testosterone
UTA urinary tract anomaly

UTD
　unable to determine
　up to date
UTF usual throat flora
UTI urinary tract infection
UTJ uterotubal junction
UTLD Utah Test of Language Development
UTM urinary tract malformation
UTO
　unable to obtain
　upper tibial osteotomy
UTR untranslated region
UTS
　ulnar tunnel syndrome
　ultimate tensile strength
　ultrasound
UTTS ultrathin-walled two-stage (catheter)
UU urinary urea
UUD uncontrolled unsterile delivery
UUN urine urea nitrogen
UUO unilateral ureteral obstruction (occlusion)
UV
　ultraviolet (light)
　umbilical vein
　ureterovesical
UVA
　ultraviolet (light) A
　ureterovesical angle
UVAC uterine vacuum aspirating curette
UVB ultraviolet (light) B
UVC
　ultraviolet (light) C
　umbilical vein catheter
UVEB unifocal ventricular ectopic beat
UVGI ultraviolet germicidal irradiation
UVH univentricular heart
UVI ultraviolet irradiation
UVJ ureterovesical junction
UVL umbilical venous line
UV/MV umbilical vein to maternal vein
UVP ultraviolet photometry
UVR ultraviolet radiation

UW unilateral weakness
UWB unit of whole blood
UWS underwater seal (drainage)
UW solution University of
Wisconsin solution

UWW underwater weight
UX uranium X (proactinium)
UXO unexploded ordnance
UYP upper yield point

V
  gas volume
  unipolar chest lead
  valine (*See also* Val)
  vanadium (element)
  venous
  verbal (comprehension factor)
  vertex sharp transient
    (electroencephalography)
  volt
V0 no evidence of venous
  invasion (TNM classification)
V1
  trigeminal (fifth cranial)
    nerve, ophthalmic division
  venous (tumor) invasion
    (TNM classification)
V2 trigeminal (fifth cranial)
  nerve, maxillary division
V3 trigeminal (fifth cranial)
  nerve, mandibular division
v
  rate of reaction catalyzed by
    an enzyme
  specific volume
  vein
  velocity
V1–V6 precordial chest leads
VA
  alveolar ventilation
  vacuum aspiration
  venoarterial
  ventricular arrhythmia
  ventriculoatrial
  ventroanterior
  vertebral artery
  Veteran's Administration
    (Hospital)
  visual acuity
V&A vagotomy and antrectomy
V/A volt/ampere
Va arterial gas volume
VAA verbal-auditory agnosia
VABP venoarterial bypass
  pumping

VAC vacuum-assisted closure
  (dressing)
VACB vacuum-assisted core
  biopsy
VA cc distance visual acuity
  with correction
VAC EXT vacuum extractor
VAD
  vascular access device
  venous access device
  ventricular assist device
VADS Visual Aural Digit Span
  Test
VAER visual auditory evoked
  response
VAERS Vaccine Adverse Event
  Reporting System
VAG vascular access graft
VAH virilizing adrenal
  hyperplasia
VAIN vaginal intraepithelial
  neoplasia
VAKT visual, association,
  kinesthetic, tactile (reading)
Val valine (*See also* V)
VALE visual acuity, left eye
VALI ventilator-associated lung
  injury
VAM ventricular arrhythmia
  monitor
VAMP venous/arterial blood
  management protection
VAN vein, artery, nerve
VAP venous access port
VAPS visual analog pain score
var
  variant
  variation
VARE visual acuity, right eye
VAS
  vagus nerve stimulation
  vestibular aqueduct syndrome
  vibratory acoustic stimulation
  visual analogue scale

V

VASC
Verbal Auditory Screen for Children
Visual Auditory Screen for Children

VA sc, VA scl distance visual acuity without correction

VASPI Visual Analogue Self-Assessment Scales For Pain Intensity

VAT
ventilatory anaerobic threshold
ventricular activation time
ventricular (pacing), atrial (sensing), triggered (mode, pacemaker)
visual apperception test

VATS
video-assisted thoracic surgery
video-assisted thoracoscopy

VAT:TAT visceral abdominal fat to total abdominal fat ratio

VB
Van Buren (catheter)
venous blood
ventrobasal
Veronal buffer
viable birth
voided bladder

VB1–3 first through third voided bladder (specimen)

VBAC vaginal birth after cesarean (section)

VBAC-TOL vaginal birth after cesarean—trial of labor

VBD Veronal-buffered diluent

VBG
vagotomy and Billroth gastroenterostomy
vascularized bone graft
venous blood gas
Veronal-buffered (serum with) gelatin
vertical banded gastroplasty

VBI vertebrobasilar insufficiency

vBMD volumetric bone mineral density

VBOS Veronal-buffered oxalated saline

VBP venous blood pressure

VBR ventricle to brain ratio

VBS
venous blood sample
Veronal-buffered saline
vertebrobasilar (artery) system

VC
vasoconstriction
vena cava
ventilatory capacity
vertebral canal
vision, color
visual capacity
visual cortex
vital capacity
vocal cord
volume, capillary
voluntary control
vowel-consonant

V:C ventilation to circulation ratio

V&C vertical and centric (bite)

VCA viral capsid antigen

VCAM vascular cell adhesion molecule

VCAM-1 vascular cell adhesion molecule-1

VCD
vibrational circular dichroism
vocal cord dysfunction

VCF
vaginal contraceptive film
velocity of circumferential fiber (shortening)
ventricular contractility function

VCFS velocardiofacial syndrome

VCG
vectorcardiogram
voiding cystogram

vCJD variant Creutzfeldt-Jakob disease

VCL volar carpal ligament

VCN vestibulocochlear nerve

VCO, V$_{CO}$ carbon monoxide (endogenous production)

VCO$_2$, V$_{CO2}$
carbon dioxide elimination
venous carbon dioxide (production)

volume, carbon dioxide (elimination)
VCP vocal cord paralysis
VCSF ventricular cerebrospinal fluid
VCT venous clotting time
VCU, VCUG
vesicoureterogram
videocystourethrography
voiding cystourethrogram
VCV
volume-control ventilation
vowel-consonant-vowel
VD venereal disease
V&D vomiting and diarrhea
V$_D$
ventilation per minute of dead space
volume of dead space
+VD positive vertical divergence
Vd volume of distribution
VDA video dimensional analysis
VDAC voltage-dependent anion channel
VDCC voltage-dependent calcium channel
VDD atrial synchronous ventricular inhibited pacing
VDDR vitamin D-dependent rickets
VDDR-II vitamin D-dependent rickets type II
VDG, VD-G venereal disease, gonorrhea
VDH
valvular disease of heart
vascular disease of heart
VDL visual detection level
V$_{DM}$ volume of mechanical dead space
VDO varus derotational osteotomy
VDR
venous diameter ratio
volumetric diffusive respirator
VDRL Venereal Disease Research Laboratory (test)
VDRR vitamin D-resistant rickets

VDS venereal disease, syphilis
VDT visual distortion test
VD:VT dead-space gas volume to tidal gas volume ratio
VE
expired volume
vacuum extraction
vasoepididymostomy
ventilation
ventricular extrasystole
vertex
visual examination
vitamin E
vocational evaluation
volume ejection
volume of expired gas
V$_E$
environmental variance
minute ventilation
peak exercise ventilation
respiratory minute volume
volume of expired gas
VEA
ventricular ectopic arrhythmia
viscoelastic agent
VEB ventricular ectopic beat
VECP visual-evoked cortical potential
VED
vacuum extraction delivery
ventricular ectopic depolarization
VEE Venezuelan equine encephalitis
VEF visually evoked field
VEGF vascular endothelial growth factor
vent
ventilation
ventilator
VEP visual evoked potential
VER
ventricular escape rhythm
visual evoked response
VERP ventricular effective refractory period
VES ventricular extrasystole
ves.
bladder [L. *vesica*]

ves. *(continued)*
    vesicular
    vessel
VESS videoendoscopic swallowing study
VET
    veteran
    veterinarian
VETS Veterans (Adjustment) Scale
VF
    left leg electrode (electrocardiogram)
    vertical float (aquatic therapy)
    video frequency
    visual field (*See also* F)
    vocal fremitus
V_f variant frequency
VFA volatile fatty acid
VFC Vaccines for Children (program)
VFD visual feedback display
VFI
    visual fields intact
    Visual Functioning index
v fib ventricular fibrillation
VFR voiding flow rate
VFT ventricular fibrillation threshold
VG
    vein graft
    ventricular gallop
V_G genetic variance
VGCC voltage-gated calcium channel
VH
    vaginal hysterectomy
    vitreous hemorrhage
V_H variable domain of heavy chain immunoglobulin
VH I very narrow anterior chamber angles
VH II moderately narrow anterior chamber angles
VH III moderately wide open anterior chamber angles
VH IV wide open anterior chamber angles
VHC valved holding chamber

VHD
    valvular heart disease
    ventricular heart disease
VHDL very high density lipoprotein
VHF
    very high frequency
    viral hemorrhagic fever
    visual half-field
VHI voice handicap index
VHN Vickers hardness number
VHP vaporized hydrogen peroxide
VI
    inspired ventilation
    vaginal irrigation
    variable interval
    vascular invasion
    velocity index
    ventilation index
    viscosity index
    visual impairment
    visual inspection
    visually impaired
    volume index
V_I volume of inspired gas (per minute)
VIA
    virus-inactivating agent
    virus infection-associated antigen
VIBS Victim's Information Bureau Service
VIC voice intensity controller
VID
    vaginal intraepithelial dysplasia
    visible iris diameter
VIED vehicular improvised explosive device
VIF virus-induced interferon
VIg vaccinia immunoglobulin
VIH Spanish and French abbreviation for human immunodeficiency virus
VILI ventilator-induced lung injury
VIM
    ventralis intermedius

video-intensification
microscopy

VIN vulvar intraepithelial
neoplasia

VIP
vasoactive intestinal
polypeptide
voluntary interruption of
pregnancy

VIP-DAC vaginal interruption
of pregnancy with dilatation
and curettage

VIP-IR vasoactive intestinal
polypeptide immunoreactivity

VIPoma vasoactive intestinal
polypeptide tumor

VIR
viral
virology
virus

vir. green [L. *viridis*]

VIS
Vaccine Information Statement
vaginal irrigation smear
venous insufficiency syndrome
video imaging system
visible
Visual Impairment Service

VISA vancomycin-insensitive
Staphylococcus aureus

VISI
Vaccine Identification
Standards Initiative
volar (flexed) intercalated
segment instability

VIT venom immunotherapy

vit cap
vital capacity
vitamin capsule

vitel. yolk [L. *vitellus*]

vitr, vitr.
glass [L. *vitrum*]
vitreous

viz. that is, namely [L.
videlicet]

VJ
ventriculojugular (shunt)
Vogel-Johnson (agar)

VKC vernal keratoconjunctivitis

VKDB vitamin K deficiency
bleeding

VL
left arm electrode for
electrocardiogram
vastus lateralis
visceral leishmaniasis

V_L
(actual) volume of lung
variable domain of light
chain immunoglobulin

VLA
very late antigen
viruslike agent

VLAD variable life-adjusted
display

VLAP
vaporization laser ablation of
prostate
visual laser ablation of
prostate

VLBW very low birth weight

VLDL, VLDLP very low density
lipoprotein

VLDL-C very low density
lipoprotein C

VLDL-TG very low density
lipoprotein-triglyceride

VLE vision left eye

VLF very low frequency

VLIA viruslike infectious agent

VLM
ventrolateral medulla
visceral larva migrans

VLPP Valsalva leak point
pressure

VLR vastus lateralis release

VLS vascular leak syndrome

VM
vasomotor
vastus medialis
venous malformation

V/m volt per meter

VMA
vanillylmandelic acid
vastus medialis advancement

V-mask Venturi mask

V_{max} maximum velocity

VMF vasomotor flushing

357

VMGT Visual-Motor Gestalt Test

VMH ventromedial hypothalamic (neuron, nuclei)

VMI visual-motor integration

VMN ventromedial nucleus of the hypothalamus

VMO
musculus vastus medialis obliquus
vastus medialis oblique (muscle)

VMR vasomotor rhinitis

VMS
Visual Memory Score
visual memory span

VMST Visual-Motor Sequencing Test

VMT
vasomotor tone
ventilatory muscle training
ventromedial tegmentum

VMU vertebral motion unit

VN
vestibular nucleus
vomeronasal

VNA virus-neutralizing antibody

VNC vesical neck contracture

VNDPT Visual Numerical Discrimination Pretest

VNE video nasendoscopy

VNO vomeronasal organ

VNR
ventral nerve root
verbal, numerical, and reasoning

VNS
vagus nerve stimulation
villonodular synovitis

VO volume overload

VO₂
peak exercise oxygen consumption
volume of oxygen consumption per unit of time

Voa ventralis oralis anterior

VOCs volatile organic compounds

VOD venoocclusive disease

VOE vascular occlusive episode

VOI Vocational Opinion Index

VO2I oxygen consumption index

vol% volume percent

vol
volar
volatile
volumetric
voluntary
volunteer

vol:vol volume per volume ratio

VOM volt-ohm-millimeter

VO₂max maximal oxygen consumption

VOO continuous ventricular asynchronous pacing

VOP ventralis oralis posterior

VOR
vestibuloocular reflex
vestibuloocular response

VORP vibrating ossicular prosthesis

VP
vasopressin
velopharyngeal
venous pressure
ventricle to peritoneal cavity (shunt)
ventricular pacing
ventriculoperitoneal (shunt)
Voges-Proskauer (medium, test)

Vp voltage peak

vp vapor pressure

VPA
ventricular premature activation
vigorous physical activity

v-PA vascular plasminogen activator

VPAP variable positive airway pressure

VPB ventricular premature beat

VPC
vapor-phase chromatography
ventricular premature complex
ventricular premature contraction
volume of packed cells

VPD
> velopharyngeal dysfunction
> ventricular premature depolarization

VPd venous dialysis pressure

V_{pe} peak ejection velocity

VPF vascular permeability factor

VPG velopharyngeal gap

VPI
> velopharyngeal incompetence
> velopharyngeal insufficiency

VPM ventralis posteromedialis

vpm vibration per minute

VPO velopharyngeal opening

VPRC, VPRBC volume of packed red (blood) cells

VPS
> valvular pulmonic stenosis
> ventriculoperitoneal shunt

vps vibration per second

VPT
> vascularized patellar tendon
> vibration perception threshold

V/Q ventilation/perfusion

VR
> right arm electrode for electrocardiogram
> valvular regurgitation
> variable rate
> ventilation rate
> ventilation ratio
> ventricular response
> vital record
> vitreoretinal

Vr volume of relaxation

VRA visual response audiometry

VRE vancomycin-resistant *Enterococcus*

VRO varus rotational osteotomy

VROM voluntary range of motion

VRR ventricular response rate

VRS
> viral rhinosinusitis
> volume reduction surgery

VRSA vancomycin-resistant *Staphylococcus aureus*

VS
> vagal stimulation

> vasospasm
> vegetative state
> ventricular septum
> vesicular stomatitis
> veterinary surgeon
> villonodular synovitis
> vital signs

V·s volt-second

vs. against [L. *versus*]

VSCC voltage-sensitive calcium channel

VSD
> Vaccine Safety Datalink
> ventricular septal defect
> virtually safe dose

VSL straight line velocity

VSMC vascular smooth muscle cell

VSO
> vertical sagittal split osteotomy
> vertical subcondylar oblique

VSP variable screw placement

VSS apparent volume of distribution (steady state)

VST visual search task

VT
> total ventilation
> venous thrombosis
> ventricular tachyarrhythmia
> verocytotoxin

V&T volume and tension

V_T tidal volume

VTA ventricular tachyarrhythmia

V-TACH ventricular tachycardia

VTE venous thromboembolism

VTED venous thromboembolic disease

V_{TG} thoracic gas volume

VTM
> mechanical tidal volume
> virus transport medium

VTO visualized treatment objective

VTOP, VTP voluntary termination of pregnancy

VTT voice termination time

VT/VF ventricular tachycardia/ventricular fibrillation

VTX vertex (presentation)

VU
varicose ulcer
volume unit (meter)

VUJ vesicoureteral junction

VUR vesicoureteral reflux (grade I–V)

VUV vacuum ultraviolet

VV
vaccinia virus
varicose vein
venovenous

V:V volume to volume ratio

vv
veins
venae

VVB venovenous bypass

VVC vulvovaginal candidiasis

VVF vesicovaginal fistula

VVG Verhoeff-Van Gieson (stain)

VVI ventricular demand pacing

vvi vocal velocity index

VVIR ventricular demand inhibited pacemaker

VVS vulvar vestibulitis syndrome

VVT ventricular synchronous pacing

VW
vascular wall
vessel wall

v/w volume per weight

VWF
velocity waveform
vibration-induced white finger

vWF von Willebrand factor

VWM ventricular wall motion

Vx
vertex
vitrectomy

V-XT V-pattern exotropia

V-Y shape of incisions in V-Y plasty

VZIg varicella-zoster immune globulin

VZV varicella-zoster virus

W
energy (work)
tryptophan (*See also* Trp)
tungsten [Ger. *wolfram*]
watt
Weber (test)
W3 World Wide Web
W-22 22 word list (Central Institute for the Deaf)
W+ weakly positive
W or A weakness or atrophy
W/A watt/ampere
WAB, WABT Western Aphasia Battery Test
WADAO weak and dizzy all over
WAF weakness, atrophy, and fasciculation
WAIS Wechsler Adult Intelligence Scale
WAIS-III Wechsler Adult Intelligence Scale-Third Edition
WAIS-R Wechsler Adult Intelligence Scale, Revised
WAK wearable artificial kidney
WALK weight-activated locking knee (prosthesis)
WAPT Weidel Auditory Processing Test
WASID warfarin-aspirin symptomatic intracranial disease
WASO wakefulness after sleep onset
Wass Wasserman (reaction, test)
WAT white adipose tissue
WB
washed bladder
weightbearing
well baby
Western blot
whole blood
whole body
Wb weber (unit of magnetic flux)

Wb/A weber per ampere
WBAT weightbearing as tolerated
WBC white blood cell
WBC/hpf white blood cells per high-power field
WBD weeks by dates (for gestational age)
WBE weeks by examination (for gestational age)
WBH weight-based heparin (dosing)
WBI whole body irradiation
Wb/m² weber per square meter
WBN wide band noise
WBQC wide-base quad cane
WBRT whole-brain radiotherapy
WBS
Wechsler-Bellevue Scale
weeks by size (for gestational age)
whole-body scan
WBT wet bulb temperature
WBTT weightbearing to tolerance
WBUS weeks by ultrasound (for gestational age)
WBV whole blood volume
WC
water closet
wheelchair
white cell
whole complement
whooping cough
worker's compensation
WCA work capacity assessment
WCC
well-child care
white cell count
WCD wearable cardioverter-defibrillator
WCE work capacity evaluation
WCH white coat hypertension
WCM whole cow's milk
WCR Walthard cell rest

361

WCS Wisconsin Compression System

WCT wide-complex tachycardia

WD
wallerian degeneration
warm and dry
well-developed
well-differentiated
with disease

W4D Worth four-dot (eye test for fusion)

W→D wet-to-dry (*See also* WTD)

WDCA well-differentiated carcinoma

WDE wound dressing emulsion

WDI warfarin dose index

WDL
within defined limits
Wood-Downes-Lecks clinical asthma score

WDS
wet dog shakes (syndrome)
word discrimination score

WDWN, WD,WN well-developed, well-nourished

WE
Wernicke encephalopathy
whiskey equivalent

WEBINO wall-eyed bilateral internuclear ophthalmoplegia

WEE Western equine encephalomyelitis (virus)

WeeFIM Functional Independence Measure for Children

WEMINO wall-eyed monocular internuclear ophthalmoplegia

W3-EMRS World Wide Web electronic medical records system

WES wall-echo shadow (sign)

WESR
Westergren erythrocyte sedimentation rate
Wintrobe erythrocyte sedimentation rate

WF
wet film
wide field
word fluency

WFI water for injection

WFL within functional limits

WFLC white female living child

WFNS World Federation of Neurological Societies (grade, scale)

WFR wheal-and-flare reaction

WFRT wide-field radiation therapy

WG Wright-Giemsa (stain)

WGA wheat germ agglutinin

WH
walking heel (cast)
well-healed
well-hydrated

W/H weight/height

wh watt-hour

WHA warmed humidified air

WHI Women's Health Initiative

WHIM warts, hypogammaglobulinemia, infections, myelokathexis

WHIS War Head Injury Score

WHMS well-healed midline scar

WHNR well-healed, no residuals

WHNS
well-healed, nonsymptomatic
well-healed, no sequelae

WHO
World Health Organization
wrist-hand orthosis

WHOART World Health Organization Adverse Reaction Terminology

WHOQOL-100 World Health Organization Quality of Life 100-Item (instrument)

WHP whirlpool (*See also* WP)

WHR waist to hip ratio

WHS Women's Health Study

WHVP wedge hepatic venous pressure

WHYMPI Westhaven Yale Multidimensional Pain Inventory

WI
walk-in (patient)

water ingestion
waviness index
weaning index
W/I within
WIA wounded in action
WIC Women, Infants, and
Children (Program)
WIP work in progress
WIPI Word Intelligibility by
Picture Identification
WIS Wechsler Intelligence Scale
WISC-III Wechsler Intelligence
Scale for Children III
WISC-R Wechsler Intelligence
Scale for Children-Revised
WISH
wearable information system
for human healthcare
Wistar Institute Susan
Hayflick (cell)
WIT water-induced
thermotherapy
WK
week (*See also* W)
Wernicke-Korsakoff
(syndrome)
work
W/kg watt per kilogram
WL
waterload (test)
wavelength
weight loss
workload
WLE wide local excision
WLI weight-length index
WLR within-list recognition
WLS wet lung syndrome
WLT
waterload test
whole-lung tomography
WLU workload unit
WM
Waldenström
macroglobulinemia
wall motion
wet mount
white matter
whole milk

whole mount (microscopy)
woman's milk
W/m$_2$ watt per square meter
WMA
wall motion abnormality
white matter (signal)
abnormality
Wmax peak work rate
WMD
warm moist dressing (sterile)
weapons of mass destruction
white matter damage
WMFT Wolf Motor Function
Test
WMHI white matter
hyperintensity
WMI wall motion index
WML white matter lesion
(cerebral)
WMLC white male living child
WMP
warm moist pack (unsterile)
weight management program
WMR
wedge matrix resection
work metabolic rate
WMS
wall-motion study
Wechsler Memory Scale
WMSI wall motion score index
WMX whirlpool, massage,
exercise
WN well-nourished
WN$_t^{50}$ Wagner-Nelson time
(drug absorption) 50 hours
WND wound
WNE West Nile encephalitis
WNF West Nile fever
WNL within normal limits
WNR within normal range
WNV West Nile virus
WO
wash-out
weeks old
wide open
without
written order
W/O water (in) oil (emulsion)
WOB work of breathing

363

WOMAC Western Ontario and McMaster Universities Osteoarthritis Index
WOMAC-PF Western Ontario and McMaster Universities Osteoarthritis Index Physical Functioning subscale and chair performance
WORC Western Ontario Rotator Cuff (index)
WOSI Western Ontario Instability Index
WP
　water packed
　weakly positive
　wettable powder
　whirlpool (*See also* WHP)
　white pulp
　working point
W:P water to powder ratio
WPB whirlpool bath
WPCs washed packed cells
WPCU weighted patient care unit
WPFM Wright peak flowmeter
WPk
　ward pack
　wet pack
WPPSI, WPP Wechsler Preschool and Primary Scale of Intelligence
WPPSI-R Wechsler Preschool and Primary Scale of Intelligence-Revised
WPT marbled pure tone
WPV within-person variability
WR
　Waldeyer ring
　Wassermann reaction
　water retention
　weakly reactive
　whole response
　wide range
W/R with respect (to)
Wr^a Wright antigen
WRA with-the-rule astigmatism
WRAIR Walter Reed Army Institute of Research
WRAMC Walter Reed Army Medical Center

WRC
　washed red (blood) cell
　water-retention coefficient
WRE whole ragweed extract
WRISS Weapons Related Injury Surveillance System
WRK Woodward reagent K
WRL World Reference Laboratory (for foot-and-mouth disease, UK)
WRVP wedge renal vein pressure
WS
　walking speed
　Warthin-Starry (stain)
　watermelon stomach
　water soluble
　water swallow
　wet swallow
　Wilder silver (stain)
　work simplification
　work simulation
　work status
W&S wound and skin
W·s watt-second
WSD
　water seal drainage
　weak syllable deletion
WSP wearable speech processor
WSR Westergren sedimentation rate
W/sr watt per steradian
WSW women (who have) sex (with) women
WT
　Wilms tumor
　wisdom teeth
0WT zero work tolerance
wt weight
WTD
　wet tail disease
　wet-to-dry (*See also* W→D)
WTS whole tomography slice
W-T-W wet-to-wet (*See also* W→W)
WV
　walking ventilation
　whispered voice
W/V, w/v weight (of solute) per volume (of solution)

WV:MBC walking ventilation to maximal breathing capacity ratio

WW

wet weight

wheeled walker

W→W wet-to-wet (*See also* W-T-W)

W/W, w/w weight (of solute) per weight (of solvent)

WWTP wastewater treatment plant

WxB wax bite

WxP wax pattern

WY women years

X

decimal scale of potency or dilution

exophoria distance

female sex chromosome

homeopathic symbol for decimal scale of potencies

Kienböck unit (of x-ray exposure)

magnification

ten (Roman numeral)

unknown quantity

x

axis of cylindric lens

multiplied by (sign)

roentgen (rays)

X′, x′ exophoria, near viewing

x′ (*var. of* X′)

X+ xiphoid plus (number of fingerbreadths)

X3 (orientation as to) time, place and person

X-A xylene-alcohol (mixture)

Xa chiasma

Xaa unknown amino acid

XBT xylose breath test

XC excretory cystogram

XCCE extracapsular cataract extraction (*See also* ECCE)

XCCL exaggerated craniocaudal lateral (angle, view)

XCF aortic cross clamp off

XCO aortic cross clamp on

XCT x-ray computed tomography

XD X-linked dominant

X&D examination and diagnosis

XDR transducer

Xe xenon

XeCl xenon chloride

XeCT xenon-enhanced computed tomography

X-ed crossed

XES x-ray energy spectrometry

XFER transfer

Xfmr transformer

XGP xanthogranulomatous pyelonephritis

XIP x-ray in plaster

XIST, Xist X inactive, specific transcript

XKO not knocked out

XL

inductive reactance

xylose-lysine (agar base)

X-LA, XLA X-linked agammaglobulinemia

XLAS X-linked aqueductal stenosis

XLCM X-linked cardiomyopathy

XLD X-linked dominant

X-leg crossleg

XLHR X-linked hypophosphatemic rickets

XLMR X-linked mental retardation

XLMR/MCA X-linked mental retardation/multiple congenital anomalies

XLMTM X-linked myotubular myopathy

XLR X-linked recessive

XLRP X-linked retinitis pigmentosa

XM, X-match crossmatch

X_m magnetic susceptibility

XMG x-ray mammogram

XMM xeromammography

XMR x-rays and magnetic resonance

XN night blindness

XO presence of only one sex chromosome (Turner syndrome)

XOAN X-linked ocular albinism

XOM extraocular movement

XOP x-ray out of plaster

Xp short arm of chromosome X

Xp- deletion of short arm of chromosome X

X

XPS x-ray photoemission spectroscopy
Xq long arm of chromosome X
Xq- deletion of long arm of chromosome X
XR
  x-linked recessive
  x-ray
X/R reactance and resistance
XRA x-ray arteriography
XRD x-ray diffraction
XRE xenobiotic response element
XRF x-ray fluorescence
XRT x-ray therapy (radiotherapy)
XS
  corneal scar
  cross-section
  excess
  excessive
  xiphisternum
XSA cross-sectional area
X-SCID, XSCID X-linked severe combined immunodeficiency
XS-LIM exceeds limits (of procedure)

XSLR crossed straight leg raising (sign)
XT, xT
  exotropia
  extract
X(T), x(T) intermittent exotropia
X(T') intermittent exotropia at 33 cm
xT (*var. of* XT)
Xta chiasmata (pl. of chiasma)
Xtab crosstabulating
XTM x-ray tomographic microscope
XU
  excretory urogram
  X unit
xULN times upper limit of normal
XUV extreme ultraviolet
xvse transverse
XX
  double strength
  normal female sex chromosome type
XX/XY sex karyotypes
XY normal male sex chromosome type

Y

male sex chromosome
tyrosine (*See also* Tyr)
yttrium

y

wave on phlebogram
yield

YADH yeast alcohol
dehydrogenase

YAG yttrium aluminum garnet
(laser)

Yb ytterbium

YBOCS Yale-Brown Obsessive-
Compulsive Scale

yd yard

YE

yeast extract
yellow enzyme

Yel yellow

YF yellow fever

YFH yellow-faced hornet

YFV yellow fever virus

YGTSS Yale Global Tic
Severity Scale

YHL years of healthy life

YHT Young-Helmholtz theory

YJV yellow jacket venom

Yk York (antibody)

YLC youngest living child

YM yeast and mannitol

YMA yeast morphology agar

Y/N yes/no

YO years old

YOB year of birth

YOD year of death

YPC YAG (yttrium aluminum
garnet laser) posterior
capsulotomy

YPLL years of potential life
lost (before age 65)

yr year

YS

yellow spot
yolk sac

YST

yeast (cells)
yolk sac tumor

YTD year to date

YVS yellow vernix syndrome

Z
atomic number (symbol)
disc (band, line) that
separates sacromeres [Ger.
Zwischenscheibe intermediate
disk]
shape of surgical incision (Z-
plasty)
zero
zone
zusammen
ZC zona compacta
Z-DNA zig-zag (left handed
helical) deoxyribonucleic acid
ZDS zinc depletion syndrome
ZEEP zero end-expiratory
pressure
ZEPI zonal echo planar
imaging
ZF
zero frequency
zona fasciculata
zygomaticofrontal
ZFP zero-flow pressure
ZG zona glomerulosa
ZI zona incerta
ZI[a] isotope with same atomic
number and atomic weight
ZIG zoster (serum)
immunoglobulin

ZIP zoster immune plasma
Zm zygomaxillare (craniometric)
ZMC zygomaticomaxillary
complex
ZN Ziehl-Neelsen (method,
stain)
Zn zinc
Zn fl zinc flocculation (test)
ZnO zinc oxide
ZnOE zinc oxide-eugenol (white
zinc)
ZNS Ziehl-Neelsen stain
ZnSO$_4$ zinc sulfate
ZP zona pellucida
ZPA zone of polarizing activity
ZPC zero point of charge
ZPG zero population growth
Z-plasty surgical relaxation of
contracture
ZR zona reticularis
Zr zirconium
ZSB zero stool (since) birth
ZSC zone of slow conduction
ZSR zeta sedimentation rate
ZT Ziehen test
Zy zygion
Z, Z′, Z″ increasing degrees of
contraction [Ger. *Zuckung*]

Contents: The Appendices

Symbols

Angles, Triangles, and Circles

$\wedge$	above	$<$	caused by
	diastolic blood pressure (anesthesia records)		derived from
	elevated		less severe than
	enlarged		less than*
	improved		produced by
	increased		proximal
	superior (position)	$\angle$	angle
	upper		flexion
			flexor
$\vee$	below	$\angle\hspace{-0.6em}\text{E}$	angle of entry
	decreased	$\angle\hspace{-0.6em}\text{x}$	angle of exit
	deficiency	$\llcorner$	factorial product
	deficit		
	depressed	$\lrcorner$	right lower quadrant
	deteriorated	$\urcorner$	right upper quadrant
	diminished		
	down	$\ulcorner$	left upper quadrant
	inferior (position)		
	lower	$\llcorner$	left lower quadrant
	systolic blood pressure (anesthesia records)	Δ	anion gap
			centrad prism
$>$	causes		change
	demonstrates		delta gap
	distal		heat
	followed by		increment
	derived from		occipital triangle
	greater than*		prism diopter
	indicates		temperature (anesthesia records)
	leads to		
	more severe than	$\Delta+$	time interval
	produces	ΔA	change in absorbance
	radiates to		
	radiating to	Δ dB	difference in decibels
	results in	Δ P	change in (intraocular) pressure
	reveals		
	shows	Δ pH	change in pH
	to		
	toward		
	worse than		
	yields		

Symbols

$\Delta\ t$	time interval	Ⓛ	left
$\Delta\ H,\ H\ \Delta$	Hesselbach triangle	Ⓜ	murmur
◯	respiration (anesthesia records)	ⓜ	by mouth mouth (temperature) murmur
♀	female female sex	√ⓜ	factitial murmur
♂	male male sex	Ⓞ	by mouth oral orally
Ⓐ , ⓐx	axilla (temperature)	Ⓡ	rectal rectally rectum (temperature) right
Ⓗ , ⓗ	hypodermic hypodermically		
Ⓘⓜ	intramuscular intramuscularly	Ⓧ	end of anesthesia (anesthesia records) end of operation
Ⓘⓥ	intravenous intravenously		

Arrows

↑	above elevated elevation enlarged gas greater than improved increase increased increases more than rising superior (position) up upper	↓	below decrease decreased deficiency deficit depressed depression deteriorated deteriorating diminished diminution down falling inferior (position) less than low normal plantar reflex precipitate precipitates slower
↑g	increasing rising		
↑V	increase due to in vivo effect (laboratory)		

↓ g	decreasing diminishing falling lowering			toward yields
↓ V	decrease due to in vivo effect (laboratory)		←	caused by derived from direction of flow or reaction due to produced by proximal resulting from secondary to to left
↗	deviated displaced increasing			
↘	decreasing			
→	approaches limit of causes, demonstrates direction of flow or reaction distal due to followed by indicates leads to produces radiating to results in reveals shows to to right		⇈	extensor response (up bilaterally, positive Babinski sign) testes undescended
			⇊	plantar response (down bilaterally, normal Babinski sign) testes descended
			⇅	reversible reaction up and down
			⇄, ⇌	reversible (chemical) reaction

Genetic Symbols

□	male		5̄	5̇	◇̇ multiple people, number known (number of sibs written inside symbol)
○	female				
◇	sex unspecified		n̄	ṅ	◇̇ multiple people, number unknown ("n" used in place of specific number)
□ ○	normal people				
■ ● ◆	affected person (with ≥ 2 conditions, the symbol is partioned and shaded with a different fill defined in a key or legend)		□─○		mating
			□─○		consanguinity

A5

Symbols

$(+)$	uncommon or uncertain mode of inheritance	⊙	carrier of sex-linked recessive
I, II 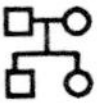	parents and offspring, in generations	▨ ∅	death
	dizygotic twins	▨ SB 28 wk ⊘ SB 30 wk ◈ SB 34 wk	stillbirth (SB)
	monozygotic twins	▣ LMP: 7/1/94 Ⓟ 20 wk ◇ P	pregnancy (P); gestational age and karotype (if known) below symbol
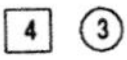 4 ③	number of children of sex indicated	↗□ ↗○	consultant (person seeking genetic counseling/testing)
⑴ ⑴	adopted people	△ male △ female ⬒ ECT	spontaneous abortion (SAB); ECT below symbol indicates ectopic pregnancy
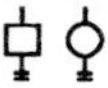 � ♀	individual died without leaving offspring	▲ male ▲ female ▲ 16 wk	affected spontaneous abortion (gestational age, if known, below symbol, and key or legend used to define shading)
□—○	no issue	⚼ male ⚼ female ⚼	termination of pregnancy
■ ●	affected people	▲ male ▲ female ▲	affected termination of pregnancy (key or legend used to define shading)
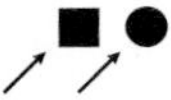 ↗■ ↗●	proband or propositus (first affected family member coming to medical attention)		
⊞	examined professionally normal for trait		
⊟	not examined dubiously reported to have trait		
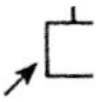 ↗⌐	not examined reliably reported to have trait		
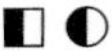 ◧ ◖	heterozygotes for autosomal recessive		

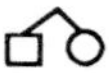

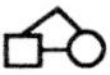

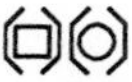

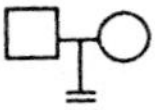

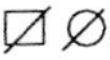

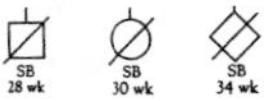

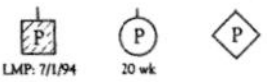

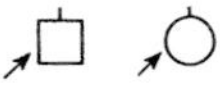

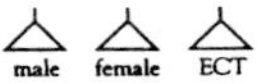

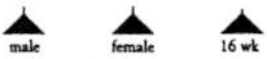

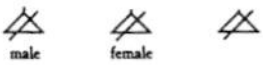

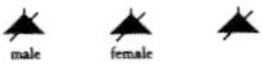

Source: Genetic symbols are public domain. We credit and gratefully acknowledge the *American Journal of Human Genetics* (56:746–747, 1995) as our source for these symbols.

Numbers

0	completely absent (pulse) no response (reflexes)	+4, 4+	normal (pulse)
+1, 1+	markedly impaired (pulse)	4+	hyperactive (reflexes) large amount (laboratory tests) pronounced reaction (laboratory tests)
1+	low normal or somewhat diminished (reflexes) slight reaction or trace (laboratory tests)	•	very brisk (reflexes)
+2, 2+	moderately impaired (pulse)	$\overline{1}$	bowel movement (numeral indicates number of stools in a given period)
2+	average or normal (reflexes) noticeable reaction or trace (laboratory tests)	1×	once one time
+3, 3+	slightly impaired (pulse)	2×, ×2	twice two times
3+	moderate reaction (laboratory tests) brisker than average (reflexes)	3×, ×3	three times, etc.

Arabic	Roman	Arabic	Roman
0		17	XVII
1	I, i	18	XVIII
2	II, ii	19	XIX
3	III, iii	20	XX
4	IV, iv	30	XXX
5	V, v	40	XL
6	VI, vi	50	L
7	VII, vii	60	LX
8	VIII, viii	70	LXX
9	IX, ix	80	LXXX
10	X, x	90	XC
11	XI, xi	100	C
12	XII, xii	1,000	M
13	XIII, xiii	5,000	$\overline{V}$
14	XIV, xiv	10,000	$\overline{X}$
15	XV	100,000	$\overline{C}$
16	XVI	1,000,000	$\overline{M}$

Pluses, Minuses, and Equivalencies

+	acid (reaction)		+++	increased reflexes
	added to*			75% inhibition of hemolysis, Wassermann
	convex lens			moderate amount
	decreased or diminished (reflexes)		+++	moderate reaction (laboratory tests)
	excess			moderately hyperative (reflexes)
	less than 50% inhibition of hemolysis, Wassermann			moderately severe (pain, severity)
	low normal (reflexes)			brisker than average (reflexes)
	markedly impaired (pulse)			slightly impaired (pulse)
	mild (severity)		++++	complete inhibition of hemolysis, Wassermann
	plus*			large amount (laboratory tests)
	positive (laboratory tests)			markedly hyperactive (reflexes)
	present			markedly severe (pain, severity)
	slight reaction or trace (laboratory tests)			normal (pulse)
	sluggish (reflexes)			pronounced reaction (laboratory tests)
	somewhat diminished (reflexes)			very brisk (reflexes)
(+)	significant		−	absent
(+)ive	positive			alkaline (reaction)
+ to ++	slight pain			concave lens
++	average (reflexes)			deficiency
	50% inhibition of hemolysis, Wassermann			deficient
	moderate (pain, severity)			minus
	moderately impaired (pulse)			negative (laboratory test)
	normally active (reflexes)			none
	noticeable reaction or trace (laboratory tests)			subtract
				without
			(−)	insignificant

A8

±	doubtful	≎	approximately equal to
	either positive or negative	=	equal to
	equivocal (reflexes, qualitative tests)	≠	not equal to
	flicker (reflexes)		combined with
	indefinite	⇔	equivalent
	more or less	⇎	not equivalent to
	plus or minus		
±	possibly significant	≡	identical
	questionable		identical with
	suggestive	≢	not identical
	variable		not identical with
	very slight (reaction, severity, trace)	≒	nearly equal to
	with or without	≐	approximately equal
(±)	possibly significant	≅	approximately
± to +	minimal pain		approximately equal to
∓	minus or plus		congruent to
‡	moderate (severity)	≑	approaches
	normally active (reflexes)	=	equilateral
#	fracture	△	equiangular
	gauge	>	greater than*
	number	≯	not greater than
	pound(s)	<	less than*
	weight	≮	not less than
~	about	≥, ⩾	greater than or equal to
	approximate	≤, ⩽	less than or equal to
	approximately		
	proportionate to		

Primes, Checks, Dots, Roots, and Other Symbols

?	doubtful	questionable
	equivocal (reflexes)	question of
	flicker (reflexes)	suggested
	not tested (severity)	suggestive (severity)
	possible	unknown

A9

Symbols

!	factorial product	√d	checked
			observed
†	death		
	deceased	√g, √ing	checking
/	divided by	√qs	voided quantity sufficient
	either meaning		
	extension	√	radical root
	extensors fraction	$\sqrt[2]{}$	square root
	of		
	per*	$\sqrt[3]{}$	cube root
	to		
	ratio	*	birth
			multiplication sign
'	foot		(genetics)
	hour		not verified
	univalent		presumed
			supposed
"	bivalent		
	ditto	°	degree, measurement
	inch		(1/360 of circle)
	minute		severity (burns, wounds)
	second (1/60 degree)		temperature
			time (hour)*
‴	line (1/12 inch)		
	trivalent	:	is to
√	check	...	no data (in given
	observe for		category)
	urine		
	voided (urine)	∴	therefore
√̣	urine and defecation	∵	because
	voided and bowels		since
	moved		
		::	as
√c̄	check with		equality between ratios
			proportion
			proportionate to

Statistical Symbols

α	probability of Type I error	$nCk; \left(\dfrac{n}{k}\right)$	binomial coefficient number of combination of n things taken k at a time
	significance level		
β	probability of Type II error	χ^2	chi-squared statistic
1-β	power of statistical test		

E	expected frequency in cell of contingency table	r^2	coefficient of determination
$E(X)$	expected value of random variable X	r_s	Spearman rank correlation coefficient
F	F statistic (variance ratio)	ρ	population correlation coefficient
f	frequency	s	sample standard deviation
H_0	null hypothesis	s^2	sample variance
H_1	alternative hypothesis	SE	standard error of estimate
μ	population mean	σ	population standard deviation
N	population size	σ^2	population variance
n	sample size	$\sigma_{diff.}$	standard error of difference between scores
$n!$	n factorial	$\sigma_{est.}$	standard error of estimate
O	observed frequency in a contingency table	$\sigma_{meas.}$	standard error of measurement
ϕ	ability continuum phi coefficient	t	Student t statistic Student test variable
P	probability	θ	latent trait
p	probability of success in independent trials	U	Mann-Whitney rank sum statistic
$P(A)$	probability that event A occurs	W	Wilcoxon rank sum statistic
$P(A\backslash B)$	conditional probability that A occurs given that B has occurred	$\overline{X}$	sample mean
		$|x|$	absolute value of x
r	sample correlation coefficient, usually the Pearson product-moment correlation	$\sqrt{x}$	square root of x
		z	standard score
		∞	infinity

---

*Do not use in written patient records (JCAHO).

Professional Titles, Degrees, and Certificates

AuD	Doctor of Audiology
ANP	Adult Nurse Practitioner
ARNP	Advanced Registered Nurse Practitioner
ATC	Athletic Trainer, Certified
BA	Bachelor of Arts
BB(ASCP)	Technologist in Blood Banking (certified by American Society of Clinical Pathologists)
BCNP	Board Certified Nuclear Pharmacist
BCNSP	Board Certified Nutrition Support Pharmacist
BCPS	Board Certified Pharmacotherapy Specialist
BSN	Bachelor of Science in Nursing
CALN	Clinical Administrative Liaison Nurse
C(ASCP)	Technologist in Chemistry (certified by American Society of Clinical Pathologists)
CAT(C)	Certified Athletic Therapist (Canada)
CCC-A	Certificate of Clinical Competence in Audiology
CCC-SLP	Certificate of Clinical Competence in Speech-Language Pathology
CCRN	Critical Care Registered Nurse
CCS	Cardiopulmonary Certified Specialist, Certified Coding Specialist
CDA	Certified Dental Assistant
CDE	Certified Diabetes Educator
CDT	Certified Dental Laboratory Technician
CEN	Certified Emergency Nurse
CCEMT-P	Critical Care Paramedic
CCM	Certified Case Manager
CFNP	Certified Family Nurse Practitioner
CIH	Certificate in Industrial Health
CCM	Certified Case Manager
CFNP	Certified Family Nurse Practitioner
CIH	Certificate in Industrial Health
CLA	Certified Laboratory Assistant
CLDir(NCA)	Clinical Laboratory Director (certified by National Certification Agency for Medical Laboratory Personnel)
CLPlb(NCA)	Clinical Laboratory Phlebotomist (certified by National Certification Agency for Medical Laboratory Personnel)
CLS	Clinical Laboratory Scientist
CLS(NCA)	Clinical Laboratory Scientist (certified by National Certification Agency for Medical Laboratory Personnel)

CLSp(CG)(NCA)	Clinical Laboratory Specialist in Cytogenetics (certified by National Certification Agency for Medical Laboratory Personnel)
CLSp(H)(NCA)	Clinical Laboratory Specialist in Hematology (certified by National Certification Agency for Medical Laboratory Personnel)
CLSup(NCA)	Clinical Laboratory Supervisor (certified by National Certification Agency for Medical Laboratory Personnel)
CLT	Certified Laboratory Technician, Clinical Laboratory Technician
CLT(NCA)	Certified Laboratory Technician (certified by National Certification Agency for Medical Laboratory Personnel)
CMA	Certified Medical Assistant
CMT	Certified Medical Transcriptionist
CNA	Certified Nursing Assistant
CNM	Certified Nurse Midwife
CNMT	Certified Nuclear Medicine Technologist
CNP	Community Nurse Practitioner
CNS	Clinical Nurse Specialist
CNSD	Certified Nutrition Support Dietitian
CNSN	Certified Nutrition Support Nurse
CNSP	Certified Nutrition Support Physician
COMA	Certified Ophthalmic Medical Assistant
COMT	Certified Ophthalmic Medical Technologist
CORN	Certified Operating Room Nurse
COTA	Certified Occupational Therapy Assistant
CPAN	Certified Post Anesthesia Nurse
CPFT	Certified Pulmonary Function Technologist
CPH	Certificate in Public Health
CPN	Certified Pediatric Nurse
CPNP	Certified Pediatric Nurse Practitioner
CRNA	Certified Registered Nurse Anesthetist
CRTT	Certified Respiratory Therapy Technician
CSCS	Certified Strength and Conditioning Specialist
CST	Certified Surgical Technician
CT(ASCP)	Cytotechnologist (certified by American Society of Clinical Pathologists)
CTR	Certified Tumor Registrar
CURN	Certified Urological Registered Nurse
CVO	Chief Veterinary Officer
CVT	Certified Veterinary Technician
DC	Doctor of Chiropractic
DDS	Doctor of Dental Surgery

DLM(ASCP)	Diplomate in Laboratory Management (certified by American Society of Clinical Pathologists)
DMD	Doctor of Dental Medicine
DNS	Doctor of Nursing Services
DO	Doctor of Optometry (seen also as OD), Doctor of Osteopathy
DP	Doctor of Podiatry
DPH	Doctor of Public Health, Doctor of Public Hygiene
DPM	Doctor of Physical Medicine, Doctor of Podiatric Medicine
DPT	Doctor of Physical Therapy
ECS	Electrophysiologic Certified Specialist
EdD	Doctor of Education
EFDA	Expanded Function Dental Auxiliary
EMT-B	Emergency Medical Technician—Basic
EMT-I	Emergency Medical Technician—Intermediate
EMT-P	Emergency Medical Technician—Paramedic
ENP	Emergency Nurse Practitioner
FAAN	Fellow, American Academy of Nursing
FAARC	Fellow, American Association for Respiratory Care
FACD	Fellow, American College of Dentists
FACP	Fellow, American College of Physicians
FACS	Fellow, American College of Surgeons
FACSM	Fellow, American College of Sports Medicine
FADA	Fellow, American Dietetic Association
FAMA	Fellow, American Medical Association
FNP	Family Nurse Practitioner
FAOTA	Fellow, American Occupational Therapy Association
FAPTA	Fellow, American Physical Therapy Association
FIAC	Fellow, International Academy of Cytology
FRCD	Fellow, Royal College of Dentists (U.K.)
FRCD(C)	Fellow, Royal College of Dentists of Canada
FRCP	Fellow, Royal College of Physicians (U.K.)
FRCPA	Fellow, Royal College of Physicians of Australia
FRCPSC	Fellow, Royal College of Physicians and Surgeons of Canada
FRSM	Fellow, Royal Society of Medicine (U.K.)
GCS	Geriatric Certified Specialist
GNP	Gerontological Nurse Practitioner
H(ASCP)	Technologists in Hematology (certified by American Society of Clinical Pathologists)
HP(ASCP)	Hemapherisis Practitioner (certified by American Society of Clinical Pathologists)

HT	Histologic Technologist (certified by American Society of Clinical Pathologists)
HT(ASCP)	Histologic Technician (certified by American Society of Clinical Pathologists)
HTL(ASCP)	Histotechnologist (certified by American Society of Clinical Pathologists)
I(ASCP)	Technologist in Immunology (certified by American Society of Clinical Pathologists)
LD	Licensed Dietitian
LMCC	Licentiate of the Medical Council of Canada
LMP	Licensed Massage Practitioner
LMT	Licensed Massage Technician, Licensed Massage Therapist
LPN	Licensed Practical Nurse
LVN	Licensed Vocational Nurse
LVT	Licensed Veterinary Technician
M(ASCP)	Technologist in Microbiology (certified by American Society of Clinical Pathologists)
MD	Doctor of Medicine
MEd	Master of Education
MLT	Medical Laboratory Technician
MLT(ASCP)	Medical Laboratory Technician (certified by American Society of Clinical Pathologists)
MPH	Master of Public Health
MPharm	Master in Pharmacy
MPT	Master of Physical Therapy
MRCP	Member, Royal College of Physicians (U.K.)
MSN	Master of Science in Nursing
MSW	Medical Social Worker
MT	Medical Technologist
MT(ASCP)	Medical Technologist (certified by American Society of Clinical Pathologists)
MTA	Medical Technologist Assistant
NCS	Neurologic Certified Specialist
NCTMB	Nationally Certified in Therapeutic Massage and Bodywork
NM(ASCP)	Technologist in Nuclear Medicine (certified by American Society of Clinical Pathologists)
NMT	Nurse Massage Therapist, Nursing Massage Therapist
NP	Nurse Practitioner
NREMT	National Registry Emergency Medical Technician Basic
NREMT-I	National Registry Emergency Medical Technician— Intermediate

NREMT-P	National Registry Emergency Medical Technician Paramedic
OCS	Orthopedic Certified Specialist
OD	Doctor of Optometry (also seen as DO)
OT	Occupational Therapist
OT-C	Occupational Therapist (Canada)
OTD	Doctor of Occupational Therapy
OT-L	Occupational Therapist, Licensed
OT-R	Occupational Therapist, Registered
PA	Physician's Assistant
PBT(ASCP)	Phlebotomy Technician (certified by American Society of Clinical Pathologists)
PCS	Pediatric Certified Specialist
PharmD	Doctor of Pharmacy
PhD	Doctor of Philosophy
PhG	Graduate in Pharmacy
PNP	Pediatric Nurse Practitioner
PT	Physical Therapist
PTA	Physical Therapy Assistant
RD	Registered Dietitian
RDA	Registered Dental Assistant
RDCS	Registered Diagnostic Cardiac Sonographer
RDH	Registered Dental Hygienist
RDMS	Registered Diagnostic Medical Sonographer
RDN	Registered Dietitian/Nutritionist
R.EEGT.	Registered Electroencephalographic Technologist
R.EPT.	Registered Evoked Potential Technologist
RHIA	Registered Health Information Administrator
RHIT	Registered Health Information Technician
RMA	Registered Medical Assistant
RMT	Registered Massage Therapist
RN	Registered Nurse
RPFT	Registered Pulmonary Function Technologist
RPh	Registered Pharmacist
RPSGT	Registered Polysomnographic Technologist
RRT	Registered Respiratory Therapist
RT	Radiologic Technologist, Respiratory Therapist
RT(ARRT)	Registered Technologist (certified by American Registry of Radiologic Technologists)
RT(CT)	Registered Technologist in Computed Tomography
RT(CV)	Registered Technologist in Cardiovascular Interventional Technology
RT(M)	Registered Technologist in Mammography
RT(MR)	Registered Technologist in Magnetic Resonance Imaging

Titles, Degrees, Certificates

RT(N)	Registered Technologist in Nuclear Medicine
RT(QM)	Registered Technologist in Quality Management
RT(R)	Registered Technologist in Radiography
RT(T)	Registered Technologist in Radiation Therapy
RTT	Respiratory Therapy Technician
RVT	Registered Vascular Technologist, Registered Veterinary Technician
SAT	Supervisory Athletic Therapist (Canada)
SBB(ASCP)	Specialist in Blood Banking (certified by American Society of Clinical Pathologists)
SC(ASCP)	Specialist in Chemistry (certified by American Society of Clinical Pathologists)
SCS	Sports Certified Specialist
SCT(ASCP)	Specialist in Cytotechnology (certified by American Society of Clinical Pathologists)
SH(ASCP)	Specialist in Hematology (certified by American Society of Clinical Pathologists)
SI(ASCP)	Specialist in Immunology (certified by American Society of Clinical Pathologists)
SM(ASCP)	Specialist in Microbiology (certified by American Society of Clinical Pathologists)
VTS	Veterinary Technician Specialist

Greek Name	English Equivalent	Greek Upper Case	Greek Lower Case
alpha	a	A	α (classifier in nomenclature of many sciences) alpha particle angle of optic rotation aromatic substituent on an aliphatic chain Bunsen solubility coefficient degree of dissociation direction of chemical bond away from viewer first in a series (general) first of a series of closely related compounds (chemistry) position immediately adjacent to a carboxyl group (chemistry)
beta	b	B	β anomer of carbohydrate buffer capacity constituent of plasma protein fraction direction of chemical bond toward viewer second in a series (general) second carbon from a functional group (chemistry)
gamma	g	Γ	γ activity coefficient

(continues)

Greek Name	English Equivalent	Greek Upper Case	Greek Lower Case
gamma	g	Γ	γ
			fourth carbon in an aliphatic acid or position 2 removed from the α position in the benzene ring (chemistry)
			heavy chain of IgG
			microgram
			photon (gamma ray)
			plasma protein (globulin)
			symbol for 10^{-4} gauss
			surface tension
			third in a series (general)
delta	d	Δ	δ
		absence of heat treatment (chemistry)	chemical shift in NMR
		application of heat in reaction (chemistry)	distance between two atoms in a molecule
		change	position of a substituent located on the 4th atom from the carboxyl or other functional group (chemistry)
		double bond (chemistry)	
		triangular surface (anatomy)	thickness
epsilon	e	E	ε
			fifth in a series (general)
			heavy chain of IgE
			molar absorption coefficient or extinction coefficient

epsilon	e	E	ε	position of a substituent located on the 5th atom from the carboxyl or other functional group (chemistry)
zeta	z	Z	ζ	atomic number symbol electrokinetic potential position of a substituent located on the 6th atom from the carboxyl or other functional group (chemistry) sixth in a series (general)
eta	h	H	η	position of a substituent located on the 7th atom from the carboxyl or other functional group (chemistry) viscosity
theta	th	Θ	θ	angle
iota	i	I	ι	ninth in a series (general) position of a substituent located on the 9th atom from the carboxyl or other functional group (chemistry)
kappa	k	K	κ	position of a substituent located on the 10th atom from the carboxyl or other functional group (chemistry) tenth in a series (general)

(continues)

Greek Name	English Equivalent	Greek Upper Case	Greek Lower Case
lambda	l	Λ Avogadro number Ostwald solubility coefficient radioactive constant wavelength	λ craniometric point at junction of sagittal and lambdoid suture
mu	m	M	μ chemical potential dynamic viscosity magnetic or electric dipole moment of molecule micro- micron position of a substituent located on the 12th atom from the carboxyl or other functional group (chemistry)
nu	n	N	ν frequency kinematic viscosity position of a susbstituent located on the 13th atom from the carboxyl or other functional group (chemistry) stoichiometric number

xi	x	Ξ	ξ ς
omicron	o	O	o
pi	p	Π	π
		osmotic pressure	ratio of circumference of a circle to its diameter, 3.14159
rho	r	P	ρ
			density
			population correlation coefficient
sigma	s	Σ	σ
		summation of a series	factor in prokaryotic RNA initiation
			reflection coefficient
			standard deviation
			surface tension
			wavenumber (frequency)
tau	t	T	τ
			protein associated with plaque in Alzheimer disease
			relaxation time
			tele
upsilon	u	Y	υ
			kinematic viscosity

(continues)

Greek Name	English Equivalent	Greek Upper Case	Greek Lower Case
phi	ph	Φ magnetic flux phenyl potential energy	ϕ plane angle quantum yield volume fraction
chi	ch	X	χ twenty-second in a series (general) dihedral angle between the α-carbon and the side chains of amino acids in peptides and proteins
psi	ps	Ψ psychology	ψ
omega	o	Ω ohm	ω

Dangerous use of Greeks: Abbreviations starting with the Greek μ should not ever be used. The correct expansions are shown here. Terms containing the Greek μ in the middle or at the end can also be dangerous, and it is best to substitute "micro" within the expansion.

μ	micron	μH	microhenry
μμ	micromicron, micromicro-	μin	microinch
μΩ	microhm	μIU	one-millionth International Unit
μA	microampere	μkat	microkatal (micromole per second)
μB	microbar	μL	microliter
μC	microcoloumb	μm	micrometer, micromilli
μCi	microcurie	μm³	cubic micrometer
μCi/hr	microcurie per hour	μmHg	micrometer of mercury
μEq	microequivalent	μmol	micromole
μF	microfarad	μN	micronewton
μμg	micromicrogram	μOsm	microsmolar
μg	microgram	μR	microroentgen
μγ	microgamma	μs, μsec	microsecond
μg/kg	microgram per kilogram	μV	microvolt
μg/L	microgram per liter	μW	microwatt
μGy	microgray	μU	microunit

Elements and Their Symbols

Element	Symbol	Element	Symbol
Actinium	Ac	Francium	Fr
Silver	Ag	Gallium	Ga
Aluminum	Al	Gadolinium	Gd
Argon	Ar	Germanium	Ge
Arsenic	As	Hydrogen	H
Astatine	At	Helium	He
Gold	Au	Hafnium	Hf
Boron	B	Mercury	Hg
Barium	Ba	Holmium	Ho
Beryllium	Be	Iodine	I
Bismuth	Bi	Indium	In
Bromine	Br	Iridium	Ir
Carbon	C	Potassium	K
Calcium	Ca	Krypton	Kr
Cadmium	Cd	Lanthanum	La
Cerium	Ce	Lithium	Li
Chlorine	Cl	Lutetium	Lu
Cobalt	Co	Magnesium	Mg
Chromium	Cr	Manganese	Mn
Cesium	Cs	Molybdenum	Mo
Copper	Cu	Nitrogen	N
Dysprosium	Dy	Sodium	Na
Erbium	Er	Niobium	Nb
Europium	Eu	Neodymium	Nd
Fluorine	F	Neon	Ne
Iron	Fe	Nickel	Ni

Elements and Their Symbols

Element	Symbol	Element	Symbol
Oxygen	O	Silicon	Si
Osmium	Os	Samarium	Sm
Phosphorus	P	Tin	Sn
Protactinium	Pa	Strontium	Sr
Lead	Pb	Tantalum	Ta
Palladium	Pd	Terbium	Tb
Promethium	Pm	Technetium	Tc
Polonium	Po	Tellurium	Te
Praseodymium	Pr	Thorium	Th
Platinum	Pt	Titanium	Ti
Radium	Ra	Thallium	Tl
Rubidium	Rb	Thulium	Tm
Rhenium	Re	Uranium	U
Rhodium	Rh	Vanadium	V
Radon	Rn	Tungsten	W
Ruthenium	Ru	Xenon	Xe
Sulfur	S	Yttrium	Y
Antimony	Sb	Ytterbium	Yb
Scandium	Sc	Zinc	Zn
Selenium	Se	Zirconium	Zr